Jessica,

It's always great to
meet a kindred soul

CB.

PARAMEDIC M.O.S.

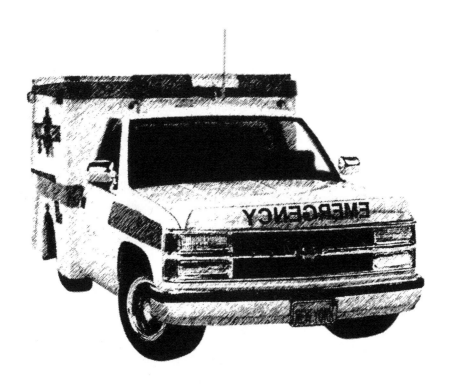

Order this book online at www.trafford.com
or email orders@trafford.com

Most Trafford titles are also available at major online book retailers.

© Copyright 2015 C.B. Garris.
All rights reserved. No part of this publication may be reproduced, stored in a retrieval system, or transmitted, in any form or by any means, electronic, mechanical, photocopying, recording, or otherwise, without the written prior permission of the author.

Print information available on the last page.

ISBN: 978-1-4907-5804-6 (sc)
ISBN: 978-1-4907-5806-0 (hc)
ISBN: 978-1-4907-5805-3 (e)

Library of Congress Control Number: 2015905448

Because of the dynamic nature of the Internet, any web addresses or links contained in this book may have changed since publication and may no longer be valid. The views expressed in this work are solely those of the author and do not necessarily reflect the views of the publisher, and the publisher hereby disclaims any responsibility for them.

Any people depicted in stock imagery provided by Thinkstock are models, and such images are being used for illustrative purposes only.
Certain stock imagery © Thinkstock.

Trafford rev. 04/06/2015

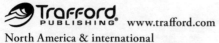 www.trafford.com

North America & international
toll-free: 1 888 232 4444 (USA & Canada)
fax: 812 355 4082

C.B. Garris

Prologue:

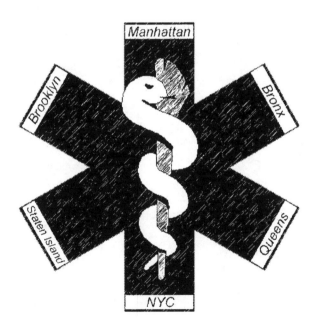

PARAMEDIC M.O.S.

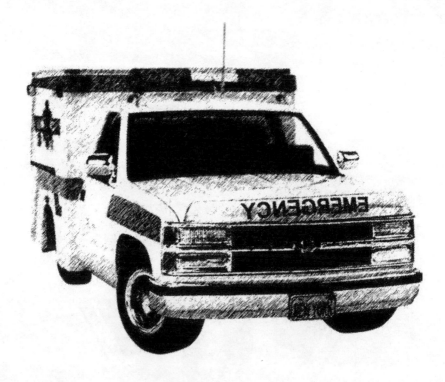

C.B. Garris

While I always wanted to write this book, I don't really think I was ever out of the thoughts in my head enough to make it happen. All of that changed on September 11th, 2001. I watched the television screen in utter horror knowing that my former coworkers were right in the middle of absolute hell; and that was more painful than I will ever be able to articulate. I have always known the response plans: who would go in the first wave, where the command post would be set up and the absolute confusion that would be taking place with the magnitude of the incident. This knowledge that at any other crisis or any routine scene of manageable chaos, I was once proud to have had intricate knowledge of. On this excruciatingly fateful day, this knowledge became my worst enemy. Having been there as a rescuer myself eight years prior for the initial terrorist bombing of the World Trade Center, I began to remember how it looked the first time.

Although I have only limited recollection of the first few hours of 9/11, a friend of mine in Los Angeles tells me that I called her five times in succession and all I kept saying was, "I can't find my friends, I can't contact them." I, probably for the sake of numbing the fear of their loss, have negated that time frame from my brain. I truly did not know what to think. I felt guilty for leaving the Service, but after experiencing my own fears of the building collapsing first hand when I was there the last time, I was somehow glad to have been elsewhere. Still, my friends were buried in ashes, asbestos, fiberglass and molten steel, some surfaced again to see the light and some will never see it again.

We live in a society that seems to judge itself by power, money, religion, and how much damage one can inflict on another. Long gone seem the days where anyone truly cares, where you can settle a disagreement with just a discussion, an argument, a handshake, a hug or if all else fails, a break-dancing session.

I had the opportunity to work with some of the best in this field and for this I will be forever proud. Before September 11th, I also suffered personal losses in the line of duty, none of them good. Some of these losses were co-workers either taken from this world or in some even more unfortunate circumstances, they took themselves. As medics we are caretakers and nurturers. We accept the sentence of what life offers. We see what it does to others everyday, irrespective of what should be. This world is not perfect by any stretch of the imagination, yet we are all

PARAMEDIC M.O.S.

responsible for ensuring that we make the best of it that we can. Helping the common person seems natural to me, some would say to a fault. No one that I ever shared an ambulance with ever wanted to see someone else hurt, rather we wanted to be there to do the best that we could when the "perfections" of life fail.

    Those that work in this profession have a silent gift. This profession is not for everyone, but for those who choose to remain offer all of us something that many cannot, and that is one last chance. I offer this book to you to share with you what it is like to be a Member of the Service.

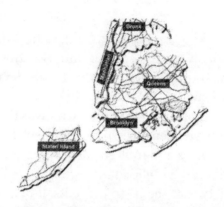

C.B. Garris

Introduction:

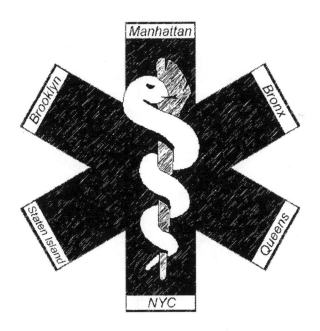

PARAMEDIC M.O.S.

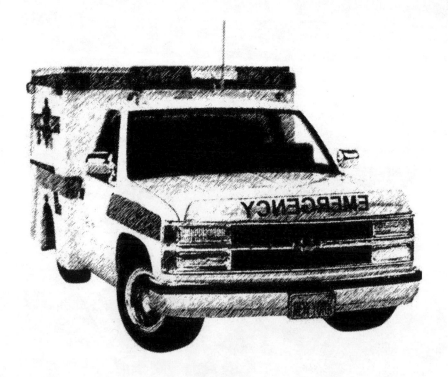

C.B. Garris

They wanted to know that we wanted the job. Our academy, which was situated on a military installation, was to ensure that the job got done correctly. There was no room for margin of error, no room for second best.

That is what made me so proud to have graduated from there. Each day began with one and a half hours of physical training including a two mile run. We had the best instructors in the world. They were tough, the most skilled at what they did and they could read people in a way that made us want to read people like they did.

This group of both men and women, of all different backgrounds and cultures shared one simple bond: to be the best damn Emergency Medical Technicians and Paramedics that lived. There was such a sense of family yet at the same time what preserved that family unit was each person being able to hold their own weight, act autonomously when necessary and know when and how to function as a team. There was no room for slackers and if you made it through the academy and earned your keep, you had every right to be proud of yourself, proud to wear that patch and proud of what you worked so hard for. The academy was only the beginning.

For us it was equal to basic training. I can remember every day and that damn two mile run – eight laps around the Heelo LZ (helicopter landing zone). You could not talk back, you could not act ignorant; what you had to do was show the instructors that you wanted it more than they loved it. PT (physical training) gave way to the showers, where we had thirty minutes to shower, shave and get prepped for six hours of didactics (classroom) work. Our medic trainee orientation group began with one hundred prospectives, we graduated a mere thirty-two; that is how rough it was.

As the days to graduation came closer, the tenser it seemed. You never knew who was going to bow out or be asked to leave. We already came in certified, but now we had to reach an even higher standard to make it through. From routine classroom exams to practical skills stations, Anatomy & Physiology, Pharmacology to Mega-Codes, PHTLS (Pre-hospital Trauma Life Support) to PALS (Pediatric Advanced Life Support) and CTC (Critical Trauma Care); you had a mere eleven weeks to get it right.

It may seem like a long time, but it is not. One of those weeks was just on EVOC (Emergency Vehicles Operating Course) alone. For this we are taken out to a large former air landing strip for 747's, where an obstacle course of cones, fake people and other objects are placed strategically.

PARAMEDIC M.O.S.

We are to navigate this course with a five-ton ambulance at the order and discretion of our instructors. If you fail, you're out. If you fail ANY of the classroom exams or practical skills stations, you may be given a chance to retest; but there is no room for second best. They wanted the best and damnit that is what we were going to give them.

It all boiled down to something very interesting. Where as people tend to judge on likes and dislikes, desires and fantasies, wants and want-nots; something very beautiful happened in the name of taking care of others. Each one of us that survived that academy, which remains the most memorable time in my life, were able to put all of our separations aside for our equal purpose: to save lives.

Whether a non-smoker was paired with a smoker, a male with a female, a heterosexual with someone who was homosexual, black with white, Asian with Latin, Irish with English, republican with a democrat, a Jewish person with one who is Muslim, short with tall, fitness fanatic with someone over or underweight, younger with older, none of it mattered. It is the most beautiful symphony of souls I have ever seen – to put aside all of those issues when our uniforms were donned and our units were called.

What we deal with on a daily basis has got to be the worst thing next to war itself. Yet in a world that is often and almost always divided by opposing beliefs, acts of violence and years of traditional thinking unchanged by modern thought, we the members of NYC EMS created a world within a world to sustain life and make life exist where it should have failed.

We all knew our jobs and we knew them well. We knew what was expected of us and that others were watching in case we lost track. We knew the dangers of what we did and got involved in. We were willing to walk into what everyone else would run from, face it and defeat it with teamwork. In those situations where death won, we hoped that at least we not only gave the individual the ability to pass with dignity and their soul with the respect that if no one ever cared about them up until that day, that we did and cared for them in the best ways possible.

For those who had to witness either the horrible trauma of what brought us to a scene, or were just the unfortunate parties to see their friend or family suffer an acute or chronic illness or trauma, we all hoped that they could go on with their lives, relieved at least knowing that there are professional nurturers out here that bring all the tools possible to help and will try with all of our hearts.

C.B. Garris

This job is not a mechanical job. While we will go into automatic mode to perform our functions, that is the combination of both professional skills and the emotional rewiring necessary to perform the tasks that our citizens and colleagues expect of us. Most of us suffered our own personal tragedies in our younger years, which makes it possible for us to walk into hell and keep right on going, often seeming unaffected to the everyday civilian. As is very common in most of society today, I would expect that many would rather keep their personal tragedies to themselves and I respect that completely. Then there are those that have come forward with story after story of intense and extreme emotional, physical and sexual abuse from their early years. Many saw their parents and siblings beaten, some saw them murdered. Perhaps they lost a parent, sibling or friend to natural causes or to suicide; perhaps they were raped once or repeatedly; maybe they just witnessed a horribly traumatic incident. Perhaps these individuals have had issues with alcohol, drugs, self esteem, sexual dysfunction, sex as a form of blocking out, perhaps some of these individuals have tried to end their lives or are suicidal. Regardless, something keeps them going and in this arena of danger.

Working for NYC EMS was some of the most fun I have ever had. The fact that we would gear up to go into the worst possible situations known to humanity and maybe even put our own lives in extreme danger was secondary to the feeling of being totally protected. We were what 911 was all about. We are the ones that go into deal with hell and we have as much backup as the US military.

One phrase over one of our radio frequencies or a push of our emergency buttons on our radios or from the mobile data terminal, and we can light up a city block causing heavily armed police officers and S.W.A.T. teams to come screaming to our rescue. We were NYC EMS.

With all that safety built in it made it easy to perform our tasks, and enjoy our work even more. We patrol the streets waiting for a call or getting flagged down for one. I laughed harder with my partners than with anyone else. Whether it was about one of our comical calls when everything went totally backwards, or some superior officer showed up on a call and embarrassed himself or herself completely, despite our efforts to save them from that embarrassment. We never knew what would happen next.

We relied on each other, even more so than a child and a parent. We were with each other eight to sometimes sixteen hours a day. We were there if we had good days or bad, lots of sleep or none, a full meal or if we

PARAMEDIC M.O.S.

were working without having eaten. If our finances got out of hand or beyond us, we bought each other dinner and never let another go hungry or unfed. We always tried to make sure that our partner was having a great day and if not we would try to find a way to help them.

If they wanted space and quiet to think, they got it. If they wanted to read our paper, it was theirs. If they were moving from apartment to apartment or for the few that could afford it, a house, we were there to pick up each sofa and chair. If in the course of our duty, one of us was injured and possibly killed, we wanted to know that everything would be done to save the other or at least help us die with dignity and love.

Pretty tall order? Not really and in fact it came pretty simple. We didn't care what you did in your off time or what kind of car you drove. We didn't care if you were Harvard educated or a master of the G.E.D; as long as you could be a part of the team you were a Member of the Service.

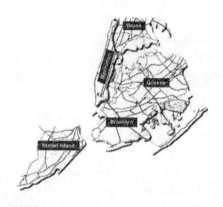

C.B. Garris

Acknowledgements:

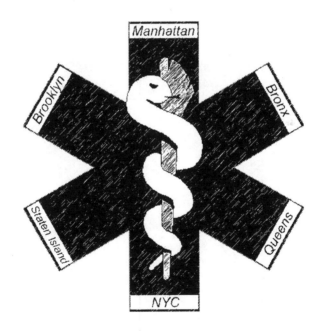

PARAMEDIC M.O.S.

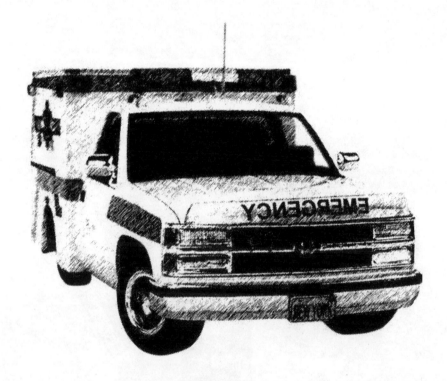

C.B. Garris

My dearest Mom, this world is a better place for the sake that you are in it. Thank you for always being there for me to help me work things out, being patient and putting up with me through the processes of life and what led up to the writing of this book. You have a gracious spirit that has been the help to many along the path of life and you are so very deeply loved. You are not just my mom but you are also my best friend. Laura & Craig, I am so very proud of both of you and you are in my heart every day. To my father and my Uncle David, thank you for your sense of humor. Boots, Jane, and Ralph (thanks for the studio time), and thanks for being my family.

Thomas & Stefanie, you will always be my life mentors and friends! Jill, Thomas, Paul, Richie, Kim, Joey, and Ron, thank you for my earliest teachings and introduction into the world of Emergency Medical Services, for adopting me and accepting me for who I am.

Jeff, Charlie, Liz, Kevin, Paul, John, "Uncle" Phil, Janice, Robert, Jace, Marylou, Pat, Debbie, Brian, Armando, Cecil, James and Christine for all of your time, teachings, trust and generous spirit that you shared with me. Robert & Mary for the eternal friendship, ears and hugs. Sean, Paul, Cookie, Carol, Andy, Hector, Scorpio, George, Scott, Rocco, Chauncey, Lionel, Geoff, Scooter, Rob, Phil, Frank, Lenny, Guy, Tony, Bobby, Raul and Ralphie for all the backup and laughs. Linda, your endearing and heart-filled care made it an honor work with you. Pauline, they broke the mold on care-giving when they made you. Will, my fellow academy brother, you always knew how to make every one laugh at the right time. Yvonne, thank you for devoted friendship, and sticking through the tribulations of life. Thank you for always being there.

Stephanie, Stephanie, Stephanie! You hold such an impenetrable place in my heart, thank you for everything. Scott and Judy (my second mom), thank you both for being such a special part of my life. Mari, Rubin & Maria, thank you for always making me feel welcome in and out of the industry and for being the wonderful people that you are.

Nick, Sol, & Thomas for your life learning lessons that provided me a framework by which to become a man and as the saying goes, the ability to change the things I can, accept those I can't and the wisdom to know the difference. Thank you for always hearing me and being there.

Janice, Richard, Valerie, Laura, Pat & Chuck, Charlesana, Lance, Jim & Louise, Elanor, Bruce & Carrie, you are all apart of my founda-

PARAMEDIC M.O.S.

tion, and one that I am very proud to know you have been for so many years. Thank you for being my extended family, and thank you for all the acceptance and laughter.

Freckles, my K-9 pal, thank you for being there with me on 9/11. Somehow you knew something was so very wrong and you just stayed by my side all day. Thank you for your grounding spirit, your unconditional love and constant comedy. You are such a special friend and I am honored to have you in my life.

Lisa, Joseph, and Michael, thank you for being the nurturing spirits that you are. Beth, thank you for all of your feedback early in the process of assembling my thoughts for this book. Meg & Brian, thank you for all of the Christmastimes. Ernest and Peter, thank you for opening your kitchen and hearts.

This book is based upon and inspired by true stories from my experiences in the line of duty. All names and locations have been deliberately altered to protect anonymity and confidentiality respectively.

For R.M., as you will forever be in my heart, soul and mind.

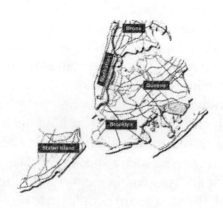

C.B. Garris

Chapter I:

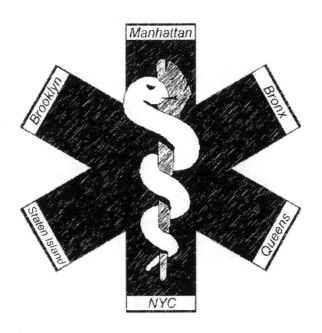

PARAMEDIC M.O.S.

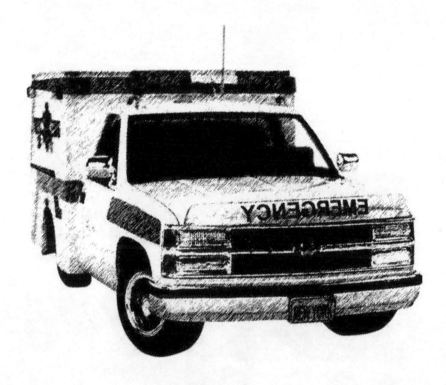

C.B. Garris

I felt the gentle pressure of Anjoline's soft, full lips touching mine before she left for work. I viewed her in uniform but I must have fallen back asleep again almost immediately. I woke up for duty around 11:00 a.m. and indulged in my normal morning fitness breakfast: eight egg whites scrambled with diced green peppers, onions, mushrooms, 4 slices of multi-grain toast, a massive glass of orange juice and a bowl of pears and apples with yogurt and honey. Everyone always asked where I put all the food.

I called the animal hospital to check on AMBU and the Vet said that she was still sedated but stable. I drove through traffic in the Bronx near the 3rd Avenue Bridge and noticed that it got hotter when I passed Yankee Stadium. I was in kind of a funk from last night. I was so scared that AMBU was killed when she was struck by that car outside the station. I got stuck in a heap of traffic near the United Nations, which put me at the station just in time to get dressed. I changed out of my watermelon colored "Black Dog" T-shirt I bought on Martha's Vineyard a year ago and also removed my jeans. I put my uniform pants on first, a white undershirt and then my level 3-A bulletproof vest. I donned my uniform shirt and checked my collar insignias to ensure they were placed properly.

Something made me stop for a second. It was like I was hit from all over with this strange sense of awareness. I looked down at the ground and then straight-ahead. I knocked on the metal shock plate of my vest three times and something said to me that I would need it tonight. That didn't stop me from heading downstairs, in fact whatever my fate would bring I would face it.

I went down and began the process of checking out my radios, narcotics and checking my Lifepak monitor in the office. Danny arrived in the office and we shook hands. He looked at me like he knew I was in deep thought, "You okay man?"

"Yeah," I said, "I just got caught in a little bit of traffic," I said as I placed the paddles back in their respective holders. The office phone rang and Lt. Alan Yobi picked it up. I could tell by his tone that the Communications Division was briefing him.

"Okay, they're going where?" Alan's voice elevated inquisitively.

"Uh, okay, I'll get them rolling." Alan put the phone down and searched his desk for papers. He looked up at Danny and me, "Oh good, you're here."

PARAMEDIC M.O.S.

"Lieu," I said with a smart-ass smile, "Where else would we be?"

Alan looked at me with an equally smart-ass look, "HA HA, check it out you two are going to Brooklyn. Apparently they are getting pounded and can't get units out fast enough. They have about 78 calls holding in the que and they need you to start picking up some slack. You might be there for awhile so I hope you remember your deployments."

I looked at Danny as he shrugged his shoulders, "Let's rock!"

"See ya," I said to Alan as we departed. I picked up my EMS portable and notified the Citywide Special Operations Logistics Dispatcher that we would be heading to Brooklyn and to let us know which calls they wanted us to pick up first. Ted, the evening Citywide dispatcher told us that most of the calls were BLS and he wanted us to get out towards Coney Island as fast as we could. Danny and I checked out our bus (ambulance) and equipment quickly: Lifepak Monitor/Defibrillator, meds bags, Advanced Airway tube kit, Advanced Life Support Trauma bags and the various necessities we would need to have on a busy night.

Danny and I made for the Brooklyn-Battery Tunnel, towards the Verrazano Bridge. I figured that at this hour of the day we would have an easier time getting into the K1-K2 area (the K stands for Kings County) from the back end.

We hit a bit of traffic but nothing that lights and sirens couldn't get us through. As we approached the exit for the Belt Parkway, we got called for a stabbing close by on Ave X at 31st Street. We went 10-63 (enroute) and were forcing our way through traffic when NYPD notified our dispatcher that it was a hoax, or what we called an unfounded assignment.

By this time we were pretty close to Station 31 at Coney Island Hospital, so we stopped in to pay a visit. The first person I saw was Julie Mednick, who when I saw her last was a mess of tears over at Jacobi Hospital after the notification of Tanya's death. That was also the night that I lost Jennifer. She saw me and ran over, putting her arms around me. She squeezed me like she did not want to let go. Everyone at the station was trying to figure it out, but just went about their business.

"How are you doing?" I asked while we hugged.

"Christian, I think I should be asking you that question. I am so sorry." She wiped her hair away from her face as tears started to fall from her eyes.

"Jesus, I don't even know what to say. I have wanted to call you but I didn't want to bring it all up again. How are you handling things?"

C.B. Garris

I accepted her hug and gave her another. "Thank you. You know you can always call and don't worry about stirring things up. It is something that has to be dealt with. Life has been different, very different. It is like there is this huge hole in my life, but I am fortunate to have someone in my life that is taking really incredible care of me. It is not that my days are not without feeling strung out, but this is an experience that I am taking day by day. Coming to work is kind of strange. There are reminders of Jennifer everywhere, especially when I get on a scene, I look up, and she is not there."

As I went to complete my sentence, my pager went off. It was Anjoline informing me that she is home safe and will be in the rest of the night. She also told me to be careful tonight.

"Is that the sparkle in your life?" Julie said quietly.

"Yes, just a check in to let me know she is there for me." I said mustering a smile through the sadness in my face.

Julie wiped tears from her eyes as she gathered herself, "Well if she is with you, I know that you are well taken care of."

The two-way portable radio on Julie's hip began to call her unit number, 31E3 (or in our service name - 31 Eddie). The radio on my hip shared the same message. Julie and her partner were dispatched to a call for a possible pin job (car accident with someone trapped inside) on the Belt Parkway. So she acknowledged the radio assignment, wrapped her arms around me gently, giving me a gentle, but deliberate kiss on my cheek and said we would speak later.

As I listened to the dispatcher on her frequency, I realized that there was no Advanced Life Support unit assigned to Julie's job, so I offered up and we were assigned. We followed Julie's unit out of the station, blasting out onto Ocean Parkway. As we made to the scene of the accident in tandem, it looked pretty bad; a Ford Taurus and a Nissan Probe seemed to have intertwined themselves. It was dusk, so as the four of us initiated patient care and pre-extrication procedures, I had the NYPD ESU units check the grassy and wooded areas off the parkway for anyone who may have been ejected from either vehicle on impact. The last thing you want to happen is to lose a patient in the shuffle of a bad scene.

Two of the three patients were in very serious condition, completely pinned under the dashboard of each vehicle. From what I could tell, it looked like one of the vehicles might have jumped the median and went head on into the other vehicle. A few more units going available out of

PARAMEDIC M.O.S.

Coney Island Hospital hopped on the call as well, so we were able to get extra hands on the scene quickly. Having the additional hands helped Danny and I concentrate on the two most critical patients.

We both initiated multiple IV's on both patients as FDNY (Fire Department, City of New York) and NYPD ESU (New York City Police Department, Emergency Services Units) started cutting the vehicles apart with their Jaws of Life. Once freed, Danny and I took the patient from the Probe; Julie and another ALS unit took patient number two. Julie's partner and another BLS unit took the third patient. We completed packaging our patient in full cervical spine immobilization and a few officers began to place him in the vehicle. Danny and I worked feverishly against the fact that our patient's blood pressure was dropping like the stock market in 1987 and that his respiratory factor was completely compromised due to severe chest and head injuries he suffered in the impact.

I began tubing the patient with a 7.0 endotracheal tube, while Danny punctured another 14-gauge catheter into his left jugular vein for IV access. He could have been bleeding internally from so many places that a patent airway and fluid replacement had to be accomplished faster than humanly possible. Once I secured the tube around his face, I notified Communications that we're enroute to Coney Island Hospital and to have the trauma teams ready. As we turned off the Belt Parkway onto a street I could not see from the rear, I heard the tech driving say, "Holy Shit, hold on!"

I heard a barrage of screeching from several directions and a thunderous, explosive bang. Next I remember an impact with incredible force and my feet coming up off the floor of the ambulance. The vehicle, Danny, the patient and I all went into a tumble, as I heard Danny scream. I tried to grab him but couldn't because of the vehicle somersaulting. I hit my head on something and I felt pressure on my back, and then everything went completely dark.

C.B. Garris

Chapter II:

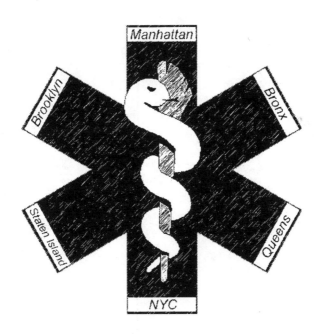

PARAMEDIC M.O.S.

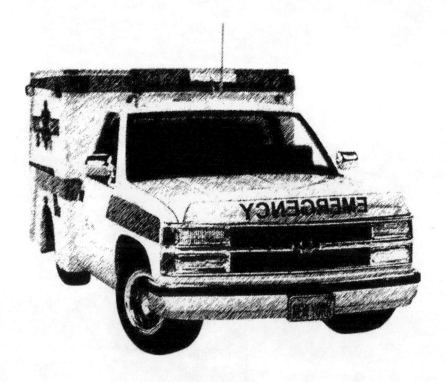

I kept hearing Julie's voice.

"Christian, Christian honey, wake up. Shit he is not waking up."

Everything was still dark. I wanted to answer Julie.

I heard commotion and bags being ripped open. In fact, I heard the sound of clothes being ripped open. The darkness was eerie, but peaceful. Since I didn't feel anything, I had no idea that I was wearing the clothes being ripped open.

"31 Eddie, get me an NYPD heelo (a helicopter) to Floyd Bennet Field now, I have three MOS's down, one in traumatic arrest, one critical and the other is stable."

I heard Julie's voice speaking these words frantically, but it wasn't registering. Another lapse of time went by and I heard rotors. I wanted to stand up and say I was fine. I had no idea what was going on.

"Damnit Christian, open your eyes," I said to myself, and still there was nothing I could do. The sound of the rotors got louder.

When I finally opened my eyes, everything was water like; I was dizzy and nauseated. I was also not breathing on my own. I looked around the room and Julie was there with Davia; meanwhile someone was holding my right hand and I realized I was hooked up to a ventilator. I could hear the familiar beeps and air suction sounds that the ventilator makes, and it synchronized with my breath. I also realized that my head was somehow strapped or taped to a wooden backboard, and I was in full cervical spinal immobilization. I began to feel sore everywhere. I could tell by the fact that my arms were pretty much taped down that I had IV's in place.

I thought to myself, "What the fuck is going on? Where are Jennifer and Danny?" I realized how hard it was to even attempt to speak with a tube in my throat. I felt this gut-wrenching discomfort in the pit of my stomach, because I remembered that Jennifer could not be in the room, because she was dead. I kept getting these visions of a funeral, a procession and her. In the darkness I experienced, I felt as if I saw her if only for a moment.

I focused on Davia and Julie as best I could, though that wasn't much help.

Everything went dark again.

At some point I opened my eyes again and this time focused much better. My sister, brother and mom were all there, along with Davia, Julie, Captain Bob and Captain Lenny, Chief Tom Conroy and of course Anjoline

PARAMEDIC M.O.S.

(AJ). AJ looked like she was holding vigil for many hours. I could finally speak and I realized that the tube was out of my throat, though my voice was rather raspy for a while (common for just being extubated).

"Hey babe," AJ said as I looked at her completely confused.

"Where am I?" I said to AJ with this grimaced face from my back pain.

"You're at Bell," AJ said as she placed her hand on my forehead. "You were in an accident a day and a half ago."

"A day and a half ago," I said as I looked at AJ like I didn't even know her. "Accident? Where is Danny?"

AJ sighed deeply and a tear ran down her face, as Davia stepped forward in a freshly dry-cleaned uniform.

"Hi sleepyhead," Davia said affectionately, "Let's talks about Danny later."

I took a second to take in Davia's discretion.

"No," I said with great furvor, "Let's talk about Danny now, where is he?"

Davia knew that I wouldn't accept a trivial answer. "Christian, Honey, with everything you have been through recently, what I am about to say may seem a little bit overwhelming."

I took a deep breath as I felt the pit in my stomach grow even larger.

Davia looked at me with sadness in her eyes.

"Christian, Danny died in the accident."

I looked at Davia with absolute numbness in my eyes.

"Your vehicle," Davia continued, "was broad sided coming off the Belt Parkway and it flipped numerous times. So far as NYPD A.I.D. (Accident Investigation Division) can piece it together, Danny was ejected out of the rear doors on impact and was subsequently struck by a drunk driver."

I felt AJ squeeze my hand hard as I just sat there inhaling and exhaling quickly. I felt as if the entire world had come down upon me and as if I had done something wrong. I began to wonder about everything and all of those around me. Chief Tom Conroy, one of my closest friends in the service reached over to my ankle and wrapped his full hand around it. He applied gentle pressure signaling that he is there. Tom and I always shared an incredible bond, where many words didn't have to be said, but we were friends since my adolescence; and he was my life mentor.

Bob, another very close friend walked up to my bedside and tapped my leg, "Yo bro, I'm sorry."

"Dav," I said with a still raspy voice, "Danny was only twenty five."

C.B. Garris

I started to cry and suddenly realized how much pain I was in when I attempted to wipe my tears. Davia just looked at me with sadness in her stare. I laid there in the hospital bed surveying all of the equipment I was connected too, respecting the bond I shared with this group of people in my life that now surrounded me, coming to be there for me in my time of need. In my sadness and frustration, I began to recall all of the events that led me here.

PARAMEDIC M.O.S.

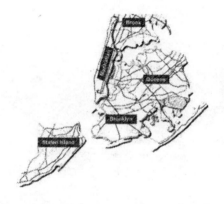

C.B. Garris

Chapter III:

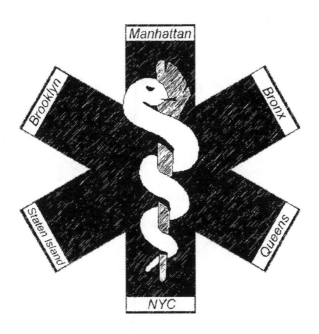

PARAMEDIC M.O.S.

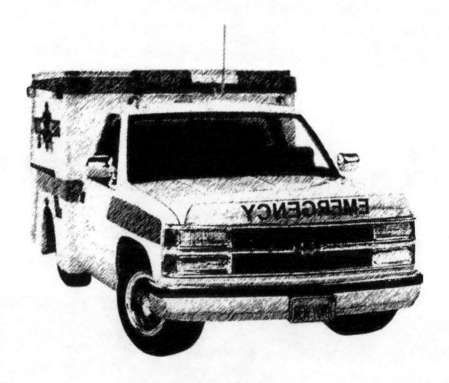

C.B. Garris

"I was looking forward to a lobster or perhaps one of those bacon-wrapped filet mignon's this time," Jennifer joked with me as we sat in the US Secret Service Advance Team Ready Room at the United Nations.

Looking in my direction, Jennifer rubbed her tummy and licked her lips while she added, "You know, the one I got with the sautéed spinach and Yukon Gold garlic-mashed potatoes when we were with the Prez two months ago."

"Sorry Jen, I believe this will be a short trip this time. Boss man is addressing the UN Assembly on his annual world hunger budget, and then he is back to Washington." I said to Jennifer adjusting my black nylon utility belt around my waist.

Jen and I were working the Medical Protection Detail for NYC EMS in accordance with the United States Secret Service. Although the president has his own physicians on staff, we are the emergency paramedics assigned to him, the Vice President or any dignitary the Federal law enforcement agencies request us to provide emergency medical care for whenever one of or all of these individuals are within the confines of New York City.

We even had the opportunity to sit down and have dinner with the President and his family on several occasions when the events would be informal.

Our bosses would have probably flipped if they knew we were eating with the President and his family.

Adjusting my NYC EMS portable two-way radio on my belt as I looked in the direction of Secret Service Special Agent Jack Trudor, I asked him, "Is this going to be one of those long speeches like the last time we were here?"

Jack was an ex-NFL Defensive Back turned Chief Security Agent for the President. He was a tall black male, standing 6'2", weighing in I would guess at about 240, all muscle. If his shoulders weren't already broad enough, the numerous weapons he had at the ready under his sports coat made him look even larger.

Though always professional, his duty-posture always eased with us around as he said quietly, "The Prez has a meeting with Congress in the morning, so he will be heading right back to the House after the speech. No press questions, no photo ops."

"Damn," I said, "and I was looking forward to good food for four days just like when he was here two months ago. That was awesome. Nothing

PARAMEDIC M.O.S.

but filet mignon, lobster, or anything else we wanted on the tab of the US Government."

Jack lightly punched me in my upper right arm, "You got the lobster too?"

I smiled, "Dude, medics gotta eat well too."

Jack, Jennifer, Michael Swarthe (Jack's right hand person) and I all laughed.

Jennifer went to the snack table and brought back a pesto chicken sandwich for herself, and for me a spicy tuna hand roll that was prepared to order, along with a couple of lemonades.

As Jack was in mid-conversation with his partner, he reached his left fingers up to his ear and stopped everything he was doing while looking around the room.

"Boss man is six minutes forty-two from finishing his speech, let's get ready to rock."

Jennifer and I wolfed down our food and were finishing up the last drops of our lemonades when the Assistant Secretary of Defense came through the doors. He nodded at Jack, Michael, Jennifer and I as we backed up four steps, making room for both doors to open. Advance Team B, the team that stood by the President inside the Assembly Room came through the doors in formation, surrounding the President who was on a cell phone.

Jen and I already had our equipment in hand: advanced airway bag with oxygen, drug bag, Lifepak cardiac monitor/defibrillator, trauma kit, suction, and Apcor telemetry communication unit so that we could talk to our 911 EMS physician or transmit EKGs if needed. As the president walked past Jen and I, he stopped and smiled.

"I was hoping you two were in this crowd; in fact I was counting on it." The President said as he extended his hand to both Jennifer and I, greeting us both with a warm smile.

He motioned for one of his agents who handed him a bag. The president reached in the brown paper bag and took out two separate ribbon decorated gift-wrapped packages.

"I am sorry that we won't have a chance to sit down like the last trip, but my country calls for me. Thank you for always being at the ready for me. The Mrs. and I want you to have these." He handed the first gift to Jennifer.

Ladies first, smart man. He then handed the other pack to me.

"Go ahead, open them, I have a few minutes," the President replied in an approving, relaxed tone. Jen and I were totally surprised, each gift contained five CDs each. Jen and I were surprised that he remembered that we were both music lovers.

"Oh my God, Andy Narell, Mariah Carey, Carly Simon, Steps Ahead and Spyro Gyra? Sir how did you know?" Jennifer blurted out as the President appreciated her almost child-like Christmas present response.

"I am the leader of the free world, I have ears and eyes everywhere." The president said with a humble smile.

I opened mine and it was the latest from Pat Metheny, Michael Franks, and some ol'school Earth, Wind & Fire, Al Jarreau and Simply Red.

Damn this guy was good.

When I looked at the President his smile was gleaming.

"If I dropped right here and my heart stopped, would you really put those paddles on my chest and send a charge through me?"

"Just like one of these fine agents defends your life, sir." I said with a smile.

A voice from behind us said, "Mr. President, we can leave at anytime sir." That voice was Jack.

"You guys are always rushing me somewhere, don't I get to just hang out with the folk?"

We all laughed as we started in formation for the egress doors.

As we fell behind in the crowd of agents, Jen said to me, "I cannot believe he did this. Inviting us to dinner the last time with his family was one thing, but he really went out of his way."

"It is pretty cool, isn't it? When Lenny hears about this he is going to shit." I said laughing.

As we all exited the doors to the main garage where our vehicles were, the President stopped until we walked up to him.

"Ya'll be careful out there." We nodded at the President and he extended his hand to do the handshake I taught him about six months ago when we had some time to chat. We slapped our hand backs together, then the front, then we pressed our closed fists together twice, then he hit my closed fist vertically on top, then I his, then we wiggled our fingers in front of the other. I thought Jen was going to pass out laughing and that Jack was going to shoot me.

We separated and made for our respective vehicles. There we all swiftly and in practiced motion placed our equipment in our vehicles; Jen and I our medical equipment, and the Secret Service agents placed their heavy weapons where it fit them. As I started the vehicle up and put it

PARAMEDIC M.O.S.

in drive in tow with the rest of the presidential motorcade, I received a message on our ambulance's Mobile Data Terminal (MDT), which is an onboard computer.

This allows us to send and receive messages to our communications division and they provide us a visual of all pertinent information of calls we are responding too.

Our on-board computer beeped once, and a message appeared in yellow Liquid Crystal Display.

The message was from Jack in the President's vehicle.

"Sorry you won't be getting lobsters this trip, and by the way, I cannot believe you taught the boss man a hand shake! You guys are an absolute riot! Have a good one and be safe out there."

Jen typed back a message. No problem, just make sure next time that our lobsters are Atlantic picked, broiled with drawn butter and lots of lemon when you come back, Jack! You be careful too. We both laughed.

As we departed from the UN, we drove off the ramp under extremely tight security, our entire path cordoned off by the NYPD. We took our place in the procession following the President, until we reached the mobilization point.

We remained in tow until we reached the landing zone of Air Force One. We pulled onto the tarmac to escort the President to his aircraft for the short flight home.

We parked in our pre-determined position and awaited our final orders.

Jack approached our unit before he boarded Air Force One.

"Hey you two, thanks a million for another job well done. We always love coming to New York, and wish we could more often. Jen, I always mistake you for one of those famous TV lifeguards every time I see you."

Jen smiled "I'll take that as a compliment!"

Jack stuck his hand inside the window to shake our hands, "You should, I think she is gorgeous."

Jen smiled an electric smile and winked at Jack, "You know, if I wasn't mistaken, I might think you were coming on to me."

Jack looked like he'd just been busted, "Uh, well, I wouldn't,"

Jen cut him off, "No worries Mahn!"

I knew that Jack secretly had a thing for Jennifer. Who wouldn't, she was beautiful. She stood at 5'3", with long brown hair and hazel eyes, with an incredible figure, and she worked out five days a week.

I shook my head and Jack saluted us. Jen and I saluted back and waved at the President, as he saluted right back.

Air Force One got underway immediately, and we rolled up our windows so that we weren't affected by the noise of the massive 747's engines. The aircraft taxied into position and lifted off. We noticed that as it reached about one thousand feet, it was joined by five military fighters in mid air formation.

Wayne Phillips, the lead advance Agent for the New York Office walked over and after making several comments into his sleeve, he thanked us and released us from the protection detail. In a matter of minutes, this airport tarmac would return to normal operations status, desolate of any sign that the leader of the free world was ever here.

As we drove back towards Manhattan, Jen and I noticed that all of our agency frequencies were very busy, typical for a summer evening. Jen sent a computer message to Communications informing them that we were clear of the Presidential detail, and that if the Watch Commander approved it, we would be happy to stay in service as a primary unit for 911 assignments.

A few seconds later our cell phone rang and I answered it, "Yello?"

"Good evening sir!" It was the Watch Commander, Captain Lenny Washington.

"Whas up, Cap?" I said with as much street as I could put into the words.

Lenny inquired, "How was the big man tonight?"

"Short stay this time," I said jokingly.

"Hey did you get my page about the river rafting trip for next week?" Lenny asked.

"Actually I did, and I'm sorry Dave broke his leg in the motorcycle accident. It is no problem to postpone it. Would you believe we got presents from the big man?" I mentioned.

"WHAT?" Lenny said laughing. "What did he get you?"

"He made a little stop at Tower records, five CD's each, gift wrapped with ribbon."

"You gotta be kidding me? What did you say?" Lenny asked like a jealous kid.

"Uh, thank you!" I said laughing.

"I should have never taken my promotion," Lenny added. "Hey if you guys want to stay out for awhile we could use some coverage. We have

PARAMEDIC M.O.S.

been getting slammed all day. Your regular unit was down mechanical earlier, so why don't we put you in as your regular 10X3 and give me a second to figure out where we can use you. Are you still in Queens?" Lenny asked.

"Actually we are about to cross over into Manhattan from the Kosciusko (bridge), but wherever you need us, just say so." I said as Jen nodded in agreement.

"We could really use some help in the M 1 (Manhattan South)," Lenny said.

I smiled, "That's our home Cap, you know we always love playing in our hood, no prob. How about we stay near the station, say Allen and South right under the FDR?" I said well aware that Lenny would agree.

As I heard Lenny get distracted in the background, he quickly mentioned to me, "Good spot ol' chap. Send a note to my terminal when you are in the area."

"Hit me on my term, a deuce (2nd alarm fire) just dropped in Staten Island."

"See ya," I said as we both hung up. As we hung up I heard the familiar three tone alert and verbal notification that would alert all specialty (tac units) and senior officials of the fire.

Jen and I drove the rest of the BQE over the Willy B (Williamsburg Bridge), hooking a left at Allen Street. We would now be only a minute from the station, so Jen asked if I would swing over to our favorite twenty-four-hour deli on Water Street. We were both thirsty, so a nice cold Gatorade would be great about now. Bulletproof vests are great, and although our bodies assimilate well to them, you can sweat more than normal depending on what threat level yours is. The stronger the impact that the vest can withstand, the heavier it is. Jen and I both had ours custom made to our bodies' specifications at Threat Level III (3)A, so they were nice and snug.

I turned onto Water Street and headed west. I pulled in and parked our bus right behind a sanitation truck. Jen walked in first and the three guys behind the counter stopped everything they were doing to get a good look at Jennifer. I walked in behind her and nodded at the guys at the counter. They were watching Jennifer so intently when she bent over to get two Gatorade's from one of the bottom shelves, someone could have robbed them and they wouldn't have heard anything.

When the guys turned back to me, they saw my look that said, "Don't take that thought any further!"

C.B. Garris

They fixed themselves right up, and the leader of the pack asked how we were doing tonight. "That's better," I said with a smile.

I paid for our drinks and we headed back to the bus.

"I think Lenny is jealous," Jen said to me proud that she received a gift from the President of the United States.

"Yeah, he mentioned that he was pissed that he left the street to take a promotion to Captain. I guess that's the price for getting your bars."

I pulled onto Water street to make a turn under the Brooklyn Bridge, that would put us right on South Street, while monitoring the Manhattan South EMS radio frequency.

As a tactical Paramedic unit, we monitor a multitude of frequencies, as we are capable of being called on several at any one time. We always monitor the sector that we are presently in, and we also monitor our Citywide Special Operations frequencies, which have the main frequency in the 400 MHZ, and then our private frequency in the 800 MHZ trunked system. We also monitor the NYPD Special Operations (ESU) Emergency Services Unit frequency. This allowed us access into the know about what was going on where and if we might be called upon. It also allowed us better up to date knowledge of what we are walking into.

Each borough has its own units and designation. Since Jennifer and I are a regular MANHATTAN tactical Paramedic unit, our designation begins with a 1, BRONX units begin with 2, BROOKLYN with 3, QUEENS with 4, and STATEN ISLAND with 5. The next number in the pneumonic of a unit tells you what general area they cover in the borough grid. Normally the numbers would go anywhere from 1-9. In this case since we were now back in regular rotation, and a tactical or specialized unit that could be sent citywide at anytime, our second identifier was the number 0. The "tactical" designation means we go wherever the service requests and we are the first line units to be either deployed to a major incident, or re-deployed to fill in if the service is getting inundated with assignments.

Members of the TAC units know the city inside and out. We knew how to get anywhere fast and without question. We are highly trained in our functions as paramedics, and additionally trained in 911-law enforcement (street combat & S.W.A.T. operations and anything to deal with situations out of the ordinary). Next is the identifier of whether they are a Basic Life Support unit or Advanced Life Support unit. If the third part of the pneumonic was in the form of the letters A-K, it was a Basic Life

PARAMEDIC M.O.S.

Support Unit. If the letter was W-Z, it was an Advanced Life Support Unit. The final segment in a designation was the tour or hours that you worked. Tour one (1) was the midnight tour beginning at 22:00 hours. The Tour two (2) segment was the daytime or business hours beginning at 06:00 hours and the tour that Jennifer and I belonged to, our favorite was Tour three (3), beginning at 14:00 hours. The first units of a new tour come out at 22:00 (Tour 1), 06:00 (Tour 2) and 14:00 (Tour 3). Units are then brought into duty at staggered hourly intervals so that there are as few gaps in resource deployment as possible. The starting time for Jennifer and I is normally 15:00 or three PM. Although due to our presidential detail today, we came in at 11:00.

We parked underneath the FDR Drive, right by the water. This put us in a great strategic spot to go north up Allen to 1st Avenue if we were needed north, west on South St. to go downtown or right to head to the Upper East Side. It was a gorgeous evening out and no reason to be driving around if we didn't have too. We were the extra unit for the time being, so we would only be called upon if we were the closest unit or if something big went down.

Jen and I both had a few rough weeks behind us, and although usually fresh and ready for anything, we were a little bit tired. We just buried one of our senior personnel who died of a heart attack at 38. He was a very well liked person and a great administrator; the funeral was a few days prior and another one of our station personnel committed suicide one day after we got news of his heart attack. Everyone was kind of wiped out. I hadn't been sleeping much, so I thought I would take time to catch up on a catnap.

I must have looked somewhat unfocused when Jen turned towards me to say, "These past few weeks have really sucked, haven't they?"

"Yeah," I said rubbing my eyes & face in agreement, "It is just hard to believe that we buried Tony a few days ago and Monica yesterday. He had a wife and four kids; and she was seven months pregnant with her second child. I feel really foul and was up the night before both funerals as I made meals for Tony's wife Terry and their kids for the week. I did the same for Monica's husband and daughter. I was up until 4am making my house recipe pasta sauce, proofing and kneading out a few pizza dough's and cooking off the linguine. I also made a huge batch of brownies for the kids too," I said tapping my right hand on the keyboard to our on-board computer.

"You are really sweet for doing that. Terry was telling me how much that will help her in this first week. I know that Monica's husband was just totally distraught and can use all the help he can get." Jen said placing her hand on my forearm in compassion. "We will all get through this."

"I know, it is just nutty." I adjusted my body sloping downward to get into a sleeping position.

"I'm going to try to catch a few Z's; could you listen up?" I said adjusting myself in the driver's seat for a quick nap.

As she unfolded The New York Times that was sitting on the dashboard, Jen replied gently, "Sure, Sweet Cheeks (Jen's nickname for me); go for it."

About an hour later, after drifting off into a great catnap, I woke up with Jen smiling on the other side of the console.

"Hello sleepy," Jen said with a warm smile, "You were out like a light!"

Jen commented as she turned the page on the Metropolitan section. Our computer beeped twice and it was a message from computer terminal WCSO, it was Lenny the Watch Commander.

Ya'll having fun out there? I see you have been in stealth mode. Be safe out there.

I swiveled the keyboard towards me and sent a smiley face back to Lenny's computer.

PARAMEDIC M.O.S.

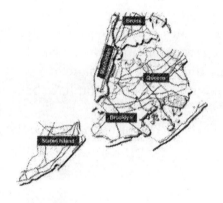

C.B. Garris

Chapter IV:

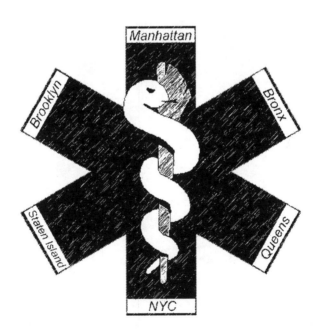

PARAMEDIC M.O.S.

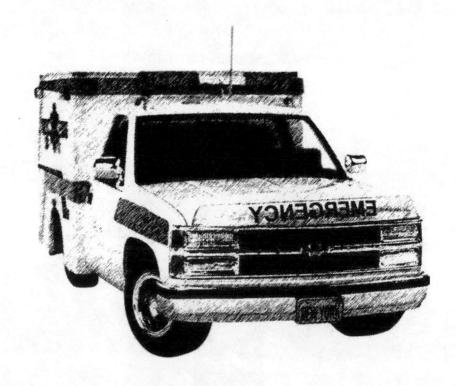

C.B. Garris

July was a fun month to be working a bus. This time of year the call volume was so large, we would often put medics not only in ambulances, but deploy additional Basic Life Support units and place Advanced Life Support medics in SUV's. This way, if the call was able to be handled by a BLS crew, it would free up the ALS unit should their particular services be needed elsewhere.

The main problem with putting medics in rapid response jeeps is that the system would get so busy, that you could not be guaranteed an ambulance when you were responding. You would get to the call in no time and initiate proper and thorough care; but you couldn't transport the patient. This could be a very volatile situation as the general public is totally unaware of our skills and equipment. They forget in their time of need, if they ever knew at all, that we bring the emergency room to them. There is so much that we can do before you ever reach the hospital.

With a gentle breeze generating off of the East River behind us, it was humid enough to have the windows open at night. As Jen and I were discussing the topic of the lack of the family unit in our society, we simultaneously heard an assignment dispatched to two Manhattan South units and also to NYPD sector car units.

"I need 12(X)ray and 11(E)ddie for a trauma," said Dana Williams, the Manhattan South dispatcher. After both units answered there call request, the dispatcher followed with "11Eddie, 12X-ray, I need you for a pediatric (child) trauma at 3rd Street between 1st and 2nd Avenue, possible secondary to an explosion. Unknown how many patients."

Manhattan like the other boroughs is split into different sections, so as to not overload the dispatchers or the units. By splitting Manhattan into three sections, Manhattan South, Manhattan Central and Manhattan North; it allowed calls to go out as smoothly as possible, while leaving enough room on the frequency for us the medics to get an emergency call in for help if we needed it.

We were in a perfect position for that assignment since we could literally shoot straight up Allen Street, which once we crossed Houston (pronounced Howstun) will turn right into 1st Avenue; 3rd Street is a few blocks in. Because of my extremely aggressive driving in a response mode, I knew we would probably beat both of the other units. I didn't even have to look at Jen when I threw the vehicle into drive, hitting the lights and sirens as I punched the gas through the intersection, heading north up Allen Street.

PARAMEDIC M.O.S.

Jennifer picked up one of the four onboard radio microphones calling the dispatcher, "Tactical X, South, we are right on top of that pediatric trauma. Put us on it!"

Without a delay in her voice and knowing we would hop on the call, Dana answered Jennifer "10X-ray I have you assigned, first unit in give me a 12 (situation report)." Dana said this with a hint of escalating worry in her voice. Generally a dispatcher would have taken the other Paramedic unit off the call, but based on the intelligence (information) she was viewing on her computer screen, this looked like a real job so whoever got there first takes it.

"10X, 12X, 11Eddie, this was some sort of explosion in a dumpster, and you have a pediatric heavy bleeder at the location." Dana said this swiftly, clicking her fingers across her keyboard as she spoke.

As the words pediatric left Dana's lips, I must have punched my speedometer to over 60 mph. Jen was holding onto the onboard computer screen for dear life as she listened to her NYPD portable against her right ear, they were just arriving when we crossed Houston. I was making so much noise with my sirens, people thought a massive truck was coming through and in fact it was, so they knew to get the hell out of our way.

As I heard the garbled transmissions of screaming from the NYPD officers on scene, "Expedite the medics, I think this kids throat was slashed by shrapnel (metal fragment from the explosion)," I felt myself go into a zone. My only focus was that child, everything else is an afterthought. Jen had seen this look on my face a thousand times before. She knew that I was aware of everything around me, though I probably looked totally untouchable by the general public. As my driving became more aggressive, my eyes sank down a bit and my breathing slowed down. Jen never saw me turn my head, but she knew that I saw every car in traffic, and every pedestrian on each corner. I was blowing through traffic like a freight train. Thirty seconds later I pulled a hard left on two wheels into 3rd Street. I saw the NYPD holding a kid in their hands at the other end of the block. As we approached I thought I saw them throw the kid into a sector car.

"CPOP central, we're taking the kid to the Mother (an acronym for one of our area hospitals)," a voice said over the PD portable radio.

I thought I was going to lose my mind.

"What the fuck is he doing? We're pulling up. That facility can't handle that injury!" I said out loud.

C.B. Garris

As I sped up, I reached over and picked up my NYPD portable saying abrasively, "EMS Paramedic Ten X-ray Central, have that Precinct unit stop his vehicle now, we are on scene and right behind him. We have to treat that child, tell him to stop now!"

The NYPD dispatcher hit a series of alert tones, "CPOP, CPOP, EMS is telling you to stop your vehicle, they are right behind you!" No answer.

I thought I was going to blow a gasket and Jennifer knew this was about to get really ugly.

I was now chasing the sector car up 3rd Avenue at what must have been fifty mph. I thought about ramming him, but that wouldn't have helped the kid.

"EMS Ten-Xray to PD Central, tell that officer to stop his vehicle now, he isn't helping the kid, that kid may have only one shot and we're it."

As the PD dispatcher went to chime in the precinct officer came up on the radio, "CPOP Central, this kid's throat was slashed and I got pressure on his neck, we ain't stopping!" I thought I was about to burst every vein in my skull.

Jennifer knew this situation was getting bad, and I was at the end of my fucking rope with this.

Cars on 3rd Avenue were making evasive maneuvers left and right to get out of the way of our vehicle's five tons of steel that I was using to chase the NYPD. The officer's vehicle pulled into the hospital ER bay. They stopped their vehicle and ran inside the ER with a bloody mess of a seven-year-old boy. My blood was boiling and I was seeing only red. I knew that what was about to happen in the emergency room was bad, but I was not stopping, as I stopped the bus with lights still on in the middle of the street, I ran in after the officer with my stethoscope wrapping me in the face, as I leaped over the bushes at the entrance to the Emergency Department. Jennifer knew that I was in a really bad place with this and was going to go at it with the officer, so she radioed Chief Davia Battieri on a private channel and told her to get over to "the Mother" STAT.

There was blood everywhere as I approached the Emergency Department, and in fact I slipped in it, just catching my balance on the entrance door. When I looked at the NYPD car, there was blood all over the back seat and the windows. A nurse exiting the E.R. bay door held it for me as I leaped through it sideways. I heard the ER doc giving orders for a PEDS CODE (Pronounced Peads Code for Pediatric Cardiac Arrest) and

PARAMEDIC M.O.S.

in between he kept yelling at the officer about why he should have taken the kid to Bellevue's trauma center.

I ran into the acute slot and viewed something horrible. A small black child, blood stained and smeared, with his throat wide open from the piece of metal that eviscerated it. His throat was so damaged that his windpipe was just about thoroughly severed. This particular hospital was not set up for major trauma, as the wounds this child suffered required a Level-1 trauma center; which consists of a complete trauma team and all of its ancillary support units ready in a moment's notice. I didn't want to interrupt the frantic, yet controlled efforts of the E.R. team attending to the little boy.

When I realized that the staff had all the hands they could use, I watched a few more seconds and then walked out when I realized that he suffered mortal wounds. I decided I would wait for the officer to reappear near the nurses station to vent my frustration. The officer appeared from a back room, pulling back a putrid yellow curtain. Something about the officer's voice was familiar as he walked around the corner. When I caught my glimpse of who it was, it all came back to me. I knew why my dander was up and why I was so angry.

Now I know why my blood was boiling and why I felt like ripping this guy to pieces. It was Officer Anthony Kertuina.

This infamous dope was the person who a collective of medics and I caused to lose his Sergeant's shield, being bumped down to an officer again. It seems that Officer Kertuina had a bad habit of beating up his fiancé on a regular basis. There were two big problems with this. One is that he was doing it. Two was that he was doing it to a fellow medic at my station.

Samantha Blangdon was a medic assigned to my station for about four years. She was one of the sweetest, most gentle persons one could ever encounter. Petite with a 5'1" frame at about 115 pounds, she was always pleasant and kind, and had a very soft way about her. She could never hurt a soul, and was great in the art of nurturing.

Her only downfall is that she allowed this guy to use her face as a punching bag. I guess for years it was mainly body blows or emotionally torturous activities such as allowing him to control her life, who she spent time with, when she could and could not go out of the house, etc. I am unsure exactly when he began beating her, but several medics and I noticed her coming into work on the midnight tour with sunglasses on regularly for about a week. At first we thought she was going through some fashion withdrawal. We knew her enough that we didn't suspect drug or alcohol involvement, as she was completely lucid and able to work with those sunglasses without a problem.

After several concerned conversations I approached her quietly, inquiring if everything was okay. At first she pawned it off to the fashion idea, but something in her demeanor suggested that I wait a few moments. I did and shortly thereafter when no one else was around, she broke down. Prefacing her statement that she would only discuss this with me because I gained her trust after being her field instructor when she first hit the street, she shared a pretty gruesome story with me. He had been roughing her up nightly, and even to the point of punching her in her sleep.

She knew that she had to get out, but she was also intent on making things better for him. I gave her the domestic abuse lecture 101 and I told her that she could not change him. I wondered why he would always drop her off at the station and pick her up like clockwork. He would pull up just short of 23:00 hours, placing her at the side entrance to the building so that she could run up to her locker being seen by only AMBU. She never made it to roll call during these times, but she was such a favorite at the station, the supervisors didn't mind. She was always there when her unit was called.

I told her that she needed to get out of that relationship, since this guy is not only a maniac, he also carries a weapon. She was reluctant to do anything for fear that he might lose his job or it might affect him somehow. I went to my locker across the hall to retrieve some pamphlets on domestic abuse counseling that we keep on the bus. I implored her to make a phone call to the agencies as a first step in correcting her situation, so that she didn't end up dead. She promised me that she would make the phone calls.

Samantha came in for next tour with a huge bruise on the side of her head, one that the fashionable sunglasses could not hide. We looked at each other with a long stare as she went to the locker room.

"I know," she said as she stood next to me.

"I will make the phone calls," she said as the hair on the back of my head stood up in anger.

Several tears rolled under her dark sunglasses as she took hold of my hand, "Thank you for caring."

"Sam, you need to call NYPD Internal Affairs and press charges. Your head cannot stand too many blows like that." I said as she squeezed my hand while crying lightly.

PARAMEDIC M.O.S.

"I know," she said, "I think I was out for a minute or two," she said as my mouth opened wide in amazement that she actually blacked out from the blunt force.

"That's it Sam, now something else has to be done. You may have trouble making the phone call, but I have no problem rearranging his face. He is a sick fuck and needs to be stopped." I said firmly, choking back my anger so that I didn't make her feel any worse than she already did.

"What are you going to do?" She asked in fear that I would follow through.

I stared at her for a long moment, "Look, you need to get the hell out of that house for a few nights until I can figure out the best course of action. Stay away from him and go visit your sister in Newark, but just get the hell out."

"You aren't going to hurt him, are you?" She asked sheepishly.

"Hurting him would be too damn nice. Don't you worry about what I am going to do, you go to Veronica's and I will figure something out."

After she went to get her gear together in the ambulance bay, I walked out to my truck. I sat behind my steering wheel for a minute and just inhaled, sitting with my anger. I drove up to Nancy's Tavern on 7th Street, just off Ave B, to meet with a bunch of the night tour medics who just got off duty.

The following night seven other medics and I were waiting for Anthony. Ten minutes to 11:00 p.m. came and in drove Anthony, with Samantha in the passenger seat. She was wearing the sunglasses. Adam Droler, "Big" Franky Lousien, Neville Michaelson, Bill Brozchek, Jose Guitierrez and I were in a closet directly behind the front door.

Flanking the fence outside out of sight were George Regiou and Phillip Haslifer. Four of the seven were 5'11 or taller, weighing in from 185 to 250 pounds a piece. Mr. Anthony, Samantha's abusive beau was a mere 5' 6" and about 150 pounds wet. He wasn't even a workout by any standard, and I wanted to put nothing but complete fear into him.

She stepped out of the vehicle as we heard him mumble. As soon as she entered the building and went upstairs, we all piled out like clockwork. George stepped in back of his vehicle as he backed up. Since George was a distant cousin to Anthony, he thought nothing of it. Next I opened the side door that Samantha walked in and I reached for the driver's door. Everyone else stepped into view as I opened it.

Anthony's eyes widened. I placed my right forearm across his throat, reaching under his left underarm and removed his service handgun, a Glock 9mm. I handed that off to Adam, who emptied the weapon as I released Anthony's seatbelt. I placed one finger in front of his face, as if to say "Shut up." As I was about to pull Anthony from the vehicle by his lapels, Big Frank said quietly, "Allow me, please." I stepped back and Frank took two really good handfuls of Anthony's chest, removing him from the vehicle as if he was a rag doll. Frank hoisted him to the back wall of the Station, not more than fifteen feet from the edge of Pier 36.

"What the fuck are you doing? I am going to arrest all of you. Do you know who I am?" Anthony made these statements in a practiced manner, as I am sure that he was one of those few cops who unfortunately gave the blue shield a bad name.

When I looked at him, all I could see is a cop who no one respected or truly liked. He was an ass-kisser, an abuser and someone who most cops would love to put away. He abused his power and influence. Maybe he was a troubled child, or had some other flaw, whatever it was I just didn't care.

"You know Anthony," I said as Frank lowered him to my height, "the trouble is I think you are the one who has to figure out who you are. You are on the right side of the law, yet you are beating up my friend and our partner. I will ask you, who the FUCK do you think you are?" I heard Adam unloading Anthony's weapon, dropping the magazine and empting the chamber so that gun would not be an issue for anyone.

"We know what you have been doing to Samantha and I know all the personal details," I said as I got right up in his face. "If I didn't have any decency, I would throw you right into the East River. But see, I cannot do that because that would be illegal."

Anthony's fierceness turned to fear as he realized he was in a completely compromised position.

"I am going to tell you how this is going to work. First, you are going to leave Samantha alone. She is going away for a few days to stay with some friends."

Anthony cut me off, "She doesn't have any friends, I am all she's got."

Big Frank pushed Anthony against the wall again. Anthony looked up at Frank without saying a word. He knew that Frank would pulverize him if he made a wrong move.

PARAMEDIC M.O.S.

"This is where you are gravely mistaken you fucking idiot. Sam has lots of friends and we are going to take care of her. When she finishes her tour later she is leaving you. She would do it now, but unfortunately she has this feeling of loyalty to you that is beyond me. If I were her, I would have beaten you with the nearest blunt object; but I am not her and she needs help. You need help too, but I couldn't quite give a rat's ass what happens to you. You won't be pressing any charges against us, because one word of this treatment you have subjected Samantha too and you will lose your rank, if not your job. You are going to respect her space and leave her be. If ANYTHING and I do mean ANYTHING happens to her, I am going to shove my foot so far up your ass, you're gonna be sneezing Nike emblem's for awhile. I will find you and deal with you myself. If you happen to shoot me, know that you have only so many rounds for your service weapon, and eventually one of us at this station will get to you. You will be in for the beating of your life." As I intensified my words, there was silence all around; though I could feel the stares of disdain being directed at Anthony.

"Adam, please place this asshole's weapon back in his vehicle unloaded." I said without even looking at Adam, staring straight at Anthony with a "Go ahead, do something stupid!" look. I heard a car door open, a gun drop along with about fifteen rounds in the backseat and then the door shut.

"Now you miserable fuck, get the hell off of my station property and don't ever show your face around here again. You are not welcome here."

I finished my statement face to face with Anthony, generating a hateful stare at him.

Big Frank lifted him up again as Anthony sighed in fear. Frank placed him in his vehicle as we all re-reentered the station. As Frank let the door close behind him, we heard the sound of Anthony's vehicle begin to start up.

"Frank," I said getting his attention, "I am not done with him. Now I am going to pay someone else a visit."

I got into my truck and drove to the precinct where Anthony worked. I walked into the main foyer of the precinct and looked around for the Captain's office. I was wearing a green scrub shirt over my bulletproof vest, while my green uniform pants gave up my professional identity as soon as I walked into the precinct.

"Hey, Christian, what can I get for you?" The desk Sergeant said politely.

C.B. Garris

"Hey Sarge, how ya doin? I need to see your Captain." I said with an angry stare.

"Chris, what's wrong?" The Sarge asked giving me his undivided attention.

"Trust me Sarge, you don't want any part of this. I need to see your Captain." I repeated myself.

"Sure thing Chris, let me get him for you." Something in the Sergeant's delivery let me know he knew this was about one of his own. The Sarge picked his desk phone up, pressed three numbers and said a few words.

Captain Bobby Hall stepped out of his office and recognizing my hunter green colored uniform pants, greeted me with a handshake.

"Hi EMS, I'm Captain Hall. I understand you want to see me? Wait a minute, aren't you the medic who saved that kid who fell four stories?"

"Hello Captain," I said with a small amount of gratitude that he remembered. "Yes, that was my partner Jennifer and me."

"You both did an exceptional job keeping that kid intact. With a look of homage, the good Captain said to me, "The surgeon's at Bellevue said it was your fast work that kept that boy alive."

"Thank you Cap, I appreciate that. I need to speak with you in private." The Captain realized that I was serious and led me to his office, closing the door behind him.

"What's up? You have confidential information on something going down?" He said taking out a pen and extending his open palm to a seat in front of his desk.

"Sorry Cap, nothing like that. I am here about one of your Sergeant's. Captain Hall's head tilted a bit as I informed him about Anthony. The head tilt turned to being straight out pissed. The Captain picked up his phone and called the desk Sergeant.

"When Kertuina gets in, he is to come directly to my office not roll call, understood?" The Captain said with quiet anger.

I watched the lines of his face stretch and settle. He was about 6'1", around 220, slightly overweight, but still maintained himself. I informed the Captain of what happened only minutes earlier, so that it was on the table. The Captain said not to worry about it, and that he was glad that I brought it to his attention.

I guess it was bad for Anthony that the Captain shared with me that he grew up as an abused child and he also watched his own mother take beatings. Needless to say, the Captain was furious enough to get out his

PARAMEDIC M.O.S.

black book for Internal Affairs. I informed Captain Hall that Samantha would not prosecute him, but the Captain said all he needs is an admission of guilt to deal with the problem in a disciplinary fashion. He had no great love for Anthony and was looking for something to get him not only out of his command, but to get his shield taken all together.

Captain Hall fixed his eyes on me to let me know he was serious, "I will call you once this thing gets underway, but in the meantime here is my pager number in case something else happens to Samantha. I wish I had known sooner. I appreciate you coming in and putting it out there. We will put a stop to this together."

The Captain sensed nothing but anger from me towards his employee, but he also established from my eyes that I appreciated his time and effort. We shook hands and I exited the building, hoping to let Anthony see me walk out of his office. While I never did see Anthony, something said that we would run into each other again. The end result of the I.A. investigation is that Anthony admitted to abusing Samantha on a regular basis. and he was given about six months on the therapist's couch. As a part of his disciplinary action he was also demoted back to an officer position, losing his sergeant's rank.

Back in the emergency room where the child had just been pronounced, I was pacing in place, ears red and pointed back, with a look of absolute danger on my face when Jennifer walked in. She was going to run into the ER, but when she saw me pacing she stopped and entered the ER slowly. She knew that look and that I was about to blow. I was so angry that I was fighting the tears that wanted to run down my face, and I was desperately trying to hold it together.

Anthony walked out of the room and I walked right up to his face.

"Are you out of your fucking mind? Did you not hear me telling you we were right behind you? You should not have brought that kid here, Jennifer and I should have transported him to Bellevue!" I said to Anthony in a fashion that made him back up.

He knew he screwed up but was acting like he saved the kids life.

"Hey punk, I did what I had to do." Anthony said to me point blank.

He tried to walk away from me.

"You tell me right now what you did that was so grand for that kid. Our job is to save lives and your job is to protect the public and us while we do our job. I know you already have issues with what your role in life is. Let me guess, you saw the kid's throat slashed by the metal and you tossed him in the car, putting your hand over his neck to stop the bleeding. That is what saved the kids life isn't it?"

Anthony looked at me "That's right, I saved his life." He was convinced he was an angel.

I don't think he knew how close to a beating he was.

As Anthony turned around walking back towards me I said, "You're an asshole!" Meanwhile Jennifer was circling us on the outer perimeter in case she had to step in. In fact the members of 11(E)ddie, 12(X)ray and a few NYPD sector cars were now piling into the ER to watch Anthony and I go at it.

"You better watch your mouth or I'm going to arrest you for disorderly conduct." Anthony said to me with a smart-ass smirk.

"Look you fuck, in your ego-driven wisdom you failed to realize that what you did out there was take that child away from the only thing that could have saved him."

Pointing my finger at Anthony's chest I continued, "Yes, you stopped the only option that child had to live!" In the background I heard the doctor asking for the time, meaning he called the code pronouncing the child dead.

"You see that, that's what I'm talking about," as I pointed into the room.

"That child is now dead because when you should have stopped for us to treat him, you decided you would try to be the hero, when your experience should have told you otherwise. Problem is when you put the kid in the sector car, you laid him on his side, closing what little was left of his airway off, and then you placed your hand or a cloth over his throat and you drowned him. That's right, you caused all the blood that was coming from the wound to fill up in his trachea and he drowned to death in his own fucking blood; because of you." As I ended the statement, my words got loud and fierce. The entire ER was quiet.

Speaking to me as if I was some third-class citizen, Anthony blurted out, "You don't know what the fuck you are talking about Mr. First Aid man."

"Oh, no. We were pulling up right behind you when you took off, your own dispatcher told you to pull over." I said as Anthony and I were now face-to-face.

Jen tried to tug on my sleeve gently to alert me that he and I were way to close; but I yanked my sleeve away. She knew that I had to get this out.

PARAMEDIC M.O.S.

She knew I was holding this in for a long time and that we both knew we probably could have saved the life of that child; and in that scenario every single second counted. I could have trached (pronounced traiked) him or intubated him and we could have raced him up to Bellevue, where he would have gone in for emergency surgery. Jen knew this was about to explode and was silently hoping that Davia arrived before it happened.

The physician walked out of the room with a look of complete detachment in his face. Validating my fury, the doc looked in the direction and asked him, "Is what he saying true?"

"Were the medics pulling up when you took off with this kid?"

"Yeah, something like that. I didn't feel like waiting around."

"What you should have done," the physician said abrasively pointing at Anthony's chest, "was let the medics treat him. They have the tools and skills to treat that type of injury. Between your piss poor decision to remove the kid from the scene and then to bounce him around in a car not equipped to care for him by a person being not trained to deal with this injury, you certified this kid's death." The room was quiet once again. The Doc walked away taking off his blood soaked gloves.

"When are you going to learn that you need to stop trying to be God and let us do what we are trained to do? What's the matter, are you feeling guilty about something you fuck?" I said to the Anthony right in his face. Anthony told me to go fuck myself and as he walked by me, put one full blood stained hand over my face and the other in my chest pushing me against the wall with force, causing me to hit my head.

"Did you see that?" I said to a nurse who nodded yes.

With that I spun Anthony around, taking hold of his lapels, getting two good fistful's of his shirt for gripping purposes and spun him around. I tossed him into mid air off of his feet, straight up into the air. I threw him about eight to ten feet into a medical triage room, with his feet completely off the ground. He slammed into a huge supply cabinet, knocking all the supplies to the ground.

"Oh, Shit!" I heard from one of the foot patrol officers somewhere in the room. While Anthony was in mid air I took off my utility belt like Superman changing into his cape, as Jen yelled my name as I stepped closer into the room. "Christian!"

Anthony stood up and after getting his composure, placed his hand on his holstered 9mm service weapon and motioned like he was going to draw on me. I heard the ER bay doors open as Anthony pulled his weapon out of his holster. Before he had the opportunity to get a fix on me, I leaped right on top of him like an orangutan at a banana-fest; taking him down and knocking the wind out of him. I disarmed him by twisting his wrist and tossing his gun to the back of the room. While we tussled on the E.R. floor, Jennifer leaped over us as did the other officers to secure the weapon.

I was in a rage and heard a familiar female voice calling me from behind, but I couldn't respond.

"You want to hit me mutha fucker, you want to draw your weapon on me?" I said this repeatedly as I laid a few punches against his jaw and body for attempting to pull his gun on me and then I pinned him to the ground.

"You want to take a shot at me, just like you beat on innocent women; you prick!"

He was no match for my defensive positioning, strength and rage. He didn't even get a chance to lay a blow into me before I was pulled off by a few medics.

The NYPD officers that witnessed me take him down just stood by and watched, which was their passive-aggressive way of saying that this guy deserved to get his ass kicked for many things they knew about, but because of his history were afraid to address. He got to his feet on his own, holding onto his jaw and rib cage gingerly with both hands as the other officers secured his weapon.

When we were safely separated, one of my EMS Chiefs was behind me; she was the voice I heard call my name. Chief Davia Battieri had never seen me like this before. I also noticed Captain Hall there as well. The physician was speaking with Captain Hall when Anthony yelled out, "I want that piece of shit arrested."

Davia and Jennifer each had a hold of one of my biceps as I was about to leap again, until Davia proudly said with a smile, "Hold on Cashus, I think you got enough shots in. Let us get this figured out."

Captain Hall looked in the direction of Anthony, "You sir need to shut the hell up!"

I turned back and glared at Davia. She could see that I was stuck in a rage, but she also knew that I was able to hear her. Jaw clenched and hands shaking, I was so angry that I was breathing deeply and even wanted to cry. Here was this little kid who got hit in the neck when someone threw a piece of dynamite in a metal garbage can. When it exploded the kid was way too close and a metal shard sliced his throat open. We could have saved him if

PARAMEDIC M.O.S.

they just waited or at least gave him a real shot. I had wanted a piece of this guy for a long time and now it was all out there.

"Chief, that sonovabitch went to draw his weapon on me! I am not through with him!" I said quietly; but it was a quiet that Davia knew she better hold on to me with all her might, because I was about to pound that five foot, six inch officer down to four eleven if she let me go.

Davia saw all of this in my eyes as Jennifer said she was taking me down the hall to get me out of the immediate area.

"Nurses lounge, now," Davia said authoritatively while looking at me.

"Christian, walk with me." Jen said softly almost coaching me as I started to back my posture down and turned to walk with her.

Davia walked in the room behind us and closed the door.

"You with me?" Davia stood before me and asked me as I stood there breathing heavy.

"Yeah, I'm with you. But not only did that mutha fucker just kill the only chance that kid had of surviving, he also assaulted me and was going to draw on me. Look at this bloody handprint I have on my face. We should have beat his narrow ass months ago."

As Davia was about to speak, the door to the office opened and Captain Hall walked in.

"Are you okay?" Captain Hall said as he approached me slowly.

"Do I look okay to you," I said as sarcastically as I could. "For the last bunch of months that sonovabitch has pressed his luck with us and now he directly interferes in a situation that was the only way for that kid to live. We get dragged through the mud enough with public scrutiny and the media. Here we had a chance to save that kid, but now he is dead and my people and I will once again get railroaded in the papers for not doing what we are trained to do. You know the routine, we do everything we can but today is the final straw. That asshole out there you call an officer stopped the only method that child had to live today. We could have damn well saved him or at least gave him a fighting chance. But now this knucklehead wants his fucking medal, so he removes this kid from the scene, causing him to drown in his own blood. We were on the block before they shoved him in the RMP (Police sector vehicle) like a rag doll. You already know of the history between me and that fuck nut out there." I stood there, exhaling and inhaling.

When I finished my words, I was sure that everyone who was not only outside the closed-door office, but even those on the street could hear me.

The Captain sat down, "I spoke with the doc and I'm sorry." I cut the Captain off as he was speaking, as Davia attempted to stop me unsuccessfully.

"Sorry? sorry? Why doesn't he go I.D. that kid and I want to listen to him call the family and say he is sorry. Then he has the fucking balls to hit me in the face and when I defend myself he goes to draw his gun? What the fuck was that?"

With one hand on my hip, the other was motioning like Yul Brenner in *The King and I*.

"I spoke with the Doc and he told me everything. Trust that I will be doing a full investigation and another disciplinary hearing with him when this is over," The Captain said seriously and compassionately.

"You will not be charged with anything. IAB (NYPD Internal Affairs Bureau) will want to speak with you though to get your clear account. Can you give me some numbers where you can be reached."

With that I took out my pocket size notepad and a pen. I scribbled down my name, serial number, badge number, rank and home and station numbers.

"You okay? Captain Hall asked," I figured you must be, cause from the looks of it you didn't let him get another shot in." The Captain said with an approving smile.

"I'll be alright" I said, "Just be glad you got here when you did."

Hall and I shook hands, and as he exited, Davia sat down next to me.

"Why don't you and Jennifer come back to the station and we'll get to the paperwork on this. I'll put you out of service with Communications. Be sure to stop and get a cool drink and your favorite quart size container of tropical fruit on the way back, maybe some Gatorade or something too." Davia put her hand on my forearm, "You are pretty hot about all this, want to talk about it?"

I sat there for a second, bouncing in place I then sat down and started to cry.

"We could have saved that one Dav, I know we could have." I said putting my head in my hands.

"I know you could have, I know." Davia patted my back as Jennifer sat there to make sure I walked out of the room calm and composed.

PARAMEDIC M.O.S.

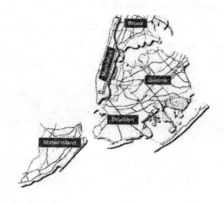

C.B. Garris

Chapter V:

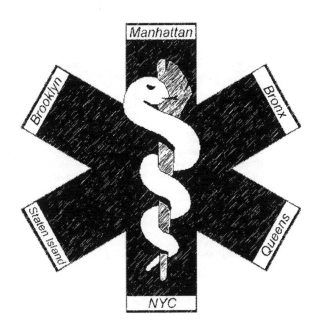

PARAMEDIC M.O.S.

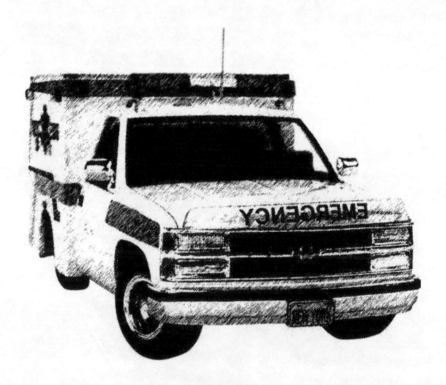

C.B. Garris

I always loved going to work as a medic in the summertime. There was something so naked about the city. Short sleeve uniform shirts, and days with the a/c on, and nights with the windows down, enjoying the sounds and scents of the city to a cold fruit drink. See in wintertime we never wanted to get out of the warmth of our trucks; the heat felt so good. It never failed that on the coldest days of the year, some nitwit would run his car into a building, forcing us to do an extended extrication. This could mean over an hour in subzero temps, trying to figure out some Einstein method of warming IV bags. In summertime, they could have sent me to a ten-alarm fire as long as I could enjoy the situation in short sleeve shirts, I was in a good place.

Jennifer, my regular partner, called me in the morning to inform me that everything went fine at the vet. Her cat "Mister" was fine, so we would be working together like normal tonight. Jen and I were both well liked by the desk lieutenants and that always had its advantages. We were usually the ones to get the new buses when they came in. Jen and I were known as two of the most dedicated members of the station, in fact we were fortunate to be attached to the best station in the city. We didn't have cliques, we just had a great group of nurturers who were incredibly technically proficient.

It was known throughout the agency that if you are going to go down in the line of duty, do it downtown. We were the medic's medics. Respectfully speaking, there was always one outpost per borough that if we had to go down in, we all preferred. Personnel from these stations were just different. We were no bullshit and we took care of each other. If there was a problem, we took care of it in the street first. If that didn't solve it, then we would take that person to the back of the garage, and if that didn't work and there was something of them left, then we sent them upstairs to see a supervisor. This was what family was all about. If you were lazy or had bad patient care skills, you were given a chance to shape up; otherwise, your ass was going to be handed to you. Never mistreat a patient, ever!

Our station was located at a focal point in the five boroughs at the beginning of two major highways that led from the South Street Seaport out of Manhattan. Our station, (also the home of the Manhattan Borough Command), was located at the corner of Clinton Street and South Street, below the elevated portion of the FDR Drive, and just a hop, skip and a jump from the South Street Seaport. This was a prime location for the

PARAMEDIC M.O.S.

units deployed from this command, as we had great access up the east side of Manhattan via the Drive, or we could access deep into Brooklyn or Queens via the Williamsburg Bridge four blocks away.

We could also head further north on the Drive to access Queens via the Midtown Tunnel at 34th Street or via the 59th Street Bridge (known by some as the Bridge named in a Simon & Garfunkel classic song, Feelin' Groovy. If we were needed way uptown in a snap, we could head straight up the Drive to get into Harlem, or into the Bronx via the 3rd Avenue Bridge right near Yankee Stadium. If we were needed on the west side of Manhattan, we would fly right past the Seaport and head to West Street, which attaches to the West Side Highway further north. We also had a great access to the Coney Island section of Brooklyn and Staten Island via the Brooklyn-Battery Tunnel at the base of West Street.

If we opted for the West Side Highway, we could just spring up the street, make a right and we could be headed uptown. This highway would connect us to the Westside, Harlem and into the north Bronx by the infamous posh section of the Bronx called Riverdale (yes, even Da Bronx has a posh section). This would also lead to the end of the city line, or the beginning of Westchester County, where I spent some years as a child. Because we had these vast array of access points, should anything go down in the city requiring tac-medics, and they couldn't find units in their own district they would always look to the medics of my station to assist because the Communications personnel knew we would.

If you belonged to my station and you were asked to head into Queens or even Staten Island you better just depress the button on your onboard computer that says 10-63(or in layman's terms, enroute). If you bitched about the distance you were being sent; you better plan on paying a visit to a trauma center when you returned to the station. Anyone who griped would be met by all of us who would wait patiently for his or her vehicle to return. It wasn't a pretty sight to return to your station to find 20 medics with their bulletproof vests off, sitting there in your honor.

My tour began at 15:00 (or 3:00pm); so I left my apartment about 12:15. No, I did not leave in fear of traffic. I had to pick up lunch and get to the station in time to walk AMBU, our station mascot. She was the best dog in the world. She was 1/2 German Shepard, 1/2 Great Dane. As big as she was, she was so incredibly affectionate and she deserved all of our love and attention. There was nothing like arriving at the station after my 1/2-hour drive into the city and being greeted by her. She would first sit

C.B. Garris

back on her haunches, and then leap for me when I either whispered her name or called her loudly. She would jump up on me and lick me, and then walk beside me to the back of my car, where I removed my bulletproof vest & a freshly starched pair of uniform shirts from the rear of the driver's side of the vehicle. She would pick up her tennis ball or Frisbee and walk with me into the station as I checked in and said hello. What more could one want in a friend?

My station sits right on the base of the East River shadowed by the elevated portion of the FDR Drive. It looks like a large tan brick warehouse, that stands four stories tall and is wide enough to fit numerous ambulances inside for maintenance. As you walk through the metal doors you will see the medics' supply room at the first door on your left, followed by the door to the gym. Walk in further and you will find a few picnic tables, which were sometimes used to grab a bite to eat, but more often than not it was used to place your equipment on top of during roll call.

Roll call was held in the next pocket of the building, next to the station supervisor's office and it was held daily in the morning at 6, 7, 8, 9 and 10. Roll call also continued in the afternoon at 2, 3, 4, 5 and 6 with the final roll calls being held at 10, 11, 12 and 1:00 am.

My station was also home to the borough tactical paramedic units. These are specialized units that are made up of highly skilled medics, who have an extra flare about them. They always go the extra mile and never mind walking into hell, and able to perform in the most extreme conditions. Personnel on these units had excellent patient care records and were known to be able to work with the most difficult patients and partners for that matter. My unit was 10X3. The one stood for which borough I was stationed in, the 0 meant we were a tactical unit, X stood for the Advanced Life Support identifier radio mnemonic X-ray, and 3 was for the tour that I worked, evenings.

I said hello to John, the station Lieutenant, and to Andrew, a medic who was on light duty after a back injury he suffered nine months ago. Andy would monitor and oversee our call reports to ensure our documentation was correct and to see that we didn't forget to write anything down.

" Yo!", I said as I opened the steel door that kept the a/c in the room. AMBU made her way in as I held the door for her.

John looked up from his desk with a look that said, "Why the fuck are you living?"

PARAMEDIC M.O.S.

Realizing it was me, John smiled and rolled his eyes in comfort, blurting out "Hey, DUDE; wazup?"

AMBU made her way over to Andy's groin. He pet her as I put down one of those 12 oz. 1950's style bottles of Coca-Cola and a NY Daily News for John, and a Nestea Iced Tea for Andy on his desk. AMBU looked up at me with those "hey, what about me" eyes, and then I pulled a bag of treats from my back pocket.

She could barely contain herself; but she sat in complete attention as I gently placed one in my hand for her; she took it, chewed it and then licked my hand with utter furvor. After the third one, she leaped up and gave me a huge lick on my face. She was happy and that's what counted. There was only mild radio traffic on the station office base station radios. It was gorgeous out and that surprised me. Nice days meant people out there; lots of locals and tourists. It meant a high call volume and probably an unwelcome amount of inflicted and intentional trauma.

"I'm taking AMBU out for a stroll, be back soon." As I said this John and Andy looked up half interested as they were both engrossed in other things.

It was all of 13:00 hours. AMBU and I walked over to her indoor doghouse and picked up her red leash. She picked it up with her teeth, completely excited that we were going to take a walk together. I was actually unsure which of us was more excited. I clicked the leash onto her collar and off we went for FDR Park. As we made our way out of the gate, 10V2 (one of the station daytime tactical paramedic units) was making their way back for supplies. As I waved, they "blipped" the siren at me and turned on their lights. Tony & Mike were smiling all the way to the station; must have just had a good job.

The entrance to FDR Park was just up the street from the station, adjacent to the overpass of the FDR Drive. The overpass begins right at South Street, where the station sits. It is an elevated portion of the roadway, that remains elevated for about 2 miles, or when you reach the Staten Island Ferry Terminal, also known as the Financial District.

On the opposite side of the highway from FDR Park was what the rich and snooty commonly call "tenement housing or projects." For those that lived there, they just called it home. Yes, twenty-three story high rise structures made of brick and metal housing an unbelievable amount of people in them. Unlike those in Brentwood or Scarsdale, the elevators rarely worked and because of close quarter living asthma ran high among children and adults. From my experience of calls in the Cherry St. Projects, which is the first set of structures, generally everyone was nice. These were people I would be proud to call my neighbors. Family values ran very high; there was this innate sense of respect and belonging. The individuals who resided here usually had very little money, but very strong character. The buildings were called projects up until 14th street.

At 14th street the tenement structures were replaced by a massive Con Edison power plant that extended about four city blocks. Once the next set of structures began again, the predominately wealthy occupants of these much nicer "tenements" came from old family money and gave themselves the luxury of re-naming their projects "co-ops."

In the daytime, you could walk the length of the park, which went to about 30th street, but in the nighttime you had better think twice. At the farthest reach of the park you had the East River, a sludge-filled Loch Ness housing depot of the nastiest water you may ever experience.

On a summer day the air was hot, but kids played & rode their bikes. You could sometimes even find the old man with the Icee cart, filled with 40 different syrup flavors. I rarely obtained one now, although as a child they were my favorite. I just had no idea where the water came from for the ice anymore. Ironically, walking AMBU made me feel like a kid: just my dog and me. Humming Simon & Garfunkel's <u>America</u>, I would stop every so often to give AMBU a treat and hug her.

By this time I knew most of the locals. We would nod our heads at one another, often we would stop and talk. Sometimes they looked at me like they knew me, but they didn't know from where. I looked a lot different in a tee shirt and jeans, then when I was in full uniform with a bulletproof vest on underneath and a sleek pair of steel-toed combat boots. Nonetheless, they recognized that I was one of the good people and that was nice.

As I walked back to the station, I heard sirens faintly in the distance, and they seemed to get closer up above. It was now about 14:05 and it must have been one of the day tour units who got a "late job." I am sure that someone was really pissed. I entered the station, letting go of AMBU's leash and then removing the collar from her neck. She nudged me and walked beside me to the stairs. As I made my way up the stairs, AMBU followed. As I approached the door to the locker room, AMBU sat down the way dogs do when they make themselves comfortable. She found her

PARAMEDIC M.O.S.

spot, and then circled in place, plopping herself down. She would wait for me to return from the upstairs locker room, after doing my super hero outfit change.

When I walked out of the door, I would be wearing the white medic uniform shirt, hunter green pants, boots and my vest. Carrying my utility belt over my shoulder, I was about ready for action. I walked back in the office and John was painfully reminding someone on the phone that he is a superior officer, and the next time they call for his coffee order, they had better get it right.

"Does your wife let you yell like that at home?" I asked.

John smiled at me, "What are you fucking kidding me, she would kick me square in the jaw if I spoke like that to her. I gotta get it out somewhere."

I rolled my eyes and laughed, since I know that John is nothing but a teddy bear.

AMBU walked to the rear of the room near the air conditioner, plopping herself down on her bed, near our radio rapid battery chargers. As I heard a dispatcher state he needed an ALS unit for a cardiac arrest in the M3, I wished that my bus was in; I would have gone.

While I waited for the Tour 2 medics to return my unit, Jennifer walked in. "Hey," Jen said as she walked over to hug me when she walked in.

We disengaged looking at each other and said simultaneously, "I'm outta here."

This was a phrase Jen and I created back at our Academy graduation together, years ago. Our Academy time was the most intensive experience of our lives, next to working the street. It was the place we had to prove ourselves beyond the shadow of a doubt, so that we could be entrusted with the lives of every person in this city. Surviving the Academy was just like graduating from boot camp. You exited emotionally whipped, beaten, strained, with all of your senses on fire; and you were all the better for it. It was a once in a lifetime experience that no one could ever take away from us. It was something I would be forever proud of making it through, no matter how much sleep I lost while there.

"What happened to Mister?" I inquired about Jen's cat.

"Everything is fine, he must have had an allergic reaction earlier this morning," Jen said.

"He got some Benadryl, which I could have given him. It's all okay now. He is home resting."

C.B. Garris

Chuckling as I looked at Jennifer, I smiled and said, "I'm just glad you came in."

Jennifer said hello to John and Andy, of course she knew to bring some bacon for AMBU who sprang right up as she knelt down to her.

10X2 drove up around the side of the building. That side of the building housed our power washer unit. Seeing our bus pulled up to it concerned me. It either meant that the bus was either filthy on the outside or worse, blood and feces stained on the inside. Either way, they were tending to it, so I was sure I'd hear about it when we changed out our narcs (narcotics). Phil Woods walked through the door, laughing loudly about his last call. Phil was about 6'5" and 260, formerly a bodybuilder, it seems he found God and his other calling. It seems that Phil's last patient decided to body check a moving city bus, causing very little damage to City property; but the same couldn't be said for him. After four IV's, 2 tubes, and a mess of defibrillation gel Phil and his partner Anjoline had lots of cleaning up to do.

I walked to the back of the rig as a wave of soapy water came flying out of the back of the rig. Looking at Anjoline inside I said with a smile, "Having a bad day?"

Anjoline gave me a sexy smile muttering, "Who loves ya babe?" Anjoline is the hottest female in the service. Born in Puerto Rico, she moved to NYC with her family as a child. After a drunk driver killed her parents when she was nine, she found herself wanting to make a difference in other peoples' lives. I knew of her family history and secretly I always thought she was reliving that moment that her parents died, making each patient she now comes in contact with her family. I know that deep in her heart she wishes she could have been there to save her parents, and in fact we talked about that topic several times.

Anjoline kept in perfect shape and was stunning even in our uniforms, let alone seeing her in jeans or an evening dress and heels. She is the kind of NY girl who makes anything she wears look good. She had a warm sensuality that only a strong heart and focused mind would allow.

AJ and I had a very interesting bond. I in fact became her Field Training Evaluator after she was on the receiving end of a very harsh situation in her early days with the service. We seemed to connect instantly. AJ had an ability to care and nurture that would puzzle me forever. She always painted her fingernails in fabulous colors and designs, and I was the only one in the service who knew that her toenails matched her fingernails always, except on Halloween.

PARAMEDIC M.O.S.

She stepped down from the side step of the bus and reached for the power dryer. As she stepped back up into the vehicle, I leaned into the vehicle to sign on the computer. Anjoline reached her right hand out and squeezed my butt gently. She did it in a way that made me happy to be alive. Her hands were soft and her touch intentional. I turned my head around looking slowly, smiling and blushing, raising my eyebrow like Thomas Magnum. She smiled that warm smile that I knew was only for me. She gently bit her lower lip, moistened it and we just smiled. I had to get my grounding since my knees became weak every time she looked at me.

As I heard Phil's feet heading our way, we returned to our official duties. Phil rounded the corner and mumbled, "All right, all right already! Will you two just get a hotel room and get it over with already?"

Anjoline looked at both Phil and I. She then said, "Phillip (as he hated being called that), I am an angel and have no idea what you are talking about. I can say however that if your summation about whatever event just happened here is correct, then Christian better have some sick time on the books because when I get through with him, he will not be walking for a few days."

Phil looked at me and said, "Damnnnnnnnnnnnnnn!" Anjoline removed her gloves and uniform shirt with princess-like fashion revealing her bulletproof vest, white undershirt, and alluring cleavage. Walking over to me, placing her left hand behind my neck and after pulling me in for a deliberate kiss from her already moistened, full lips AJ looked at Phil, smiled, sighed and walked away.

Phil looked at me, the one who had a permanent smile stuck on his face and a dazed look in his eyes; and then he watched Anjoline as she walked in the building.

"Bro, I guess you just got it like that," Phil remarked.

Still coming down from that kiss, I looked at Phil and mumbled, "Yup!"

C.B. Garris

Chapter VI:

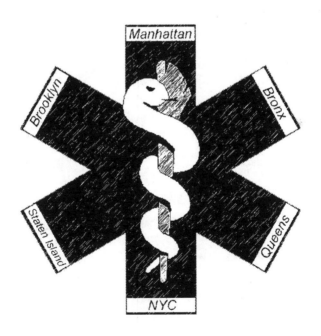

PARAMEDIC M.O.S.

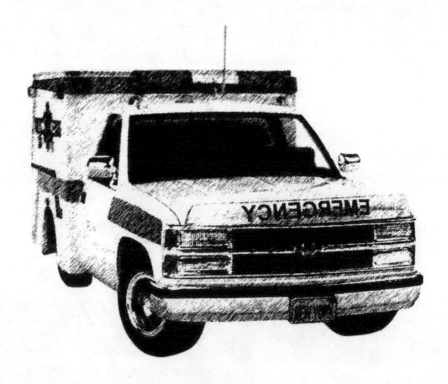

C.B. Garris

Jennifer and I checked out the rest of the vehicle, replacing a few lines of NS (Normal Saline) and a few LifePak batteries. With Jennifer driving, we headed up the FDR for Houston and then towards First Avenue. We were on Tactical assignment in lower Manhattan, which gave us the run of everything below 40th street.

Just as Jennifer made the right onto 1st from Houston, our dispatcher called us, "10X-ray & one-two boy."

I let the BLS (Basic Life Support Unit) chime in first, "2 B", as I followed with "tactical X-ray."

As the dispatcher began to inform us that we were both going to a shooting at 31st St. and 2nd Avenue, the job hit my computer with two distinctive beeps. I began reading the text which contained the call type "SHOT", as well as the address and any pertinent information the call receiving operator felt compelled to kindly share with us. This area was mainly apartment residential with a few markets and local businesses. We rarely if ever got a shooting on this block, which is why I was puzzled that it was happening in the middle of the afternoon.

As I was reading the text, the PD radio became a flurry of activity, breaking the silent spell of earlier. The comments over the NYPD portable were in reference to the call we were enroute too, something about shots fired, multiple victims and a hell of a lot of blood everywhere. Two units out of Station 13 (Bellevue) hopped on the call, having heard the shots from around the corner at their station.

As we arrived and Jen parked the bus, I saw Nancy Graglio from 13X leaning down between two parked cars while NYPD Emergency Services Truck 1 was getting into tactical gear. I saw Nancy's partner stick her head up and point in front of her when all of a sudden gun shots rang out and I saw a series of muzzle flashes from all different directions. Jennifer dove under our bus, and I back flipped under another car as an NYPD tactical sergeant returned fire with a semi automatic MP-5. I looked at Jennifer underneath our bus and she motioned that she was fine. After a bunch of rapid bursts from his weapon, I called Nancy on my radio to ensure that she was okay and that she was not pinned down by crossfire.

Nancy replied to my inquiry as shell casings fell from the sergeant's high powered weapon in rapid succession right in front of my face. First two, then three, then four more. Having worked the street with Nancy often in the past, I was able to tune out the high pitched pinging of shell casings and make out her vocal denomination as she spoke to me. While

PARAMEDIC M.O.S.

civilians dove for cover anyway they could, Nancy said she was fine and that she and her partner had three head shot patients, two of who were DOA (Dead On Arrival). They were heading for the bus with one they felt was viable. The tactical Sergeant was standing above me with his legs in a Tae-kwon-do stance, knees bent giving him superb power of reason. The sergeant (Jason Fassutig) leaned down and tapped me on the shoulder "Chris, you are clear, Intel states we got a trail of blood going into the bank on the corner."

I got to my feet as Jennifer made her way to the gear. Sirens, both PD and EMS were wailing in from all over the place as cops and medics were walking in between cars and checking vestibules for any other victims. I grabbed my ALS Trauma Bag and Airway bag, along with a BLS crew I knew under the tactical designation of 10D, Ed Munch and Billy Danip. After Jen grabbed the monitor and the drug bag, we headed towards the bank with the NYPD ESU S.W.A.T Team from Truck 1 and Truck 3.

We approached from the northwest sidewalk, and from the amount of blood on it you would have thought there was a slaughtering in progress. We entered the bank in formation, two S.W.A.T members, two medics and two more S.W.A.T members and two more medics. We made access keeping two perfect symmetrical lines, following the blood trail from the base of the door, through the office space to a long corridor that led to the bank vault. As we turned the corner to the corridor, the blood became more pronounced and darker in color.

There was a long smear of blood on the floor, and blood splattered all over the walls. I swallowed in concern and then thought to myself, "I should have called in sick today." As we inched our way into the corridor, the two S.W.A.T members behind me were whispering on their head microphones to the incident commander outside and they both locked and loaded their weapons. Now is the time that I really hoped I had a change of underwear in my locker back at the station. As we approached the vault door, I realized that the S.W.A.T teams were using our shoulders as a balance for their weapons, I got a chilling feeling as I looked to my left and right to see two ends of high powered weapons at either ear.

Two feet from the vault door, the door opened almost as if in slow motion, and into view came the double barrel of a shotgun, I mumbled to myself, "Ahh SHIT!" I spun around grabbing Jennifer and somehow without getting any blood on either of us, we knelt down under the legs of the

S.W.A.T members and the other medics and bolted out of the corridor, leaping over the desks in the office space and laying flat on the ground. I then heard about two other pairs of feet follow behind us, each one of the medics following me in succession by diving over a desk and taking out the computer on top of it with a horrendous crash. A huge bay window that faced the street gave everyone a front row seat as four EMS medics dove for cover, wrecking the inside of the bank in the process.

It was at this point that it was easy to tell the veterans from the rookies. The veteran EMS medics and POs outside that saw me dive for cover, dove for cover themselves. The rookies outside just stood there, clueless as to what was happening or what to do about it. I heard a short burst of weapons discharge and a PO said out loud "EMS WE ARE CLEAR. WE GOT TWO DOWN IN HERE, NOT OURS!"

We all got up and headed back for the corridor. One of the victims was an obvious DOA as his head was splattered everywhere. He was one of the perps. The other victim was the bank security guard, a former Marine Sniper. This explains why both the two DOA's (also perps) in the street ended up like they did and why the third victim (the ringleader of this sad ass excuse for bank robbers) that Nancy and her partner would transport, died.

The security guard, whose name was Frank, had been shot three times in the chest. Frank was the one holding the shotgun when the vault door opened. Dazed and confused from the loss of blood he experienced after being shot, Frank actually thought that we were the perps coming back to finish him off. He and the perp in the vault with him were at a standoff, and according to Frank, the last words from the perp when he heard footsteps heading for the vault door were to the effect that his buddies were coming back for him and they would all finish Frank off.

Well it so happened that the S.W.A.T leader put a very quick and decisive end to that hypothesis. It seems that the perp raised his .45 caliber weapon a tad bit too late and ended up with a face full of lead.

As I gave the word that the perp was now the property of the NYC Medical Examiners Office, calling out the time for DOA confirmation and identifying that his new name was Stubby; I quickly but gently laid Frank flat on the ground. Frank was having obvious difficulty breathing and was spitting up pink, frothy sputum. I had one of the NYPD's finest hold traction on his neck after I put on the blue "ceremonial" gloves. Okay the gloves weren't so much ceremonial as they were the best barrier between me and the various bodily fluids I come in contact with daily.

PARAMEDIC M.O.S.

Jennifer and Ed started cutting away Frank's clothing so that we could better assess the damage, and damnit if he didn't have an exit wound. Actually, all three 45 bullet's entered his front chest area with bad grouping. One hit his vest, one entered and probably went the way all bullets tend too, towards the path of least resistance. The other entered his right clavicular area, exiting out his lower right flank. He lost a lot of blood, but by the grace of someone up above he was still able to remain pretty lucid. I told Frank that he needed to stay calm and just put up with what we were about to do to him, and that he would be fine. As I reached for my radio, I heard Billy behind me opening the 1000 ml {1 Liter} bags of Normal Saline (NS).

I called over my portable radio, "10X, priority!" The dispatcher acknowledged me, "all units stand by for priority traffic," he cleared the frequency for me, "10X c'mon with it."

I chimed back in, "Call Bell and tell them we are bringing in a 55 year old male, shot times three with one exit. He is mentating and we are working on vitals, full ALS workup. We are literally across from the Trauma Center but in a precarious situation, possible tube, and Vladamier tell them to STAT that trauma team now."

My buddy Vladamier the dispatcher, with his thick Jamaican accent replied, "I got it Chris, on the phone with them. Units, unless you have a priority message for Central Dispatch, stand by."

Ed placed the C-collar on him while ESU brought in my backboard. Placing Frank on his side before securing him to the backboard, we held him for a few seconds so I could get a good glance at the damage from the projectiles. These are situations where you have only a few seconds to view, just enough so you can paint the picture for the trauma team as you are heading down to OR (Operating Room).

Frank had a hole in his back about the size of a cantaloupe, and I said to myself silently, "FUCK!" As we rolled him on the backboard he started to spit out even more blood. Frank's consciousness disappeared and his pulse oximetry started to fall. I said to Jen, "I am going to attempt one tube and we are outta here." Jen placed three NS IV's in Frank's arms with absolute precision while I went for the tube, and she even took 60 CC's of blood for cross, type & match. It would take about ten minutes to get the Trauma Team out of their beds and through the maze of Bellevue's facility, so I knew I had one shot. I put my hand in the air and Billy tossed my tube kit right into it on instinct, without either one of us having to look. Smiling internally at the silent, yet consistently demonstrative connection I maintain with my co-workers, I thought to myself; this is teamwork at its best.

I removed the C shape blade called the Macintosh and clipped it into the battery pack for light. I placed the laryngoscope into Frank's mouth and saw too much blood. Ed handed me the suction as they secured him on the board. I suctioned out about 30 cc's of blood from his throat and once cleared I bagged him with 100% O_2 ten times rapidly in prep for the tube. I placed the scope back in his mouth, resting the blade on his palate as I lifted his head up gently so I could see his chords. I passed a 7.0 through his vocal cords, waiting for that familiar sensation and final slurping sound, the one that is like when you open a bottled beverage.

"Jen, sounds." I said as I began to tape the tube to Frank's face. Jen whipped out her scope and check the left and right sides of his chest, otherwise known as bi-lateral. Then as I bagged one final time as she checked to make sure I didn't go to far and hit the stomach.

"All good," Jen said quietly, as I secured the tube to Frank's face. As we lifted Frank to the stretcher I bagged him every three seconds.

We placed him on the stretcher as the Detectives looked to me and said, "Is he likely (In NYPD terms this means likely to die)?" I replied, "not with this team he isn't. We are headed for Bell's OR now and he cannot talk to you presently." I said this because the detectives do their best to get as much information in situations like these, as even a dying declaration is admissible in court. Sometimes I have to be the guardian. As we started moving towards the door, Frank opened his eyes and looked at me, frightened as all hell. After all, in the last fifteen minutes he was held up, shot up, lost at least one to one and a half liters of blood, stuck with three IV's and now awoke to this huge lump in his throat that is in control of his breathing pattern. Yeah, that would fuck my day up too.

"Frank," I said, "I know this feels crazy, but I need you to trust me and stick with me. We are taking you across the street to Bellevue, and I promise you that I will not accidentally drop you off in the psych ward." I could see Frank almost smile with the tube in his mouth; and as we rolled up to the ambulance he looked at me and gripped my right forearm with his right hand. I looked at him intensely and I knew that was his way of saying thank you. We put him in the back of someone's ambulance and made the roll down the hill to the ER.

The Bellevue ER bay was like a long loading dock. Today it was bright and sunny and the Trauma Team was waiting for us like a pack

PARAMEDIC M.O.S.

of wolves that hadn't eaten for a week. As the BLS crewmember parked the bus, the door was opened from the outside. It was Pete Motengena, the Chief of Trauma Surgery for Bellevue.

Pete was a cool fellow. He stood about 6'2", moderately stocky, and he looked very studious in scrubs, wire rimmed glasses and his blue scrub kango. He was always serious and I had the fortune of seeing him on my most interesting cases. He said "Wadda ya got?" Without ever taking my eyes off of Frank's eyes, which were looking at me for complete support as I held the balance of his life in my hands, I said, "Doc Pete, this is Frank. He's a 55 year old male shot times three, one bullet stopped by his vest. He was the security guard at the bank on the corner. All three perps are dead, I believe that you already met one of them. Vitals 90/60, 110 on the pulse and respiration are being assisted at 16, extensive cantalouped flower damage to the right posterior flank, and one entrance no exit."

The crews were now rolling us out of the bus as I followed holding onto the tube. "He had one witnessed focal seizure during assessment, and positive LOC(Loss of Consciousness). Rule out for this one is a hemo-pneumo(Bleeding into the lung cavity secondary to the GSW(Gunshot wound)."

"Frank," Pete said confidently, "my name is Doctor Peety and we are going to fix you up. Besides I have an account at that bank and I want you back on duty as soon as we can get you there."

Pete smiled, and I even saw Frank smile again, working a smile around the tube I had just jammed down his throat. As I handed the tube over to the Respiratory therapist, Pete looked back at me, pointed and then lipped with a smile "U DA MAN!" I smiled and headed for the scrub sinks.

What originally began as a day with a crisp white uniform shirt, in one call turned into my cleaner's nightmare. Covered in blood, I removed my uniform shirt, revealing my dark blue type IIIA bulletproof vest (capable of stopping a high-powered rifle from 10 feet, but trust me you do not want to be on the receiving end of that concussion) over my under-shirt. One of the BLS crewmembers of 10 David drove our rig down to the Bellevue for us. I was so glad that we transported in someone else's unit. Transporting in someone else's unit meant that the cleanup was someone else's problem.

I took one of the Povidine scrub brushes out of its protective sheath and stepped on the hot and cold foot pedals at the sink. I ran the warm water over my forearms and began to scrub gently but vigorously. I lathered up so much in the anti-bacterial soap that you would have thought I was trying to get a part in a Calgon commercial. I wasn't anal-retentive about things, but body fluids were flying everywhere during that call. Around the corner came Victor Diego, our patrol supervisor.

"Looks like you had a hell of a first call tonight! I heard you did a hell of a job; how is he?" Victor said in camaraderie fashion. I thought for a second before I answered. "I think he is going to make it; he was a Marine you know."

Victor smiled and said "I guess all those days in basic training will get him through the post-op."

As I scrubbed up and down my forearms in circular motion, I stepped on both foot pedals to get both hot and cold water to rinse. I stepped to my left, placing my foot on the pedal that opens the biohazard red waste container and dropped in my used scrub brush. I pulled out about seven towels and began drying from my forearms to my hands. As I stepped over towards Victor to pat him on his shoulder, I noticed he was reading the NY Daily News, financial section. There was some article about a financial analyst ending up back in jail for the tenth time.

Jen walked in and said "Hey, I'll put your shirt in the bus. I called the Communications Division and told them we have to go back to the station 10-62 (out of service) for a uniform change. Gina said it has calmed down now and also that she just absolutely loves your voice."

Jen and I walked out to our bus #851, one of the brand new ones in the fleet. Since we just got the vehicle at the station last week, I knew it was only a matter of time before one of us indoctrinated the vehicle into the EMS ambulance casualty list. Usual casualties were dents or fender benders, some of our more illustrious medics found it necessary to actually overturn the ambulances or better yet and my all time favorite, drive right through a store. Now that is precision!

As we departed from the ambulance bay, I tapped the spacebar to the onboard computer, to ensure that our status was correct. The onboard computers were actually kinda cool. We received all of our pertinent information about the assignment including the location, time the call was received, the actual call type or classification and then all the text that the 911 call receiving operator and dispatcher received and entered. The lower left corner of the computer was the status area, which said 10-62 in yellow liquid crystal display.

We drove out of the Bellevue campus, across First Avenue heading towards 2nd Avenue. We usually take this route to stop at a little grocery

PARAMEDIC M.O.S.

store just before we turn onto 2nd. A cool drink today would be the best; iced tea, lemonade or grape juice perhaps. In the winter those drinks commonly came as coffee, hot cocoa with the little marshmallows or hot apple cider. Usually from the heat of wearing our vests it was straight for the Gatorade aisle.

Normal protocol to restock your vehicle was to go to the closest EMS station; there is one at Bellevue, but that would be for things like Oxygen, medications, IV bags, backboards, or a broken Lifepak cardiac monitor/defibrillator. Anything related to uniforms or personal stuff sent you back to your original station. The quicker route would be to have hooked a right onto 1st, then a right on 34th, and another right on the Service road to the FDR.

We used to be able to do this regularly until about a year ago, when one of our Tour 1 (midnight) crews decided to drive onto this exact spot on the FDR during a major overhaul of a support bridge. One thing to know about these ambulances is that ours weigh just over 5 tons, not the amount of weight you want to bring onto an unstable elevated platform. The ultimate fate of what we eventually named the EMS Minnow, was that they accessed a portion that was clearly cordoned off by signs for construction that they ignored and when they struck a plate, the entire area collapsed sending the vehicle down 1 and 1/2 stories back onto the service road.

Now one would think that with such absolute disregard for the safety of the public and for the damage caused not only to the construction project and labor time lost, but also to the vehicle that was completely destroyed, the employees would have been fired. If I remember correctly both of the medics were checked for back injuries, administered Preparation H for a year, placed on modified assignment, and then promoted.

The one downfall about civil service status is that when you have someone or a group of people who are unfit for duty, for reasons they exhibit clearly there are many loop-holes they can hide behind. This causes them to remain on payroll endlessly, for twenty years or more. I am all for everyone being able to do their part, but you should have to earn your keep, not be able to stay because the government feels the need to just put bodies in jobs.

Enroute back to the station I asked Jen to stop at the precinct down the street-home of the NYPD police academy. While putting our equipment back together, I found a shell casing in one of my bags that I was restocking from the bank robbery assignment. It appeared to be NYPD issued. I was certain that with the media frenzy that was already in motion over this incident, Internal Affairs wanted complete accounting for all casings. We turned onto 20th street, and there were the NYPD ESU trucks Adam-1, Boy-1 and David-2, reloading all of their weapons. NYPD has several types of Emergency Services Trucks. There are the Atom trucks and the BIG RIGS. Both are vital in our rescue and tactical system.

REP trucks carry two special operations police officers with tools for auto extrication(jaws of life), and tactical gear in case a S.W.A.T. operation has to be initiated on the double. They assist in setting up perimeters, and if the situation goes bad rapidly, they can at least lay down a cover of weapons fire so that we, the medics or their own colleagues have a chance of getting out somewhat intact. They are out there 24 hours a day.

The BIG RIGS carry the same equipment, and also carry water rescue rafts, scuba gear, heavier weapons, bomb detection and deactivation equipment as well as much more that remains classified. The BIG RIGS are as big as a FDNY heavy rescue unit; and that is big! Because of their size, they are harder to manipulate down the little streets throughout the city; so the R.E.P. trucks are extremely important in those situations.

I walked past Sgt. Jason, who conveniently laid down the cover fire to protect us at the bank incident, and shook his hand.

He smiled and said "Good thing for you that I leaped out of my truck with the MP-5," as Jason cuffed the barrel tightly. "I had a feeling about that situation, there was too much information being provided by someone at the scene. We actually were looking for these fuckers about four months ago. They fit the M/O of a group that was pulling jobs out in Flushing and College Point. Is that guard going to make it?"

I nodded, "He is in surgery now and judging how he arrived still conscious, I'd say he has one hell of a chance."

Jason placed a cartridge of bullets into the bottom of his MP-5, and slapped it with the bottom of his hand, loading the weapon.

As Jason placed the weapon back in its holding bracket, he smiled at me and said, "What brings you by here?" I reached into my back pocket and pulled out a sandwich-size ziplock baggy with the shell casing now visible. I handed it to Jason, "I discovered a shell casing when I was restocking over at Bell. It looks to be one of yours."

Jason opened his eyes wide and smirked holding the bag up to the sunlight, "yup, looks like ours. What frightens me is that you have seen enough of these in street combat to know it better than my people do."

PARAMEDIC M.O.S.

Jason shook the bag, rolling the bullet to where the NYPD identifier is and said while squinting his eyes in amazement and frustration, "Fucking Crime Scene Unit, they shouldn't be missing these things. I already got a call from the SOD Lieutenant telling me he wants the detectives to have all the paperwork on this immediately so their reports are in order. IAB (Internal Affairs Bureau) is going to be so far up our asses for the weapons fire exchange."

I shook my head in disbelief, "Jason, that was an entirely uncontrollable situation in which you did what you had to do, you know that!"

He smiled "You want to talk to Internal Affairs on our behalf?"

I smiled gleefully, "Why sir, I'd be happy too! Now the public needs you Superman, you better go back out there. I gotta drop these off upstairs, so I will see you out there; and damnit be careful." Jason patted me on the back as I walked past him.

The entrance to the precinct was like any other precinct for the most part. Baby blue frame doors with green lantern outside on the upper left wall. As I walked through the double doors, a gentleman in a blue pin-stripe suit in his mid 40's walked past me in the opposite direction then turned around and faced the inside of the vestibule yelling "You haven't heard the last of me, I am getting my attorney. You can't impound my car because I was buying coke uptown", as if no one would hear how ridiculous he sounded.

"I will make it so you can't work again," he directed towards the Sergeant at the desk.

I looked at him with the interest of a snail, and when he caught me he said "What the fuck are you looking at?" I returned the eye exchange and thinking for a moment I replied, "Apparently someone who is not only ignorant, but who is less one car."

I smiled as I continued on my path. He looked at me puzzled as I kept going. As I entered the precinct, Sergeant Jefferson, a very strapping, tall black man who looked more like a linebacker than a police officer was leaning over the desk demonstrating the alphabet to a full grown adult. The desk officers were abstractly shuffling paperwork, drinking coffee and answering phones. There was always a lot of activity behind the desk.

Sergeant Jefferson looked up from his desk and nodded, "Hey Chris, I hear you really know how to leap in a single bound!"

I looked at him sheepishly, "HA HA HA, everyone is a fucking joker around here," I said cynically, "I hope you are still married."

The smile swept from his face as he said, "Say man, that was low."

C.B. Garris

I smiled and we clasped hands like two army buddies who hadn't seen each other for awhile. "I know," I said "I'm going upstairs to see those crack detectives regarding evidence submission from that earlier situation."

He looked puzzled and interested, "No shit, wadda ya got?" I showed him the plastic bag and he pointed upstairs.

When I returned from logging the evidence with the detectives, I came back down the stairs getting ready to salute Sergeant Jefferson. He looked up and used his hand to call me over to the desk.

Leaning towards me he said quietly, "Check it out. We got some guy down the hall we just collared (arrested), who is mumbling something about he's sick and wants to go to the hospital. Can you check him out or do you want me to give communications a call?"

I picked up my radio and called Jen on the private channel, letting her know we got something inside. Jen acknowledged, notified communications and met me inside. We walked down the corridor to the jail section. As we walked down the cobblestone ramp toward the jails, Sergeant Jefferson informed me that they picked this guy up after he attempted to feel up some 8-year-old kid. Seems the kid had some lessons in karate and was able to deflect the attack. The kid was physically fine but a little shaken.

"We ran him through BCI (Bureau of Criminal Investigation)", said Jefferson, "and he has a wrap sheet of previous convictions including armed robbery, stalking, attempted vehicular homicide, and we got a hit that he may be a sex registrant out of Michigan. If this is the guy we think it is, the feds have been looking for him for about two years. During the collar he was uncooperative, resisted arrest, kicked one officer in the cajones, and was an all around piece of shit."

When I approached the cell, where this guy was by himself; I heard someone mumbling to himself and I could only imagine how the next few minutes would go. Jen and I rounded the corner to find a male in his late 20's. He looked like the Sergeant described, like a left over piece of shit. He was about 5'9", and 220, and when he saw both the sergeant and I round the corner, he had a few choice words to say.

"What's your name sir," I asked professionally.

He looked up at me with his beady little eyes and said "Ah, fuck you!"

I raised my eyebrows "Now I don't know what happened before I got here, but the nice sergeant here informs me that you are feeling ill, my name is Chris and I am a paramedic, maybe there is something I can do to help."

PARAMEDIC M.O.S.

He squinted his beady little eyes again and said, "Man, you all the same, mutha fuckas with badges. Why don't you come in here if you so bad!"

The Sergeant looked towards me and said "I tolllllld you he might have an adverse reaction."

As the Sergeant finished his words, 'beady eye' spit in our direction, hitting the sergeant right on his left cheek. I grimaced at how utterly foul that looked, while Jen silently mumbled to herself, "See now, you shouldn't have done that."

Beady eye was about to discover what kind of a bad ass this Sergeant really is. I placed my hand around the Sergeant's bicep, which was twice the size of mine and said "Sergeant, let me handle this."

"Guard," I yelled, "Open 21," and the door clanked really hard as I let it open all the way.

I stepped inside and beady eye swung at me really hard. I backed up and let him throw himself down to the ground from the motion of his swing. He got up and backed up saying, "What are you gonna do, kick my ass?"

I looked at him and said, "Looks to me like someone did enough of that long ago. I will describe to you what is going to happen over the course of the next few minutes."

I took off my utility belt, handing it to the Sergeant on the other side of the bars. This way, if he and I tangoed inside the prison cell, I had nothing from my belt that he could use as a weapon if it got loose.

With my eyes still locked on beady eye, I yelled to the officer at the gate control "GUARD, close 21, HARD!" The door clanked again and made a reverberating loud slam when it was finished.

Beady eye looked at me with absolute confusion realizing that it was just he and I in the cell together now. Maybe he wasn't such a bad ass after all. I could see several thoughts going through his mind: why did he take that equipment belt off and hand it to the officer? Why did I swing at him? Why did I spit at the cop? What is about to happen to me? As I got real close to him, he winced, grimaced and even cowered at my approach as the next look from his eyes said it all, *I want my momma!*

Looking at him closely and in a very calm, firm and focused voice I said, "You better hear exactly what I am about to say to you before we go any further."

I paused and almost like a priest giving counsel to a parishioner I said, "I am here to help you, which is what the nice Sergeant asked me to do. He wants me to evaluate you to see if you need medical treatment since you said you are apparently so sick. I will not tolerate you being disrespectful or acting inappropriately towards me or my partner as long as we are respectful towards you."

The next statements I said slowly and deliberately accenting the last three words, "If you spit or swing in my direction again or even think of kicking me, I will have you handcuffed, then I will take you by the scruff of your neck, drag your silly ass outside and use the curb to bust your head down to the grey meat you beady eyed fuck!"

The whole room went quiet as a few officers peeked in to watch our little dance. The Sergeant kept his parental look of disappointment on beady eye, as Jen took the baton that the Sergeant was gripping tightly, out of his hand.

"Now you already got caught attempting to ass-jack a child today, so as far as I see it your day is going south real quick; and I have no patience for the shit bag you have already proven to be. It would be in your best interests for you to control your urges of expression so that you live through the next few minutes."

There was nothing but silence in the room now.

"That said," I continued, "what seems to be your problem today?"

The eerie silence already in the room now echoed as beady eye made for his bunk like a child who had just been caught red handed. Beady eye realized that I was more than capable and willing to rearrange his body parts as I saw fit, and if the occasion presented itself. He realized that even though he outweighed me by at least sixty pounds and a few inches in height there was a beast beneath the bulletproof vest that he never saw the likes of before.

He looked at me, "Yo man, I don't want no trouble from you. I'm a diabetic." I looked at him like I was waiting for the answer to a difficult Jeopardy question when I said "Okay, you are a diabetic and?" Beady eye started to shuffle in his seat and said, "Well you know man, I gots ta eat man or my shit gets all messed up."

I raised an eyebrow and moved closer to him, "Okay now we are getting somewhere. Do you take medication for your diabetes?"

Beady eyed started sweating on my approach and said "No."

I asked him if he ate today, he replied he had. In fact through a barrage of the best questions we are trained to ask, he had no specific reason why he needed our assistance.

PARAMEDIC M.O.S.

"Look, you want to go to the hospital, not a problem. If it is that you are a diabetic, then I will do all that is necessary to help you which involves putting you on a cardiac monitor, sticking you with IV's and taking blood for a sugar count and probably administering meds if necessary. If you just want us to take you because you think that taking a ride to the hospital will shorten your jail time or give you an opportunity to bolt while in the ER, think again. You will be handcuffed at all times and have an armed police officer who, if you try to bolt from the ER will be happy to shoot you wherever he or she desires too. Now there are plenty of people out in the streets who really need us, people like kids getting hit by cars or adults getting struck by trains, fathers and mothers having heart attacks, and even people getting stabbed and shot. You seem awfully well enough to swing at me and spit at the sergeant, so I suggest you tell me the truth about this now."

Beady eye thought to himself for a second and staring at the ground said "Yeh, just wanted a ride to get out of this shit hole man. Fuck all the idiot cops who wanna treat me bad."

I looked at him and said, "Signing this piece of paper makes it official that you are lying to the cops and us. Further it states you have no need for medical attention, releasing us from any liability if you are bullshitting us. If you made this whole situation up, then sign at the X. Otherwise, I will begin to do a full medical work up on you right here and right now."

Beady eye thought to himself again and said he would sign. He looked at me with this devious smile and said "You know I couldn't help myself earlier," referring to the child. As I rose up and called for the guard to open the cage door I said to beady eye, "I bet you couldn't and someday that is going to get you killed." The smile disappeared from beady eye's face.

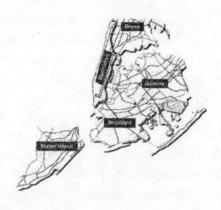

C.B. Garris

Chapter VII:

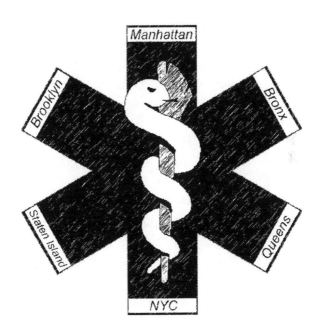

PARAMEDIC M.O.S.

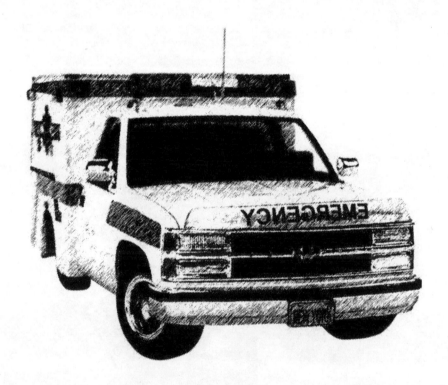

C.B. Garris

Jen and I returned to our truck, making sure to shake the hand of the good Sergeant on the way out. As Jen and I exited the same blue doors we entered through, Jen said to me, "You know that schmuck is going to start whimpering once he gets down to the Central Booking."

I pushed the door to open it and looked back out of the corner of my eye saying, "Yeah, what a world, what a world."

As I got in on the passenger side of the vehicle, Jen already hit the ignition; and our vehicles always sounded like you were starting a truck when you activated them. I put my NYPD radio on the inset of the door handle next to me. There was a little suitcase like handle attached to the door, and it always fit perfectly there. We carried the NYPD portable radio's since we worked side by side with them. Since both EMS and NYPD patrolled the streets, we were there for each other when it got hairy. If a cop went down or if we got into a jam, we didn't have to wait for the call to go to our respective dispatchers, so it could be disseminated and then reprocessed with the other agency.

When you are caught in a cross fire or your life is on the line, every single second counts; and it only takes one event for you to realize that. If it went down on either front, we could each call for help. Since all 911 calls were fielded by the NYPD first, it also gave us a head start on the calls in our area, since they would be dispatched to the patrolling PD units before our Communications personnel had a chance to interrogate the caller to classify it properly.

I picked up Jen's EMS radio, which was resting face up in top of the monitor and waited for the hospital notification that my bud John was giving off of 12E3 (pronounced 12 Eddie 3). Seems their patient fell three stories from a window washing scaffolding, and the impact did not agree with his body. Surprisingly he was still with it, or at least still breathing on his own, but sounded like the rest of him took a hell of a beating. John finished off his notification stating that this gent was C-collared and boarded, ALS on board and the ETA (Estimated time of arrival) at St. Vincent's was approximately 3 minutes. His transmission ended with silence, as they always did with these new noise-canceling 800 megahertz radios we were using.

Gina, our beloved dispatcher, keyed up, "12Eddie, got it and on the line with Vinny's now. All units unless you have a priority message stand by."

I waited for Gina to come back on a minute later clearing the channel by saying, "12Eddie, Vinny's awaiting your arrival, other unit with a message?"

I keyed up my radio, "Ten X-ray, tactical X."

PARAMEDIC M.O.S.

Gina replied with a joyous and almost alluring tone, being sure to slow down the descent of her remark, "The pride of the City, Tactical X-Ray, go ahead."

I pressed the button on the handset, "Good afternoon Gina, show us sixty-two heading back to eleven for a uniform change."

Gina was gone for a second and when she replied I heard her fingers clicking across her keyboard in front her, "Tactical X, 10-4, your out sixty-two and a pleasure it is to have you with us today."

Our on-board computer beeped twice as Gina finished her words: "Are you both going to get all spiffied up?"

Jen and I both smiled, and I keyed the radio before putting it down again replying "Thank you central, the feeling is mutual and yes."

The computer beeped twice again this time with a smiley face that Gina sent along with the next message.

"It has quieted down so just let me know when you are ready to come back out to play."

I leaned over the keyboard and typed a message to Gina with a special command that allowed only the tactical units to be able to send messages to the dispatchers.

This message would say: How are the expectant mommy and the expected doing? As Jen made a left onto 3rd Avenue our terminal beeped again, "Good, just the mornings are still a little funky." Jimmy asked me to ask you to call him about the protection unit. I picked up the radio and said over the air, "10-4 on the sand box."

This meant that I got her message. For those of us who work the special protection detail, we have an entirely different code system than most of the service. Gina is one of our Special Operations Dispatchers who works those details with us; so she is in the know.

Jen hooked a left on St. Marks, took it down to 2nd Ave. and made a right.

Jen looked at me and said, "Mike's?"

She was referring to the Station's favorite spot for the best burgers and black and white shakes in the city.

I said, "Well, let's go clean up first and stop back on the rebound."

Jen looked at me with those hungry puppy eyes and said, "Dude, you know that we are gonna get busy in awhile!"

She continued the rest of her words in her best James T. Kirk impression, "And if we get busy, we just…. don't… eat!"

C.B. Garris

As we passed by Mike's I said, "Civic duty my dear, it always comes first. Besides, I got a whole bunch of protein bars in my sack!"

Jen looked at me and said "Protein bars? Did you bring me any?" Jen asked in a grunting voice, like a person who hadn't eaten in weeks.

"Hey, I eat, you eat. You know the drill. Anything I got is yours." I said with a smile.

Jen smiled and patted my hand as she changed lanes on 2nd Avenue, "You're so good to me!"

Jen began to tell me the recent events in Artie's life, her brother. Artie was always a comical character and great for a laugh. In fact, he and I could have passed for brothers and Jen got a real kick out of it. Where as I come from a very mixed background, Artie was straight up from Puerto Rico. He had very short hair, Navy Seal cut like mine, brown, with a fair skin tone. He was a tad bit more caramel in his complexion than I am, but the only difference is that he had hazel eyes; mine are brown. Women always flocked to him, but they didn't know what Jen and I know.

See, about four years ago, after Artie was promoted to the much sought after Detective Grade shield in the NYPD, he decided that one particular night was the big night for he and his lady friend. His lady friend too decided that night was the night. What Artie didn't know was that she was fertile enough to bear quadruplets from that one night of passion. Monica, now his wife, was one of our trauma surgeons from Saint Vincent's Hospital and she is a great woman. She had earned enough time so that she could take off awhile to get the kids started and she and Artie had a great relationship. They were really good to each other and nothing beat going to Artie's house and seeing the circus that would always erupt with four kids. They are great parents to the little ones, and being that they are two good-looking people, they spawned some adorable children. Jen loves being the Aunt to all the little ones and has always taken great pride. She especially loves Christmas time with them all.

We turned left down Houston towards the Drive (FDR Drive), and made the right onto the Drive itself. It was about 1800 (6:00 PM) when we turned into the station, and Lieutenant Jimmy Mctiernan was washing his patrol supervisor's vehicle. Also brand new, he got the nice and shiny Suburban. All decked with emergency lights that made it look like a Christmas tree when everything was activated, he joined us many times doing mach ten down some side street hauling ass on a hot job. Even the bosses, whose job function while operational was also now administrative, couldn't get the itch out for a good job.

PARAMEDIC M.O.S.

With Jimmy in possession of the new vehicle, it was only destined to enter the EMS vehicle casualty list soon like ours. Jimmy just finished soaping the unit down with the power washer when he looked at the inside of our vehicle, and noticed both of us were wearing our bulletproof vests without our uniform shirts. Judging by the way his eyes popped out of his skull, I presume Jimmy got a stronger look at Jennifer.

He took his hands off the soaper and walked over smiling as he leaned on the vehicle, "You know guys, when we said you were a tactical unit, we were trying to keep the tactical thing incognito. You keep driving around with vests exposed like that, and I am going to think you are going to ask for weapons next."

I smiled my smart-ass smile and said, "You know Lou (short for Lieutenant), we would not be opposed to the idea, since every little bit helps."

As I made my remarks, Jen smiled.

Jimmy said, "I will never understand you two. By the way, you guys do move quickly. By the time I got to the scene of that bank job, you were pulling into Bell."

Jen looked at me and I nodded. Jen looked at Jim, and laughing hard she said, "Yup Lou, that's why we are working the street and you are the boss." While I could see Jimmy trying to contemplate as to whether that was a compliment or a professional dig, we all smirked and Jen pulled the bus around to the back of the station near the oxygen tanks.

As we exited the vehicle I sat back down inside and sent a message to Gina again, letting her know we were at the station. AMBU walked out of the garage, looking at me first and then placing her paws out in front of her as far as she could for a serious stretch. She then made her way over to me as I watched her approach. As I stepped out of the bus, she immediately placed her nose in my flank and blowing out from her nose she then inhaled, recognizing my scent.

"How you doin' girl," I said to AMBU. When AMBU stood up she was as tall as I am, and she proved it once again with a reach up to my shoulders and a smooch from her on my cheek. Jen went to restock a few things from the meds supply room as I went up to the locker room. I heard the pitter patter of little paws coming at me grunting. As I turned around, I knew it was AMBU with a huge yellow ball in her mouth. She dropped it in front of me, signaling that it was time to play with her. She was really looking out for my emotional state of being. Taking a moment to enjoy a game of catch with AMBU put it all in perspective, and her affection in the midst of all the shit that we would see was priceless. No matter how many times we got shot at, assaulted, or no matter how horrible of an incident we just left the scene of, knowing that she would always greet us when we returned was a reason to think clearly out there. She depended on us to take care of her, but more so than that, to take care of ourselves.

I bent down and picked up the ball while AMBU snuck in a lick of my ear. I picked it up and faked it, watching AMBU lurch forward and then do a sound like Scooby-Doo while I still had the ball in my hand; "Harumph!" AMBU remarked with the ball still in my hand. I then tossed it to the end of the station and she took off like a bat out of the cave for a night.

I opened the steel door to our stairway towards the locker rooms on the third floor. When you walk in our locker room, it is a basic industrial type locker room, painted white with four rows of huge tan lockers spaced evenly with nice wooden benches in between to sit on as you change for tour. Along the south wall of the room was another set of lockers. At the end of that row were the decontamination showers, the toilets and the sinks.

We had an IA (Industrial Assistant) more commonly known as a janitor. Adam kept the place in pretty good order; that is when he showed up. He was the son of a city official, not that bright and neither was Adam.

My locker was in row 4, and as I keyed into it I noticed a very distinct smell. I had to stop it was so powerful. This smell always seemed to overcome me and turn me introspective. This smell is one that was with me everywhere: in my car, taking a shower, or one of the umpteenth times my life would flash before me in the line of duty.

This smell was Anjoline's perfume, and it was perfectly annointed on the dozen Fire and Ice tulips she left in my locker for me. I stood there for a second, feeling this incredible warmth come over me, and wishing she was near. Azymuth was her perfume and it was so powerful it was almost haunting. What she meant to me was something so visceral that I am unsure if words could place it correctly.

The note attached said, *Hi gorgeous, just wanted to let you know I am thinking of you. Why don't you come to my place after your tour, I will be waiting for you in nothing but a T-shirt; and perhaps less than that.*

Love & hugs,

AJ

I met AJ about eighteen months ago just after she had just graduated the academy. She was an "intern" working with a crew of medics as all medics do for the first six months. AJ became a medic from a rather

PARAMEDIC M.O.S.

unusual background; she obtained her MBA from Pepperdine University in Malibu, California.

She stands at 5' 2", with a flawless light caramel complexion, long straight hair that was the color of a rich dark chocolate(almost black) and down to the bottom of her shoulder blades, high cheekbones, deeply penetrating black eyes that light danced off, very muscular legs, and luscious, full pouty lips. The dialect in her accent spoke proudly of her Puerto Rican heritage, and if she ever became annoyed which was rare, her dialect also told you that she came straight from the streets of San Juan. AJ's elegance, demeanor and poise is that of a debutante, yet she maintains enough street in her to make attackers think twice and men trying to get over on her think three times. Her alluring natural beauty was a combination of stunning features coupled with confidence, exotic mystery, longing, and a yearning innocence to share her heart with only her equal.

One look at AJ and high maintenance is all one would figure. I was the only person who ever had the fortune of knowing how vulnerable she is, and how simple she wants and makes life. I had a penchant for seeing and revealing the part of her that she never showed to anyone. Her past rendered a tough woman, with the soul of a frightened child. Like me, although she had a bevy of bad relationships, she treated herself well, very well; since those around her never did. The men she dated wanted only to conquer her, make her the proud trophy. Anjoline's heart was the trophy.

Her character spoke in novels. Anjoline was so used to men in the mono. One of the many things that she said attracted her to me was that although I was only 5 '7", I walked tall and in stereo. I had a silent but very deadly presence about me. Most couldn't understand it, but they knew it existed and it made AJ very safe and comfortable. Many might have thought they would step up to me to challenge me for AJ because of my quiet poise and muscularly, slender frame, but when my eyes locked on theirs they always turned away. AJ admired the look in my eyes that said, "You may swing at me once, but you won't use that arm again."

AJ's presence was such that her alluring qualities made not only men stop in their tracks, but she made many a female fan as well. We shared the same sentiment in that we preferred a walk on a private Caribbean beach together holding hands rather than anything else. I was the recipient of her trust even more than I knew, and she told me early in our relationship that she realized very early that she would always be safe with me and I would never do her harm. I was stunned when one day she told me that I was all she ever wanted but was previously unable to receive tangibly. She commented on my being strong, caring, more loyal than a Labrador, of great work ethic, mysterious, private, highly intelligent, and she loved how much I adored her.

She was very empty inside after a bunch of unrelentingly bad boyfriends and one horrific engagement. She witnessed paramedics work on someone in a restaurant in midtown, and coupled with how she felt about the death of her parents, she decided she wanted to try this line of work. Usually you are paired up with a direct partner as your evaluator, but her training partner attacked her. Davia put her as a third medic on a unit for a while, like all brand new medics, until she was seasoned.

PARAMEDIC M.O.S.

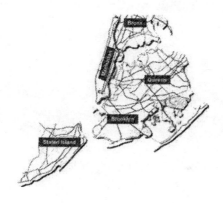

C.B. Garris

Chapter VIII:

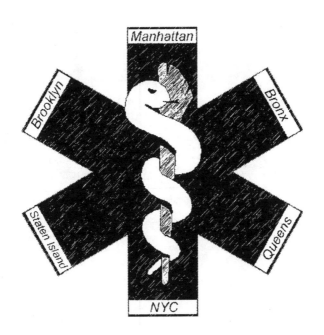

PARAMEDIC M.O.S.

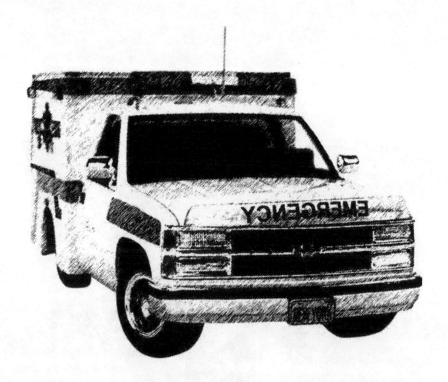

C.B. Garris

I had been working overtime on the day I met AJ. I was the borough logistical support unit, which means I did ancillary functions for eight hours. I drove around from hospital to hospital, retrieving backboards and c-spine immobilization equipment that were removed from patients hours after they were seen in radiology. When I pulled into St. Vincent's Hospital I saw several ambulances parked outside. I exited my supervisor's SUV and began to walk inside. I heard the annoying and often painful voice of Eddie Von Furstenberg speaking to someone in a very smooth tone.

I knew Eddie from a number of negative situations that always seemed to involve him, but he always came up clean after the investigations. He was your typical male chauvinist pig, with misogynistic tendencies and even known to be an all out racist. The problem is that situations occurred where people were afraid to say anything.

As I rounded the corner to enter the Emergency Room, Eddie was in the back of the bus, awfully close to some gorgeous female that I had never seen before who was wearing one of our uniforms. I had to catch my breath so as to not stare at her. The female who would later turn out to be AJ smiled at me in a way that made every cell in my body tingle. Whoever this girl was I thought to myself, when she smiles you listen.

As I entered the ER, Eddie said, "Yo, wasup Chris?" It was obvious that he was trying to impress this girl, as I had no love for Eddie at all. He was a sleaze and there was something about him I never liked. If Eddie was saying hello to me in an excited fashion, he wanted to make it seem like he knew everyone, as if he was "THE MAN."

I returned outside from the ER a few minutes later with a few backboards. The boards were totally covered in blood and brain matter, so I decided to do decontamination with peroxide before I put the board in the back of the jeep. While Eddie tried his smooth talking self on AJ, I placed the boards against the brick wall over a subway grating. I turned each upside down so that I could just douse the head areas of the boards with a gallon of peroxide each and then wipe them down. Per protocol and common sense, I gloved up first and realized that one of my gloves was ripped. I walked over to the rear of the vehicle. The doors were somewhat closed in a triangle fashion which was strange, but I pulled one open to get a pair of gloves from Eddie's vehicle and also ask what was all the brain matter from on the boards.

As I reached for the handle I thought I heard the female voice say, "Can you get off of me please?"

PARAMEDIC M.O.S.

I swung the door open and Eddie shuffled back to his side of the bench. "Hi guys," I said while surveying the situation, "Mind if I snag a pair of gloves? By the way, what did you have on your last call that caused all this brain matter?"

Eddie was looking at me like I had just interrupted his chance at getting some. "Uh, we had couple of pedestrians struck by a car, one was DOA. Hurry up man, I'm taking care of business here. I'm trying to show this new Latin wonder here the ropes." Latin wonder looked at me with this look that said, "I am so glad you are here, would you please shoot this fool!"

I looked at AJ and her eyes were intense as was the rest of her.

I extended my hand introducing myself to her, "Hello, my name is Christian and you are?"

She looked to her left at me and smiled a million watt smile saying "Hi, I'm Anjoline but I like for my friends to call me AJ, so please call me AJ."

I smiled, nodded, and said "Nice to meet you," as she did the same.

Eddie looked at AJ saying, "Hey I'm your training partner, why can't I call you AJ? I'm your friend too."

I motioned for Eddie to come out of the rig to help me with something. AJ just smiled and each time she did I was becoming addicted. If I wasn't so professional, I am sure my jaw would have dropped at first sight of her, along with my tongue rolling right out of my mouth and she would have figured out that I was about to pass out at her presence. I pulled Eddie to the side and inquired as to why he called her the "Latin Wonder". Pretty much within earshot of her he said, "Have you seen how hot this girl is? Did you see the size of those fucking melons man? I gotta get me a piece of that!"

I looked at Eddie long enough to decide exactly where my fist was going to connect with his lips.

I thought to myself, "Shall I go for the bicuspids or the molars?"

I inhaled deeply and punched his upper chest firmly "Eddie, shut up. Are you out of your mind to be addressing another co-worker like that, let alone addressing a female that way? Why did she ask you to get off of her?"

Eddie stepped back defensively, "What are you talking about man, she didn't say that?"

I looked at Eddie, "I was right there when she said it, which is why you leaped back into place when I opened the rear of the bus."

Eddie shrugged his shoulders, "Aw man, nuthin happened. You know how these hot Latin bitches are. What are you afraid she is going to start talking about that bullshit sexual harassment stuff?" I was about to smack him.

"Should I be Eddie?" I said with fierce concern. "Look, you need to stop this course of conversation now, because I am not going to continue it with you. What I will tell you is that you better calm your fucking jets, and I better not hear any complaints from her about you."

Eddie said, "Man she is my student and I am just teaching her the ropes."

I looked at Eddie firmly, "Just make sure that YOUR rope stays behind its zipper." Eddie backed down, "All right man."

Eddie went inside to use the bathroom, and I walked back over to the vehicle. AJ was reading over her call report when she looked up. Her stare had me mesmerized, and I had to find a way to remain composed. I asked her if everything was all right. AJ said it was, but her answer came too quick. When I had asked my question, it looked like I scared her.

"How is your training going? Is Eddie giving you any problems?"

AJ looked at me with this look like something was up, but she wouldn't talk about it. This was instilling no confidence in me about how her training was going. AJ informed me that her regular training partner was out sick for about four days, and that she was stuck with Eddie. She just wanted to get through it and didn't want to make any waves.

I didn't want to push her, so I told her what unit I was working, what station I was from and that if she had any concerns to reach out to me. I didn't know how to be sincere without looking like I was trying to pick her up.

Something in her look said she understood that right away. I excused myself and put a phone call into Chief Davia Battieri, our Borough Commander; as I think I needed to chat with her about what I witnessed. Unfortunately, she was in an OPS (operations) meeting that was going to last for hours, so I left her a message to contact me as soon as possible.

Later that evening after I finished my retrieval duties, Jen and I hit the street together working our regular bus 10X3. We had just finished dropping off a patient suffering from insulin shock to Bellevue. We were outside the ER bay chatting with a few police officers from Midtown South when 13X3 drove in and began to back up. I knew it was 13X3 because of the vehicle identifier 175 on the sides and rear of the vehicle.

Each unit was assigned a regular ambulance, so unless the vehicle was taken out of service for preventative maintenance (oil change, etc.....), you

PARAMEDIC M.O.S.

could expect the crew to be in their proper vehicle. It was common practice for us to help other units unload their patients if our hands were free when they backed into an ER bay and just the same to give the ER critical notifications if the dispatcher was too busy to pick up the hotline.

I opened the door to 13X3 to find an absolute mess in the back of he rig. Eddie was back there again with AJ. As I viewed the rig, Eddie was sitting in the Captain's seat (the seat that faces out to the rear of the vehicle, which is directly behind the driver's seat inside the box), while AJ sat on the main bench.

The patient appeared unconscious, but he was huge. I looked at the Lifepak, which told me he was pulsing short of bradycardia (slow pulse) of about 54, with some ectopy (what we generally call FLB's, funny little beats).

I looked at Eddie who had this huge smirk on his face, as if he was "The Man," and he barked at AJ, " Well, didn't I tell you to push all of that Narcan? Do it now!"

Eddie's tone was anything but constructive, and although I could see that AJ was calculating everything in her head, I suspected she was new and that Eddie was trying to win her over with his abrasive attitude. Last time I checked with my female confidants, they were not too hip on being treated like a piece of dirt.

Giving AJ a momentary reprieve from Eddie's attitude I chimed in, "Wadda ya got?" AJ looked at me and I thought I was going to faint. I could see that she wanted to clock the shit out of Eddie, and knowing Eddie I was confident that she had good reason.

Eddie said to me "Yo, Chris, I'm teaching this J-A-F-O (Just Another Fucking Observer) here how to treat an overdose patient."

He tried to step past her and yelled, "Well c'mon girlie, you can do it." Now I was about to clock the shit out of him.

Eddie's partner, Myron turned the vehicle off and came around the corner saying, "Hey, what's up Chris?"

I smiled and patted his shoulder without taking my eyes off of AJ or Eddie, "How you doin' Myron."

Just as I saw AJ go to push a bolus (a full prefilled syringe or equal to 2 mg of Narcan I stopped her, "Hold on a second."

AJ halted everything she was doing and I could see her breathe a sigh of relief for the first time since I opened the back doors to the unit.

I asked AJ, "How much Narcan and Lidocaine have you pushed so far?"

Eddie blurted in, "Hey man, I got it, this is my patient and she is my student." AJ didn't move.

"Eddie," I said, "if I want answers out of you, I'll give them to you. First of all, this is not just your patient, because we work as a team. Second, the only reason she is your responsibility for the day is because her regular training partner was out sick, so save your lack of ego for later as I am not impressed. I should not see ectopy on that monitor right now."

AJ looked at me and smirked under her breath. I leaped up into the vehicle as Eddie jumped out the side door.

AJ looked at me and said, "We only gave him .4mg so far, I wanted to push more at a slow push but he kept telling me to push it bolus."

I shook my head and said to her, "If you push that bolus with a heroine addict, he is going to not only wake up and puke all over you, but he will be the most belligerent son of a bitch you have ever seen, since you'll have ruined his high. Push slowly to 1 milligram in .2 milligram increments, and watch his vitals improve. As long as his rate(pulse), BP, and respiration's increase, you are home free and you can administer the rest slowly. What Eddie was telling you to do is called hot-shotting, and you don't want to do it unless you have to."

She pushed an additional .6 mg of Narcan slowly, as Eddie lit up a cigarette outside. I peeked my head out "Hey you're not done, put that shit out and get over here."

Eddie looked pissed off, like I ruined his chances with AJ. The unconscious one's vital signs increased like clockwork. We slid the stretcher out, as AJ looked for the call report.

A calm voice from the two-way radio on my hip said, "10X-ray, tactical, are you 81 (still at the hospital) or 97 (available)?"

Good old Marcus the dispatcher checking in. I pulled the portable radio off of my belt, "10X, we're here at Bell, 10-97. We are just helping 13X with a patient, but if you need us, send it over."

Marcus came back after a brief pause " 10-4 10X, thank you. All's quiet Chris, but I'll hit ya up if I need ya."

I smiled at our camaraderie and keyed up my radio once, which will give Marcus a momentary signal telling him I got the message. I walked in with the crew of 13X and when Eddie stepped away from the nurse's triage desk, AJ walked over to me and said softly, "Thank you, again."

PARAMEDIC M.O.S.

Her approach was so warm and genuine, I thought I was going to faint again. "Has he been treating you like this all day?" I asked as AJ looked frustratingly at me.

Looking like she was about to have a fit, she said "I have been on since 15:00 and he has been embarrassing me in front of patients all day. I just got to this station a week ago and I just want to do what is required of me."

Something about her look concerned me. I could tell that there was more going on there, but that she was trying to be tight lipped about it.

I said to Eddie firmly, "You discuss the patient with the charge nurse, I'm going to help AJ put the bus back together. Don't forget that he was given an additional 1mg SLOW before we entered."

Eddie snatched the paper out of my hand, "I can take care of my student and my bus, why don't you get out of here."

As Eddie started to speak I was walking away, but as he made his arrogant comment to me I turned back around and said, "You will stay with your patient, and you and I will speak after this call."

I gave Eddie one of my do-not-fuck-with-me-tonight looks and he heard it crystal clear.

"I get the impression that there is more to this story than you want to speak about," I said to AJ as we approached the bay doors to the ER. The doors opened thanks to the infrared seeing-eye, as she breathed heavily.

"Look AJ," I said with a caring but firm tone," What I witnessed was very inappropriate on his part, so if there is something else going on this is the time to tell me and deal with it."

We stopped at the bus and AJ went to open the rig, remembering that Eddie had the keys.

"Damnit!" she said with a large amount of frustration.

I reached for my kubaton and pulled out my fleet master key, which gave me access into any vehicle in the service.

"How did you get a key to our ambulance?"

I smiled and said, "I work for the Special Operations Division, and I am also the senior training medic for the borough." She looked up at me and replied, "So you would be someone to talk too."

We started red bagging biotoxic needles that she used on the patient, "AJ I don't know you from a hole in the wall, but I do know Eddie."

She sat down on the bench and began to cry, so I said, "Come with me."

C.B. Garris

Closing the doors to her ambulance I led her to my vehicle that only my partner and I have keys too. I had her get in and sit on the bench, then I closed the doors. The windows to the rear and side of the ambulances are tinted, so she could cry in privacy and I could get to the bottom of what was going on.

I grabbed some tissues and gave them to AJ, keeping my distance while not being too far away.

She sat there and cried for a few minutes.

"AJ, obviously you are upset and something happened. Whether I hear it from you or I go in there and I have a talk with numskull, I am going to find out what is going on and it will be dealt with. We are a family here and there is no reason why," AJ cut me off saying, "I don't want to lose my job."

She sniffled and wiped her nose.

Looking at AJ as if I was counseling her on getting out of an abusive relationship, I continued, "The only way we keep each others back around here is if we are here for each other. Now you may only be months out of the academy, but you have every right to wear that patch that I do. If you don't want to talk to me for any reason, that is totally fine. I don't know the whole story, but if you are more than comfortable speaking with a female, I can reach out to our best chief who is available right now. I want you to be comfortable talking about this."

I knew this was going to be bad and my blood started to boil. I was hoping it would not be as bad as I suspected.

AJ looked at me and said, "I feel like an absolute fool here."

"What do you mean?" I asked.

Sniffling a little more, "I have been here for two months and I, I , I am afraid that if I say anything that I will be labeled."

I handed her more tissues.

"When I got to the station originally, I had a pretty good instructor, or at least he wasn't hounding me. Every time I get Eddie as a preceptor, he is arrogant, rude, and nasty." I looked at her like I was trying to make wine from a rock, "What else AJ, what else is there?" She looked at me and I could see the emotional detachment taking place in her face as she looked away from me and looked out the rear one way windows, "And he has tried to feel me up from both ends on calls."

It was as bad as I thought. I felt something in my stomach turn and I had to get hold of myself, since something was telling me that she was totally honest.

PARAMEDIC M.O.S.

AJ looked at me slowly, "I haven't said anything because I thought someone might say that I was just trying to make trouble." I sat there in silence with her, as I felt her humiliation everywhere. "I just want to do my fucking job," she said angrily.

I asked AJ if she had mentioned this to anyone and she said no. I asked if she kept a running record of what happened and she informed me that she did in her personal journal.

I said, "That's good enough. I don't need your permission to investigate this, but I would prefer having it. I will contact Chief Davia Battieri and inform her of this as soon as I leave this hospital. She will decide how to best handle this, but in the meantime if you have any more incidents of a sexually harassing nature then I want you to contact me immediately via Communications. If you want or need to, feel free to contact me at Station 11. If I am not there, the station boss will reach out to me right away. Are you assigned to 13 regularly?"

AJ looked at me with a swollen nose from crying and remarked, "Yes, I start at 14:00 on B Platoon."

"AJ," I said assuringly, "we are going to get to the bottom of this and most of all it is going to be dealt with. You are not alone out here and your job is NOT going to be in jeopardy for saying anything to me or anyone else. You are protected by a stringent set of regulations for coming forward in a situation like this."

She nodded quietly, "Thank you. Why are you doing this for me?"

I smiled a confident and caring smile saying "Because we look out for each other out here, because you earned that patch on your right shoulder, because I know enough about you in the first few minutes to know that you would do the same for me if I was in a similar position, and most of all, because NO ONE should have to put up with that shit, ever!" She looked at me like I just revealed all of her secrets, "How do you know what you do?"

Smiling a smile that said I have been around the block many times I looked her straight in her eyes, "One thing you will learn about this job is that you have ten seconds to size a person up and decide whether the scene is safe. I can see your character quite vividly and feel all the better for being able to recognize what it represents." Now I thought AJ was going to pass out. I got the impression that she is unaccustomed to being dissected, but it helped to establish a trust between us. I could see her warm to my observation of her.

"I am not trying to mess with anyone's job," she said gently.

I said, "I didn't think you were, and for that matter if anything happens to Eddie's job as a result of this situation, then that is Eddie's fault not yours. The best thing you can do is what you have done, to tell somebody. While it is the responsibility of the senior ranks to deal with the issue and to make final determination, it helps them if we bring this stuff forward. It does nothing for our morale or our patients if we have abusers out here working on patients, or if we have medics scared to come to work. I have worked too hard in this field to see someone go through this. In fact what Eddie will get from Inspectional Services (EMS Internal Affairs) and management is going to seem like an all expense paid vacation to Disneyworld compared to what he has coming from me."

AJ looked at me with relief and fear. She recognized immediately that I was caring and concerned, but there was a protective streak in me that attracted all of her senses and attention full bore.

"Do I want to know what you might do," she asked.

I looked at the floor for a few seconds then raised my eyes slowly until our eyes locked, "Don't worry, it's nothing that an operating room can't correct."

I heard Eddie's loud mouth heading for the electronic doors, so we exited my vehicle and continued cleaning.

Eddie said, " C'mon you two, you have been out here for twenty minutes, what's taking so long?"

I smiled at Eddie. To Eddie it was a buddy smile. To me it said I am going to kick your ass all over this bay in about ten seconds. I motioned for Eddie to walk back inside with me and he did.

As we re-entered the ER together he said to me "Why'd you jump all over me in front of that babe man; she's hot for me."

Approaching the sinks I remarked "I got the impression you were setting her up to get hurt in there and that wasn't cool."

He patted my shoulder and said, "C'mon dude, you know how these Latin bitches are, cause they're so fucking hot they think we are going to be all googily eyed and nice to them. Fuck that, when was the last time one of these ho's gave me some. She has to lick my boots for as long as she is on my truck."

As I scrubbed my hands with a pre-packaged surgical brush, I considered about seven different untraceable ways that I could end his life.

"Eddie," I said, "does that have anything to do with her skills?"

PARAMEDIC M.O.S.

Eddie became puzzled, "C'mon man," he said, "I know she got the skill's, she passed the academy, but unless I clear her evaluation, she ain't gonna make it. It's beautiful."

As I stood there looking at him, I considered the eighth method of death. "So what your telling me is that because you have an issue with your inability to get a date, you are going to make this girl's life a living hell, regardless of how qualified she is." Eddie smiled and raised his eyebrows several times like Groucho Marks. I was now on the eleventh method.

As I dried my hands, Eddie said, "She wants me man, I know she does. What, did she say anything to you?"

I looked at Eddie like he had four heads, "Say anything to me about what?" Eddie studied me for a second, "Man if that bitch says anything to get me in trouble," I cut Eddie's words off, grabbed him by his uniform shirt and slammed him into the wall next to a supply cart, "YOU WILL WHAT?"

Eddie looked at me like he knew he crossed the line. Nurses all around looked as Eddie's body hit the wall, and Jennifer came around the triage desk and watched. "Look you piece of shit, you have been given a student to evaluate. I don't know who you blew to get a spot with the academy, but you have a standard to uphold."

Eddie started to sweat as my hands gripped tighter on his uniform shirt, "You will evaluate her on her skills based on her performance and that is all. If you have any social plans for her, I just canceled them. I better not see any other incidents like I saw tonight, because she could have been permanently injured or killed if that overdose patient went off. Your job is to guide and protect her until she is confident enough to do that for herself, just as you would for any MALE medic intern. You got me?"

I let Eddie's shirt go as his feet hit the ground. "Hey man, I got ya. I don't know why you all in my face man."

I turned back to him and Eddie flinched like I was going to strike him. "Eddie, what is my title?"

Eddie looked like a scolded child, "Tac medic," I cut him off, "no you idiot, the rest of it."

Eddie looked at the floor, and then me "You are the senior training medic for the borough of Manhattan."

I looked at him with one of my most serious looks, "What you did out there aside from putting AJ's life in jeopardy, is you could have killed a patient."

As the next words left my mouth AJ appeared in the corner of my eye, "and I am going to be watching you like a fucking hawk."

I left Eddie standing there, feeling embarrassed and checked in place. I said good night to AJ in a business fashion so Eddie would not get suspicious, and also said goodnight to the nurses at the triage station and the trauma surgeons who were filling out charts and drinking coffee. I didn't know that we had such an audience.

As we left the ambulance bay, I sent a confidential message to Chief Davia Battieri's onboard computer telling her that I needed to meet with her. Davia knew that if I was sending it in that terminology, that it must be serious. About thirty seconds after sending it I received one back on our computer screen, "Hey you, where would you like to meet?"

I asked her to meet us at the comic shop across from Tompkins Square Park, at the intersection of 9th street and Ave A. The comic shop while home to many super hero friends, was my favorite for the ice cream sodas and the icees. Their icees were a close second to my all time summer icee spot The Lemon Ice King in the Corona section of Queens. Sitting in a panoramic position at the corner of 108th Street and Corona Ave., you will not find a better Italian icee on the planet. When Davia drove up Ave. A, she parked her Chief's vehicle (a white caprice classic with our agency's orange and blue stripe on the side and our insignia on both front doors), right behind us. I came out of the comic shop with three ice cream sodas: a strawberry for me, vanilla for Jen, and a chocolate for Davia.

She stepped out with a smile and said, "Hey, what's going on?"

She smiled when I handed her the beverage, "Aw, thanks! What do I owe ya?" I rolled my eyes and said, "Chief puhlease, it's on the house; you work hard for us."

She knew my smile, and we always got along well. I was very fortunate to have her respect from my earliest days at the station. Our mutual admiration was spilling out everywhere.

"Your office or mine," she said to me.

Jen and I sat in Davia's department vehicle, while the air conditioning in our bus kept everything cool. I informed her of the events that just unfolded in front of me regarding AJ. Davia listened intently, sipping her ice cream soda like a child. As I spoke there was minimal radio chatter, and I was hoping that we didn't get a call. Davia could have put us off service for our meeting, but that is not how we worked. She respected me for that, and it also helped keep it confidential. By the time I finished the story I thought she

PARAMEDIC M.O.S.

was going to take off with us in her car to find Eddie and beat him severely. The cool thing about Davia is that like me, she too is a Scorpio. We could read each other's eyes in an uncanny fashion. What appeared as innocence to many, said something entirely different to me. She was one of the best administrative bosses I ever had and I was proud to be under her command. She asked for my gut feeling on this.

"Chief," I said, "I sat there and watched AJ cry. If that wasn't evident enough, when I got into some dialogue with Eddie, he gave it to me on a silver platter and said everything but that he was planning to force himself on her or at least create a horrendous situation." She nodded while looking at me.

The one thing about Davia is that she was aside from being my boss, she was also a stunning woman. She was tall at about 5'10", with long straight brunette hair and deep hazel eyes. She was 41 but looked like she was all of 24. She worked out on a regular basis, but did indulge herself in a cigarette every once in awhile. She was intimidating in that she was in a high-ranking position and also very attractive; this tended to throw many off. She had a demeanor that always made me feel safe and one where I knew that she would listen to me, valuing my opinions.

"How do you wanna handle it?" She asked as she slurped out the end of her soda.

"Chief, I know that there is a jacket (confidential file) on Eddie and that he has never been caught. I also know that I am not supposed to know that. I know that his jacket has several unsubstantiated situations like this, and I think we can catch him on this one. I want to! Especially if he is fucking with students who are just coming out here. If that is the case, he is ruining careers before they get started."

Davia looked out the rear view mirror and said, "Tell me about her."

I pressed my lips together and paused, "She seems genuine and from her descriptions of events, I have no question about her qualifications. I want to hang in the M3 (13X-ray's primary area of response) and step in on a few calls when they call for backup. I want him to know he has been caught and I want her to know that we take care of each other out here."

Davia nodded slowly, "I like it and your idea. One thing is that you will not be alone in tailing him. I will also put a call into ISU Inspectional Services Unit (Internal Affairs) right now."

I smiled and said, "I thought you would."

C.B. Garris

Davia looked over to me, "Why don't you head up into the M3, I'll send Marcus a message that you are being redeployed; and call me the moment this fucker acts up again." I said goodnight to the Chief and stepped towards my vehicle in a good place.

As Jen and I got back into the bus, I sent Marcus the dispatcher a message that we were heading up into the M3, and his reply to my computer was, "I just got the message from Car 10 (Davia). Do I want to know?"

I smiled that we knew each other well enough to know that something was up. I transmitted back a simple "No."

About twenty minutes later 13X got a cardiac arrest at 34th street and 9th Ave. in an apartment. 13Boy was sent as the BLS backup and Jen and I headed in that direction in stealth mode, never to be heard or seen. I sent a message to Marcus that we were going to stop in on 13X-ray's call to see if they needed a hand, but that we were available. When we pulled up, 13X and 13Boy were already parked and upstairs.

Jen and I entered the building. This area, which was right across from Penn Station, was more businesses, but had some residential apartments. The apartment was on the 4th floor, and for a cardiac arrest that was good, considering that most were on the seventeenth floor when no elevators were available. Jen and I stood on opposite sides of the doors, as you never stood directly in front of any door you were knocking on.

I tapped three times with my flashlight, and a police officer from Midtown South opened the door. "What is this, a fucking medic convention," the officer said to me since there were now seven medics with us entering the room. I smiled as we walked past him patting him on the shoulder. You need or I should say prefer at least four medics on a serious call, because a multitude of things may have to be done expediently.

IV's have to be initiated, endotracheal intubation has to be initiated, cardiac monitoring has to be set up, oxygen needs to administered and medications have to be decided upon and delivered. Two medics can do this, but it is more beneficial to the patient to have more hands on. When all is said and done, someone has to carry your equipment, and this is where the NYPD comes in.

As I surveyed the room, one member of 13Boy was bagging the patient in prep for a tube, Eddie's partner was initiating IV placement into a forearm vein, the other member of 13Boy was opening IV bags of D5W (5 % dextrose in water), and AJ was doing chest compressions. Eddie was fumbling with his Lifepak Monitor. Just as I was about to step out of the

PARAMEDIC M.O.S.

darkness to ask if I could help, he took out the monitoring cords placing three electrodes on them, and then did something that made me want to nail him right there.

Instead of putting the electrodes on the patient's chest from the side where he was initially or from the head of the patient, he crouched in behind AJ while she was committed to performing chest compressions. Her positioning for this was with her butt out in the open, and as if he was trying to set up to enter her from behind, he leaned into her butt slipping the electrodes under her arms during compressions. This made not only his groin connect, and I do mean connect with her butt, but also gave him the ability to cop a feel from her breasts with his hands and forearms.

He was so close that you couldn't get a piece of paper between them. I don't think the family noticed, but I saw AJ's eyes open wide and I hoped she would have kicked him straight in the nuts.

She was the professional I thought she was and maintained herself, so that patient care could continue. Twice he leaned in repeating his actions, claiming that he was checking the electrodes. Eddie had no idea we were there or watching.

Officer Graves from the Midtown South leaned over to me and said, "Not for nuthin, but is that normal?" I looked at him out of the corner of my eye and said, "Not at all."

After a consult with our EMS physician at EMS headquarters and two rounds of first line meds and a dopamine drip (we generally gave dopamine when a patient is circling the drain. It is a last ditch blood pressure effort medication to get some kind of reaction; though if we are in dopamine it ain't looking too good).

"Hi." I said to the group, "can we help bring your equipment down?"

Eddie started to stutter as I picked up his drug bag, while AJ smiled continuing chest compression's without interruption. We helped lift the patient downstairs, and Eddie thought Jen and I would disappear after that.

I looked at AJ and said, "I saw everything."

She looked at me like I had just saved her kitten from a tree. They transported down to St. Vincent's, and we were in tow. As both units pulled into Vinny's, Jen and I pulled in behind a few other ambulances, and we watched from the cab of our vehicle. After turning the patient over to the ER staff at Vinny's I saw AJ come out and then I saw Eddie moving abruptly towards her. I had a distinctively bad feeling. I told Jen to send a message to Davia to head in this direction with ISU. The bay at Vinny's can only hold two ambulances, but it leaves a walkway on the Greenwich Avenue side of the bay. I walked up slowly and quietly as I heard Eddie chewing AJ out.

"What the fuck is your problem," I heard Eddie's voice say.

"Can you just leave me alone," AJ said frantically. Then the whole bus seemed to move with a thud. I heard both doors slam shut and I took out my keys.

"Get off of me you piece of shit," I heard from AJ. I keyed the door and opened it to find Eddie on top of AJ on the bench, trying to pull her pants down with AJ squirming for some footing.

I reached in and grabbed him by the back of his neck and seat of his pants, throwing him out of the back of the ambulance into the ER bay. Eddie's face and chest landed against a brick wall in the bay.

Eddie got up stunned saying, "Yo, man, what the fuck is your problem. You trying to save this Latin bitch from what she really deserves?"

I looked at Eddie while grabbing him by his throat and lifting him off of the ground, "Eddie, you have gone way over the line and now your ass belongs to me. Go ahead, give me a reason to have you admitted to this hospital."

Seconds later the crew from 13Boy walked out to find AJ on the floor of the ambulance with a bruised arm, trying to fix her pants, me with Eddie in the air, and I heard the familiar footsteps of Chief Davia and Jen running into the bay.

"Hey, what is going on here," said Davia.

"Chief," I said "I caught this waste of a human being trying to force himself on the student, and she was screaming for help. He attempted to force her pants off while he laid on top of her. He had closed the doors to the vehicle specifically after she told him to vacate the area."

Davia said to me with absolute disdain, "Hold him right where he is."

She approached AJ and kneeling down she said "AJ, I'm Chief Davia Battieri and I want to know if that mark on your arm came from this scuffle."

When Davia called AJ by her first name, AJ looked at her with complete confusion since they had never met before.

Obviously AJ realized that I followed through with my promise to speak with the Chief.

PARAMEDIC M.O.S.

AJ got to her feet and said, "Yes Chief, this mark happened when he forced me to the bench."

I thought Davia was going to take a gun out and shoot Eddie. Since she didn't have a gun, she picked up her radio and switched to the Citywide Special Operations frequency, "Car 10 to Citywide," she said firmly.

A deep male voice came right back over the radio, "Car 10, proceed."

Keeping her eyes locked on Eddie, Davia said, "Car 10, have P.D. respond to Vinny's for an assault on an MOS, and place 13X, 10X, and 13Boy 10-62 administrative my authority. Have 13 patrol respond to Vinny's."

The citywide dispatcher came back with, "Car 10, 10-4, any injuries to EMS personnel?"

Davia keyed her radio again and said, "Car 10 that's affirmative, I'll landline (telephone) you with the info. Do me a favor and have ISU respond here as well." Davia looked at the crew of 13Boy, which both members were in utter shock not knowing if they should duck, run or hide. Davia was as sweet as a button on a regular basis, but do not piss her off.

"Tony and Jim," Davia said speaking to the crew of 13Boy, "take AJ inside and sign her into the ER for treatment." Both crewmembers rushed into the vehicle and walked her inside. I informed Davia of what Eddie did to AJ on the last call, that a P.O from Midtown South witnessed it and Eddie's mouth dropped when he realized that we witnessed the whole thing.

Davia approached Eddie, whose throat I still had in my grip, "And as for you mister, now you will find out what happens when you cross the line with me and this time you will not be getting away with it."

Davia reached over to Eddie's shirt and removed his shield, demanding that he turn over his ID card. Now that I let his feet touch the ground he was able to orient himself. He reached in his left breast pocket and took out his photo I.D. card. He handed his I.D. card to Davia as six marked NYPD sector cars, 3 unmarked patrol cars and two ESU trucks converged on the ambulance bay. Even if call for assistance is one that is not urgent, we always tend to flock towards the incident...... just in case.

Car 11(Chief Wallace) was in the immediate area and pulled up, right on the sidewalk to Vinny's. A uniformed sergeant walked up and knew right away that something was grossly wrong.

"What's up," said Sergeant Mckinna." Davia looked right at Eddie, "This individual attacked his partner, injuring her and we have witness accounts that there was some type of attempted forced sexual attack. The victim is inside the ER getting evaluated." The sergeant's look said it all, "Damn, why did I have to come to work today."

Eddie was taken into police custody and ultimately jail.

PARAMEDIC M.O.S.

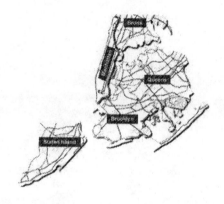

C.B. Garris

Chapter IX:

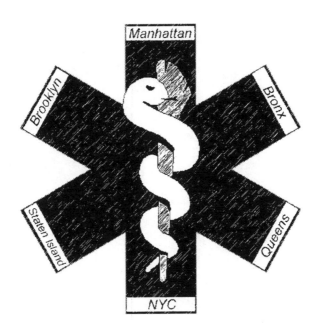

PARAMEDIC M.O.S.

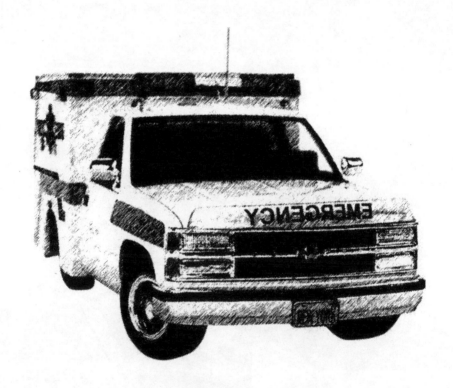

C.B. Garris

The fact that I was the luckiest guy in the world resonated through my entire body. To have AJ's affections and heart was something too special for words to make into common sense. Most people never understand what intimacy is about, so they never understood our bond. We really did make a cute couple. It wasn't so much that it was how we looked together, but anyone could see how close we were.

Yes I admit I was the googily-eyed one around her, because I was the guy with the girl who is exceedingly intelligent, caring, sexy, smart, utterly adorable, insatiable and I let her know everyday how very much I appreciated her in my life. Ironic that I found the flowers in my locker, as I already sent her 1 dozen Hawaiian Orchids of the deepest maroons, pastel blues, oranges and yellows, and they would be at her home waiting for her.

One of the patients I saved about a year ago was the owner of an international flower company. He came from Molokai where in his beliefs since I had saved his life, he owed me his. This guy had a major heart attack at Tavern on the Green, and after we revived him, he found out who the lead medic was and came down to my station.

He introduced himself to me and I recognized him right away. We talked for a while, which I must say it is wild to speak with a person who by all means was clinically dead a month before. He gave me his card and said anytime that I needed flowers for someone to give him a call, it was on the house. I couldn't accept the gift of something free for doing my job, so I asked him would he just be kind enough to let me know when these particular orchids come into season, and I would pay for them. He was a little confused but understood.

He called me every few months to let me know when the orchids would be coming into season, and even drop me a card whenever he would go home to Hawaii. He did of course invite me to visit and bring anyone I wish to his estate on the Big Island. I told him that if I was ever in town I would let him know. Tiko Clarence Muhaitian was his name and he seemed like such an absolutely genuine fellow. Widowed a few years ago, I hated to see someone like that alone. I get the impression that he made his money earning it and building a business. He is one that you want to see succeed and be happy.

I took a freshly starched shirt out of my locker and put it on over my vest. I looked to the right of the flowers and there was a tape entitled, *Me for You*. This was obviously from AJ also. The inscription read: Something

PARAMEDIC M.O.S.

for your drive home. It was a combination of Harry Connick, Jr., Al Jarreau, Michael Franks, Earth, Wind & Fire, Lenny Williams & Tower of Power, Anita Baker, The Style Council and Simply Red – some of my favorites.

I always looked forward to going to AJ, anyone who knew the depth of her care would. If guys saw her on the street, one of a few things happened. They would be intimidated by natural beauty, so they would stumble if they even attempted to approach her. The other is that she really knew how to dress. When she was out shopping it never failed that some suit would approach her, talking some smack about how high up on the corporate ladder he was or moving. A few even went so far as to ask if she wanted to join them on their private jet. She would make them falter so hard that it was painful to watch.

Our relationship was based on a connection not ruled by possession, but by mutual respect and an absolute desire to take solid care of one another. AJ was a person who looked deep into character and could size you up in a second. We are very much the same and it was like a cosmic hit when we met. It was almost as if we knew right away. She was sweet as a James Taylor composition, soft as a Roberta Flack lyrical melody.

It took time for us to be at a point when we could be there for each other, but when it happened, it put everyone else to shame. She didn't need money or materials to make her happy, and neither did I; especially on my salary. What we did have was a deep sense of mutual love for each other, coupled with a strong need and want for affection, great music, great food (she loved the fact that I was also a professional chef), endless games of Scrabble on rainy days, the Caribbean and being there for one another.

As I found myself caught up in a deep thought of her, Jen knocked on the locker room door and stuck her head in. "Hey sweet cheeks, I'm going next door to the Borough Command to log in some narcs from one of our calls from yesterday."

I finished buttoning my shirt and said, "Cool, I'll be right over." I touched the flowers, smelled them and thought of AJ. "Just a few hours my dear and I will be with you," I thought to myself.

As I walked out of the locker room, I made a right towards the Command office. I walked in and Erin Dericky was at the console. Her job was to monitor the entire borough of Manhattan to ensure all of the units were getting into service on time. She was also the receptionist for the Borough Commanders when her Partner Nick Friederland was off duty.

Erin said, "Hi!" as she leaped up and gave me a huge hug.

Should all hell break loose, Erin would make notifications and back up communications however she could. She was 5' 11", about 160 lbs., long blonde hair with brown eyes and a smile that was kinetic. Jen asked her for the narcotics logs, and I took up a seat next to her.

Clasping my hands on her desk while looking at the computer display of all the 911 activity in the City I said, "Hi Ya! Last time I saw you, both your legs were wide open!" Jen heard this and instantly fumbled the clipboard all over the place, looking at the two of us like we had eight heads. Jen momentarily forgot that three months prior I had the immeasurable pleasure of delivering Erin's baby boy at her house in Queens when I was working overtime. Complications during her delivery almost ended her life, and this call is one that will stay in my memory forever.

On the day of Erin's delivery, I had just pulled out of Station 46 (Elmhurst Hospital), after picking up some of the call volume slack in the Q6. I looked at the address and knew it sounded familiar. I looked up at the tinted portion of the windshield repeating the address over and over again in confusion when it hit me.

The job came in as an OBCOMP (Obstetrical complications), and I looked at my partner, Woody and said wildly, "Go man go! That's the house of a M.O.S. (Member of the Service)!" Woody punched the gas with his right foot, lurching us thorough the intersection.

He made a hard right evasive maneuver to avoid hitting a car as I picked up the radio and called our dispatcher, "10X, 10X, Queens check that address on file and start a patrol boss."

Woody made a hard left again to get us out of the fishtail. The dispatcher must have been new because she questioned me in the confusion.

Doing my best to keep the anonymity of my fellow co-workers I keyed up again, "10X Queens, start the boss my authority, they will understand when they arrive, conditions to follow! I don't have time to discuss this with you"

After a pause, Lieutenant Pino Delilugi came up on the frequency, "40-Patrol, Queens, put 10X-ray's assignment on my screen. I'm coming out of 46 now."

There was a pause on the air and then, "Yes sir 40-patrol, " said the dispatcher.

I re-keyed the radio, "10X Queens, start me a BLS back also!" (A BLS back is a Basic Life Support backup unit. By protocol, both advanced

PARAMEDIC M.O.S.

and basic units are to respond to high priority assignments, but high call volume dictates otherwise often).

The dispatcher returned immediately, "None available 10X." I returned before she even finished her message, "Well find one Queens!"

What was a two-minute response felt like twenty. It was actually a very messy delivery as she hemorrhaged more than expected and went shocky on me. We delivered the baby fine, but her vitals bottomed out post-delivery. Here I was in my friend's house, where I ate dinner countless times and where I helped train their Labrador puppy, Wiggles; now I am faced with her life in my hands. Her placenta had just delivered and simultaneously a clot the size of a ripened mango shot out of her vaginal cavity. Erin turned ashen gray, then sheet white. I knew the look. I dreaded the look. It was a look that I'd seen on a thousand patients before. It was a pre-death look.

"Erin!" I said forcefully getting no response. I checked her carotid pulse, which was very weak.

"Fuck!" I said to myself. Keying the mike as I propped her legs up, "10X priority, I need that BLS backup STAT, be advised this is the house of a MOS!"

The closest BLS unit was 46David out of St. Johns, and they were there in no time. I guess letting them know it was a MOS made them press that accelerator a little more. My partner Woody put Erin on the monitor and she was taching (pronounced tacking, which is short for tachycardia, a rapid heart beat) away at about 140. The blood clots kept coming out. I slapped two Normal Saline lines into either antecube (the anterior portion of the elbow joint, the opposite end from where the pointy bone is.) I titrated her IV's wide open for a fluid challenge. Her breathing went to shit on me, so I had no choice but to tube my own friend.

I remember setting up for the tube, and all of a sudden everything went into slow motion. I couldn't think of the possibility of losing her. With Robby her husband standing right in front of me, I placed the tube into her vocal chords. I told 46David to move with the infant to St. Johns, we would be close behind. Robby stood there crying, not knowing if he could collapse or how to be strong. He knew that the medics of 46David would treat his newborn son like their own, and since he was stable he stayed with Erin. Hard call to make, as a husband or a father.

NYPD ESU (Big) Truck 4 heard the call about the MOS go out over the EMS Citywide Special OPS frequency and responded. They asked if

I needed anything, and as I retrieved the stylet (a hard metal device that helps you maintain the rigidity of the tube while being placed) I replied, "Go to my bus and get my backboard, and make me a straight shot to St. Johns, NOW!" This meant that all available NYPD precinct units in that sector, Highway patrol units, ESU Special Ops units and EMS Units would respond in and shut down the streets in our path for the hospital. Between EMS and NYPD, we could effectively shut the city down in a matter of seconds if we wanted too. Membership has its privileges.

I got her tubed and as we packaged her for transport, her vitals improved, but not to where I was comfortable since she was still unconscious. We placed her on the board and headed for the bus. As I squeezed the ambu bag repeatedly (an ambu bag is a device used to ventilate a patient either with or without a tube in place) in my right hand, I held one end of the backboard in my left and between my teeth I held the two liter bags of Normal Saline that were attached to Erin's IV's. As we manipulated the backboard out of the narrow front door, I saw a stream of red and white lights everywhere. When my boots hit the sidewalk I heard an NYPD Highway Lieutenant yelling into his radio, ordering units to shut down Queens Blvd. at 58th St., both directions. We were moving swiftly but gingerly to the bus. Neighbors kept peeking out or walking out to the street to see what was going on.

On the way to St. John's I talked to Erin's unresponsive soul as I bagged her through the tube. "C'mon Erin, C'mon Honey, I know you can hear me. Girl you got a lot out here that we need you for, so keep doing what you're doing. Baby Robby is fine and he cannot wait to put his little arms around you."

No response from Erin. My heart was sinking into my boots as we drove. I picked up my radio and called out, "10X priority and I want the mixer off!"

The mixer is a device at the communications center consoles where when activated by a dispatcher, it keeps the conversation between the unit and the dispatcher only. Under normal conditions, all units in a zone can monitor all transmissions; this secured the channel so that no one else could hear what was being said.

Frank Dietz was dispatching and had already cleared the channel in anticipation of my call, "Mixer's off, X Go wit it!"

I adjusted Erin's tube again and keyed the radio, "St. Johns ETA 2 with a 27 year old female, hemorrhagic shock post delivery. BP 80/60,

PARAMEDIC M.O.S.

sinus tach at 140, intubated and unconscious. The neonate delivered successfully. Tell St. Johns I want that surgical team out of bed and ready, I don't want to hear any excuses about diversion." Diversion is a courtesy that if the hospital is filling up with patients, they can request we take the patient to a different facility. Too many times this is abused by many of the hospitals so they don't have to work. This jeopardizes the patient's health and our sanity.

Frank chimed in, "Tac X, St. Johns was on the landline with me during the note, they got the notification and they assured me that they will be ready!"

I keyed up my radio for a moment, "10X, 10-4!"

"Stay with me Erin," I told her. "Stay focused," I told myself.

As we were pulling into St. Johns I glanced out the back and saw traffic stopped in every direction. As we pulled into the bay I was relieved to see ten people in scrubs waiting for us. As we exited the back of the bus, you would have thought that the President of the United States was being brought in. There were NYPD units all over the place, and I think I saw about eight ambulances blocking traffic as well. We wheeled Erin inside as I gave the rundown to the Chief of Surgery.

"Chief of Surgery," I thought to myself, "I guess they know my wrath!" Erin went straight to OR(Operating Room).

Settling into her position once again, today was Erin's first day back to work since that the night she hemorrhaged.

Jen just finished her logs for the narcotics administration as Erin put her arm around me affectionately and squeezed my biceps and said, "Someday some lucky girl is going to get a hold of you and not let go."

I must have started blushing as she backed up a bit and Jen acknowledged, "See what you did Erin, you made him red."

She looked at me deeply and said "Is there finally someone in your life?" I smiled with that AW SHUCKS-GOLLY GEE look.

She continued softly, "Your not going to kiss and tell are you?"

I looked at her out of the corner of my eye with a smirk as she said, "Damn you Scorpio's, you did it to me every time. You and my husband are exactly alike. I never mentioned to you that Robby cannot thank you enough for what you did." The only ones in the service that knew of my relationship with AJ were Jen, my buddies and former partners Chief Tom Conroy and Captain Robert Jansen, and our station mascot, AMBU. I knew that AMBU could keep a secret. Before I said anything else I picked up a finger to tell her to hold that thought. It was now 18:15 and I reached for my radio saying, "Tactical X, 99 (available) at the station."

Some new dispatcher obviously in training came back at me over the air and said "which unit, X who?"

Having been a Dispatch Instructor for the Service, I knew what those new days were like. I re-keyed the radio and said in a relaxed voice, "Tactical X, 10-Xray, we are ninety-nine (available) at the station if you need us."

There was a pause, "Uh, Uh, okay Tactical X 10 ray."

Erin looked at me "Do you want to call Gina?"

I said, "Actually yes, I get concerned when this newbie can't figure out who we are on their channel when our unit designation is on his computer screen in front of him."

Erin handed me the phone and she depressed one button for the centrex line to the Communications Manhattan board.

"Hattan", said a pleasing female voice. "Hey you," I said, "who is the new guy?"

Gina laughed, "I had a feeling that you might call, Christian, meet Ray Delipri, he just came out of the last dispatch class."

There was a moment and then, "Uh, hi Christian." said this distracted male voice.

"Hi Ray. I'm Christian from Ten X. I know this is all new to you, so just know that if you need a medic unit we are out here. We will be in the M2-M3 (dispatch sectors of Manhattan) most of the night. Don't worry, you will get all this dispatch stuff; it takes some time to get used too. You have the absolute best trainer there in Gina." They both chuckled and we said our salutations.

As I was handing the phone to Erin, Jen said, "Not for nuthin, but I am still a little lost on the entire open legs incident you referred to a few minutes ago. You were referring to the baby thing, right?"

Jen and Erin laughed, as I smiled. I asked Erin if she wanted anything from Mike's, and she said to pick her up a loaded burger.

I said to Jen, "Lets head back out and try to get to Mike's before we get another job."

PARAMEDIC M.O.S.

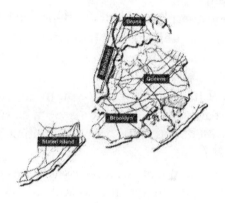

C.B. Garris

Chapter X:

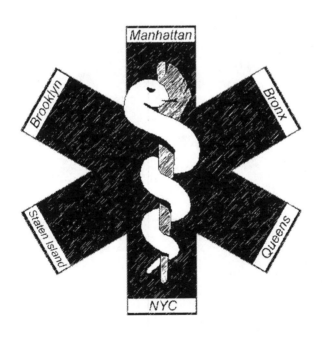

PARAMEDIC M.O.S.

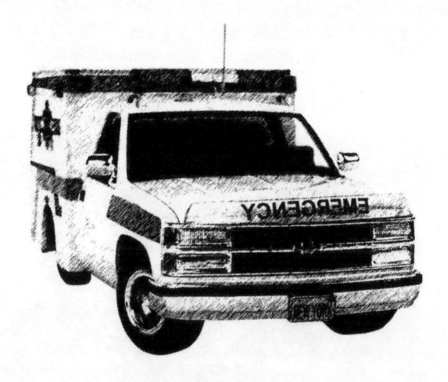

C.B. Garris

Jen was just rounding the corner of 2nd Avenue at 8th Street to park next to Mike's, when I heard 12 Frank (12F3) get a "Man Under" (person hit by a subway train and now stuck under it) at Delancy & Essex on the E Line.

The dispatcher said almost in a state of imminent confusion, "12 Frankie, I'm trying to find you an ALS from the M3."

Since we are the extra ALS unit in the sector, and the closest to the call I picked up Jen's radio saying, "Uh,10X, Tactical X put us on the back of 12 Frankie; we are about two minutes out."

Surprised and almost elated Ray the Dispatcher came back with, "Tac X, 10-4 thank you. 12-Frankie, you got 10X on your back (as your backup unit), please give a 10-12 (situation report)."

12-Frankie consisted of Connie Bover and Anita Sylindi, and Anita said to me over the radio, "Chris, we are coming from the station, we'll let you know."

"Gotcha Ani," I replied, "we are enroute from Mike's, we'll make it there first."

I then reminded the dispatcher, "10X, be advised that the E Line at Delancy & Essex is three sub-basements down, so a 10-12 will be impossible. Have 12-Frankie bring their suction, backboard and Airway bag, we will grab the rest."

Poor Ray, before he got a chance to let us know that he would relay the message, Anita said, "10X got it, see you soon."

As we approached Houston at some ridiculous speed, the dispatchers next message was crystal clear, causing Jen to head eastbound in the westbound direction of traffic on Houston. "10X and 12Frankie, Transit PD confirming you have two, that's two under and they are screaming for a rush on the bus. The power is still active, I repeat the grid has not yet been shutdown."

Ray's reference to the "grid" is the power supply of some 75,000 kilowatts of electricity that power the subway system via the third rail. It will kill anyone instantly; which brings me to my next point. One person under a train is enough of a fiasco, two people is just ridiculous.

These scenes which happen more often than most think they do, require specialized heavy rescue resources, a lot of patience, precision, a large amount of luck and rapid organization. Since we had two confirmed hit by the train, I picked up the radio and said, "10X, with two confirmed at Delancy and Essex, start me an additional BLS and ALS if

PARAMEDIC M.O.S.

you can find them, get me a boss, and also ensure that transit PD ESU is enroute."

Transit PD is exactly that, the Transit system Bureau of the NYPD, responsible for law enforcement operations on the mechanized transit system both in subway and on buses. This used to be a very lax segment of the department through most of its years, but since the late 80's and forward administrations of others who recently commanded the department, the enforcement has improved immensely. Transit PD ESU like the surface PD ESU carries heavy rescue equipment, and in this case has specialized lifting bags that we utilize to raise the trains up, if someone is trapped underneath.

Performing this operation of joint-agency collaboration usually turns into an utter nightmare, because the MTA (Metropolitan Transit Authority) routinely shuts down the wrong power grid so that we cannot enter the area. The other fundamental breakdown comes when they activate the power supply right next to us when we are under the train performing patient care. That sound when the grid activates is a sound you will always remember once you have experienced it.

There is this distinctive " HUMMMMMMMMMM," that accompanies the powering up of the grid, and with so many volts activating next to my face, I swear that every single hair on my body stands straight up.

Jen hooked a left onto Delancey that had us on two wheels, and me wondering if we would stay right side up. I trusted Jen's driving like I did mine. It may be a tad bit unorthodox and indigestible by the general public; but we have a job to do. As we approach Essex I saw four Transit PD cars parked in separate, abstract positions, totally disjointing traffic. As Jen looks for a place to land our vehicle, I pointed to the sidewalk. She smiled and shrugged, putting us right next to a market. I hit the 10-88(onscene) button on the computer letting our dispatcher know we arrived.

Depressing any of the status buttons on our computers changes our status on the dispatcher's computer. If I hit the enroute button(10-63) it makes us orange, if I depress the 88 button, it makes us magenta. As I opened the passenger side compartment to grab my Trauma bag, Airway kit and Lifepak Monitor, Jen, in synchronization with me, went to the rear of the vehicle obtaining a backboard and cervical spine immobilization equipment. As we were about to descend into the subway system, I saw my buddy Captain Bob Jansen pull up in his department issued unmarked car.

C.B. Garris

I heard Connie and Anita approaching, my guess was they were about 40 seconds out. NYPD ESU (Big) Truck 1 and R.E.P. (a smaller ESU truck) Boy-1 pulled up alongside. Truck 1's crew went for their lift bags and Boy-1 for their Hurst Tool(Jaws of Life). Even though these are the surface PD units, when someone is hurt and in need of us, we all work together better than a finely tuned machine. In most municipalities, it is generally the fire department that is responsible for rescue services. Don't get me wrong, F.D.N.Y. is there if they are needed by us. I presume that the political powers that be wanted to leave them solely for fire suppression unless specifically called to a scene. The city houses about eight million people, and you need every single firefighter on duty to make that system work.

The community surrounding Delancy & Essex is of lower income, working class people. It was an area that was often dirty, with vacant lots on one side of the street and tenement housing on the next. Like the Cherry Street projects, there are a lot of families here and people trying to survive an often difficult existence in a city of such vast caste systems.

Just a few blocks away was a methadone clinic, the two blocks north on Delancy housed the area OTB(Off-Track Betting), and there were a number of social service outfits for unemployment and people who have been through hard times. Many people in this area grew up here and either couldn't or chose not to leave the community. Some have never been out of Manhattan, even though Brooklyn is just a stones throw away by the Williamsburg Bridge three blocks south. Traffic off of the Willy Bee (Willamsburg Bridge) was at a stand still as Connie and Anita approached from the east off Rivington Street.

Jen, Bob, me and what must have been a regiment of police officers were bolting down the subway stairs, as we had to get to three sub-basements below grade with time running out. The subway system underground was filled with people either running at the site of so many police officers entering the station, or just trying to get home oblivious that anything was going on.

As I reached the bottom of the stairs with Jen in tow, we heard several Transit Police officers yell above us, "MOVE, MOVE, MOVE!" A number of civilian stragglers were frozen on the stairs at the sight of so many uniformed emergency service workers with so much equipment, hauling ass straight down the subway stairs in the shadows of intermittent lights and siren sounds.

PARAMEDIC M.O.S.

About seven officers and I approached the token stand where you obtain passage into the subway system, as the token clerk looked up at our approach while he dished out about $30.00 in tokens to a hard looking guy with tattoos. Without stopping his counting process, the token clerk reached above his waist, depressing a button that opened a special door for emergency personnel. He apparently has done this many times before. One officer held the door as the token clerk and the officer nodded at each other. We all ran through in single file headed for Level Two, in loose tactical formation as we have been trained.

Once in the subway system we have no more radio contact, so we are on our own. The FDNY and NYPD radio's worked just fine, but whoever handled the budget for our agency did nothing to ensure that we had subterranean radio capabilities. With forty pounds of equipment on my arms, I leaped over some guy who was asleep in the middle of the platform; I felt my heart start to beat harder and harder. How mangled would these two people be when we got there? Would there be anything left of them or would they be splattered throughout the station? Would they be children or adults? Would they be a mother, father, daughter, son, sibling or even one of my own family members who was at the wrong place at the wrong time?

We reached the third sub-basement stairwell where there was at least 70 people huddled along both sides of the stairwell. As we hoofed the last four steps to the E train platform where I planted my feet with a long leap, a voice from the civilian audience said, "Took you fuckers long enough!"

"Can you believe this guy," I thought to myself. I just did a Jesse Owens remake down those stairs hauling all this equipment, with my partner putting our lives in danger getting to the scene, only to have to deal with the horrifying events I know are about to unfold, and that's what this bystander who isn't doing anything to help the injured is saying? There is always one in the crowd. If I weren't so intent on getting to the victims and saving them, I would have turned around and introduced him to my fist.

Sergeant William Downing of Transit District 2 came running over to me. I have worked with Will for years and he never runs, so I know this is bad.

"Chris, one is DOA, and the other is a still underneath. The DOA is a female in her 30's, or so we think since all we have found is her head so far. The rest of her we hope is underneath. Lifting OPS have started as you can see. There is a male under the fifth train, but as you can see us overweight types can't get under there."

C.B. Garris

I knew exactly what that meant. Being 5′7″, 160 lbs. and in prime physical and athletic shape, I was one of the more agile members of the service. As a result, I was now going to be the one going underneath to access and extricate (remove) the patient. Why did I have to always be the one?

The Metropolitan Transit Authority supervisor confirmed and swore on his grandmother's grave that the power grid was off. This meant I had a 95% chance of being electrocuted. The train was just about all the way into the station, so I took off my uniform shirt and vest, handing it to a transit officer and hopped down in front of the train.

The next few minutes would make anyone want to just say, "You have got to be kidding me!" I took one final look at the platform and made my descent. I began by placing myself at dead center of the train, making sure that I was between the rails. This way in the worst-case scenario, if the train started to roll I had a chance at living, suffering probably only an unwanted haircut. The worst part about this is when you advance up the middle of the tracks, it is generally filled with nasty, murky water with creatures in it that have not been identified by science and the CDC (Center for Disease Control) refuse to work with. The creatures love to sit idle in the water until agitated by movement, as I have found on occasion. I figured they were part of some city science experiment.

I began crawling with the use of my elbows, similar to the obstacle course training used for military Special Forces where you have the barbed wire above your head. My barbed wire was in the form of thousands of tons of steel, powered by 75,000 kilowatts. I think I would have rather been on that military course. By the second car I could smell the blood, warm and pungent. As I moved past the second car I found what appeared to be maybe a pelvis, crushed and blood stained, with all the skin sheared off. Must have been the DOA's. A few more feet and I found part of what appeared to be a lung, and a rat the size of house cat noshing on it.

Having done this routine with Jen so often, I knew that she was following the sound of my boot kicking the train. She knew where I was at all times. When I found the rat I screamed up to Jen on the platform, "Jen, I got unfriendlies down here."

That was just to let Jen know that I had rodents in the area. As I approached the fourth car, my forearms and t-shirt were covered in black murky water, blood, bone fragments, splattered organs and flesh. Next I found two things that were totally disturbing. One was the heart of the

PARAMEDIC M.O.S.

female victim, still intact resting on the third rail. Almost as if in slow motion I said to myself, "Hollllly shiiiit!"

Then I saw the next immediate phase of my evening. I found the male victim, barely conscious. He was missing one leg up to the knee, and both of his hands were gone; his chest was open and his face totally mashed, but he was breathing. "Jen I got him, get this train up now!"

Then I heard it. HUUUUUMMMMMMMMMMMM. MTA activated the grid and I felt my hair stand up on edge. I stayed absolutely still as I watched the heart, that was now resting against the electrified third rail, sizzle in bright phosphorus light.

The smell was awful and next I heard Jen scream, "Boriquah, what the hell is that smell?"

I replied in an unsurprised but pissed off tone, "Jen tell MTA to turn off the power grid now! Everything down here is starting to cook except me."

I heard a few words then a loud scuffle on the platform and I thought I heard someone get decked, then several bodies hit the platform. Next I heard someone say "Okay, okay! I'll have them shut the power off as soon as possible."

The heart exploded in front of me, all over my face and hair as I heard another something on the platform get hit again as Jen screamed, "Look you piece of shit, I don't care what problems this is causing the transit system presently, that is my partner down there, turn off the fucking grid or I will end you right here!" Jennifer may have been very prim and proper, but she grew up on the street and I would not want to set her off. I am just sorry that I could not be on the platform watching this exchange.

I heard the jingling of police utility belts and keys, and another scuffle, and I was still frozen in place. The blood from the heart was dripping down my face, off of my chin. Thank god I had my eye shields and mask on, but I was going to need a serious shampoo after this call.

I heard someone say, "Keep her away from me!" This time the voice was muffled, like the person had swollen lips.

The bodies on the platform seemed to move in unison as if trying to act as a blockade as I heard a female voice say, "C'mon, you waste of a civil servant, you got less than a minute to shut that grid off; nothing better happen to my partner!" As the words were being said, I felt the hair on my body rest, and the pieces of the heart that were burning stopped. I spit on the third rail and nothing happened; it was finally off. I moved quickly towards the male victim.

I saw what looked to be his leg under the platform, but there was too little light to make it out. I reached for his carotid pulse and he actually had one. He was taching away at about 160, which told me he lost a lot of blood and we had maybe minutes to do this.

I yelled at him, "Sir, can you hear me, what is your name sir?" Figuring that getting an answer out of him at this point was a moot gesture, I decided to rename him Mr. Sir, to add some dignity.

All that "Mr. Sir" could do was mumble, so that was futile. The heat from the mechanical portions of the underside of the train was so hot, that I felt as if I was in the Delta. I placed an Oropharygeal Airway in his mouth, and he had little if any gag reflex; another really bad sign for the position we were in. Jen slid down a few extrication collars, and as I let one hand go through the pile, I found my favorite, NO-Neck. The purple collar NO-NECK was a great default when someone's neck would not fit in any other collar.

While whispering to myself, "C'mon Mr. Sir, hang on just a few more minutes," the train began to lift above my head. They lifted the train until they could tilt it properly, allowing us to get a backboard and more personnel in the pit. If you have never seen this done, it is like being on a ride at Universal Studios, you won't believe it until you see it.

They lift the entire train, and support it at the closest points as it is tilted, this way it does not come crashing down on us. Jen was now getting him situated on the board, while the Transit cops were retrieving his leg for us. Two police officers were off in the distance, joining numerous members of the crowd in the game of who could vomit farther at the site of this twisted body.

We got him on the platform as I yelled to Sgt. Will to have his dispatcher call Bellevue and inform them we are coming in with a replant candidate, lower right leg, and possible imminent traumatic arrest. A replant candidate decision gives us medical-legal leeway to transport this patient by ground or helicopter to a Level 1 Trauma facility that can perform replantation of appendages.

It is a split second decision that has to be made. If the person is too unstable, that pretty much defines to in cardiac or traumatic arrest at the time of transport, then we have to transport to the closest 911 receiving hospital for stabilization. As long as we can initiate ALS in the field and the person is in any other state then cardiac arrest; since our tools are the same ones in the Emergency Room, we have standing order medical authorization to make the call.

PARAMEDIC M.O.S.

Once on the platform, Jen went for the tube, which she did like magic every time. Watching Jen tube was like Zen and the art of intubation. When I looked up to see the MTA representative, it was apparent by the knots on both sides of his forehead and the swollen lip that he went a few rounds with Jen and lost. I worked on establishing four IV's on Mr. Sir with a combination of trauma fluids (Normal Saline) all initiated with 14 gauge catheters.

Catheters come in various sizes, and are used in conjunction with the amount of fluid you want to administer. The smaller ones that rarely hurt are commonly known as butterfly needles. The smaller the numbers get, the larger the bore of the needle. Thus a 22-gauge needle is pretty small. The ones we usually use on patients for medical conditions or as a route for medication only remains in the 22-gauge, 20-gauge and 18-gauge arena.

If we have a trauma patient or a medical patient who needs large amounts of fluid, as in a person who has non-traumatic gastro-intestinal bleeding, we go for the gusto: the 16-gauge or 14-gauge catheters.

It is a good thing this guy was barely awake, since I started two of the IV's in his Jugular veins (neck), and the others in his arms. I heard a voice in the crowd remark that watching Jen, Anita, Connie and I working together was like watching Leontyne Price and the Metropolitan Symphony Orchestra at their best. We didn't speak to one another, because we didn't have too. Everything flowed like water from a waterfall. It was just that simple. This is what being a MOS was all about. We trained for this, night and day.

Jen set the tube in place, Anita packed the stump at the lower right leg, Connie was monitoring vitals and set up my Lifepak (cardiac monitor), as I finished securing the IV's. This entire procedure once on the platform took less than one minute.

The transit cops assembled our equipment and made a hole through the crowd, trying not to slip on the vomit-laden stairwell. Six officers grabbed the backboard as Jen ventilated "Mr. Sir"; I re-checked the titration of IV's and watched the monitor; Connie was checking vitals and Anita was making a B-line for one of our ambulances to get it set up and ready to go when we hit the surface. There we were with this forty year-old male missing appendages, covered in wet and dry blood, with tubes in almost every orifice of his body, on a backboard with IV's swinging in every direction, a tube jammed down his trachea to ensure proper ventilation and wires from a Lifepak Cardiac Monitor monitoring his heart.

There was a rumbling of feet and keys and the crackling of radios as bystanders looked on in both amazement and horror. Once again, they thought that with all this activity we were treating the President of the United States.

In fact, one of the transit officers said to me going up the level two stairwell, "Man I haven't seen this much activity since the President was in last week." I looked up at him after checking my footing and said, "When we arrive, everyone is the president!" The officer raised his eyebrows as he pseudo-slipped up three stairs. I caught his end of the backboard.

When we hit the surface, Anita had pulled my vehicle around in a great position. One problem with this though; it was MY vehicle. As I leaped inside ahead of the stretcher, Anita had already laid out my first round meds (medications) for a traumatic arrest on the side console.

As they wheeled him into the vehicle, Anita leaned over to me as Jen jumped in the back with us and said, "We are using your vehicle for this one, since you used mine on that stabbing two weeks ago that had me cleaning for two hours."

I smirked while putting on a scrub covering over my white undershirt and said to Anita, "I love you too!"

Anita smiled.

Bagging the victim with my right hand, I picked up my EMS portable with my left and called our dispatcher, "10X, 10-82 (enroute to the hospital), hospital 02 (Bellevue). I need a trauma stand-by and a notification when you're ready to write."

There was a pause and then a clicking of a keyboard, "10X, c'mon with it," said a husky male voice.

"X-Ray, they should be expecting us; 45 year old male, man under, replant candidate for right lower leg, multi-trauma, ALS established eta 5-6 minutes."

The dispatcher acknowledged as Connie started driving. I heard all kinds of sirens outside as I bagged "Mr. Sir," and looking out the back window I realized that the NYPD came through again. They shut down all traffic for our route to Bellevue, from Delancey to Allen, then 1st Avenue right to Bellevue. For more than thirty city blocks, we had a police escort all the way. I trust that Mr. Sir would have been proud to know how we honored his situation.

As we approached 11th Street, and being proud of how our dedication to our patient's safety can set so many things in motion, I thought of that old Toyota commercial, OH WHAT A FEELING!

PARAMEDIC M.O.S.

"Mr. Sir" went into cardiac arrest, as Jen administered 1mg (milligram) of Epinephrine (also known as Epi) and 1mg of Atropine in his IV injection port. Ani initiated compressions without me even to having to ask. I thought about calling EMS Telemetry (our department Emergency Physician on duty 24-hours a day for the purposes of clinical treatment consultation.) The deciding factor on that idea was that by the time we actually establish our connection, since the agency has this long procedure to get him or her on the phone we will be pulling into Bellevue's ambulance bay. Since we already have standing orders for this situation, that is we are cleared to apply certain treatments without the necessity of contacting a physician, I scratched the idea of Telemetry and maintained Standing Orders Protocols. Continuing CPR, we still got no response after the meds were administered, so Jen dropped a second Epi (Epinephrine) and we got a pulse back with a pressure.

"Hot Damn!" I thought to myself. We rounded 28th street into the Bellevue campus. When we approached the ER bay, another pack of hungry wolves was waiting for us.

Needless to say when that call was over, the one place I could be found was at the scrub sinks. Jen was sweet enough to join me, as she also offered to remove the chunks of heart out of my hair.

"Only you," Jen said as she flicked a big chunk into a red bag. We cleaned up the best we could there and once again, Jen and I went out 10-62 back to our station for clean up. On our way back to the station we stopped at Mike's. I actually called Mike's from Bellevue so our order would be ready when we got there. I went in and picked up.

Mike was a great fellow. Born and raised in Colorado, he decided to make a break for the big city, and that was fifteen years ago. Mike was about 5'9" and wiry, with a mustache and a smile. He was always glad to see us when we arrived, and always made us feel at home. I think he realized the same thing that we did – that the meal we eat at his establishment could be our last if things got funky out there. Mike was a fighter pilot in the Air Force, and always loved to hear our scuttlebutt (shop talk). I picked up our orders, shook hands with Mike and then Jen and I made for the station.

As we pulled in Jen said, "Well that was an interesting evening. I trust that you are going to see AJ tonight."

I smiled looking over at her, "But of course."

"Have her give me a call tomorrow, so that we can decide what restaurant we are all going to critique next." Jen said with a smile rubbing her tummy.

"Gladly, think I have the new Zagat's at home; we will break it out. Anything in particular you up for this time?" I said making a few notations on our unit run sheet for the night.

"I hear that there is a great place up on 11th street called Aramanthe, we should check it out. I was by it yesterday and I saw some pretty good looking seafood." Jen said as she took a bite of her burger. She then informed me that she was going to her niece's school in the morning. It seems that a teacher may have hit her niece this morning in school, and she told Artie that she wanted to be right there in the Principal's office when they confront the teacher.

I waited for AMBU to appear but she didn't.

"Hmmmm." I thought to myself. The Lieutenant's door opened and out she flew, right at me. It seems Ms. AMBU was enjoying herself some air conditioning.

John walked out of the office and said, "Man, you had some kinda night!"

I laughed and said, "Damn Skippy, but it was nothing compared to your first marriage."

He laughed saying, "Well, you gotta point."

"Hey," Jen blurted in with a smile, "I'm getting thirsty, let's head over to the place."

We said goodnight to John, and made for South Street. I turned the bus towards the Brooklyn Bridge and we pulled up once again to our favorite deli. We both went for Citrus Gatorade, one for now and one for later. The guys behind the counter went to make their perverted stare again, and then realized I was walking in also; they stopped.

As I picked up our respective bottles of Gatorade, a voice from my right hip squawked, "Ten X, one-zero X," a very strong male voice said over the radio speaker.

Looking at Jennifer kind of puzzled, I picked up the portable radio to answer. First, we weren't in rotation for any line assignment since we were the Tactical Unit, and more puzzling was that the voice I heard was that Watch Commander, not the Citywide Operations Dispatcher.

"Ten X, go Citywide." I said clearly and with authority.

"Ten X," the male voice said again and now I knew it was Lenny, "Ten X, Chris are you in the M1?" There was a lot of two-way radio traffic in the background back in Communications.

The area in the Communications Division known as Citywide is where all major incidents are coordinated. When a major incident is not

PARAMEDIC M.O.S.

in progress, it is used as a monitoring resource, ensuring that all EMS 911 Operations were being handled appropriately. The Watch Commander is also in direct contact with them so that he or she can make all pertinent decisions from this area. We operate in a para-military structure and always very official, as all of the senior ranking officials for the agency are monitoring this frequency twenty-four hours a day.

If Lenny is calling me on the 800 MHZ radio, it means whatever is going on is serious, and if he is using my first name it also means that something hot was about to drop. It told me without even having to know what was going on, that they were doing crisis plotting in the "War Room" as we called it.

"Ten X-ray, we are in the M 1 (lower Manhattan). What can we do for you Citywide?" I said with an inquisitive and humorous tone.

"X-ray," Lenny again answered, "you are in perfect position. I'm assigning you a job at the Wall Street Heliport. You're gonna eighty-five (our terminology for meet with) a U.S. Coast Guard Search and Rescue "Heelo" (short for helicopter). Further information to follow."

For one brief moment Jennifer and I looked at each other with a look that said, "Coast Guard Search & Rescue, what the hell is this about?", and we then made a B-line for the bus. As I turned the bus on, Jen punched up the call on our on-board computer. I popped the lights on and tapping on my siren, drove up to Whitehall Street and made a left near the Staten Island Ferry Terminal. I looped around heading the north on South Street, next to the elevated entrance to the FDR. Not more than a thousand feet and we were at the Heliport. I pulled the rig right onto the property and did not see a heelo.

Jen read the job out loud to me as I looked, "Well my dear, looks like we are headed out to sea. It says here fifty year old male, multiple seizures on board an inbound car freighter that is possibly fifty miles offshore."

As Jen finished her statement we both looked at each other.

"Fifty miles out to sea?" I said with my eyebrows up. Jen gave me her "I dunno" look. We were used to doing Med-EVACS (helicopter evacuations) of trauma patients with the NYPD Aviation heelo's; but with the U.S. Coast Guard, that's a new one. As we got out of the bus to start compiling our equipment, our department cell phone rang.

As I put the phone to my ear I heard, "Yo, Chris," it was Captain Lenny. Lenny had a hint of hurried excitement in his voice, "Check it out, I already know what you're thinking so let me brief you." Your Heelo will be arriving in approximately 4 minutes off the Verrazono Narrows. They are coming in hot so be ready. Coast Guard got a distress call from a vessel that may be about fifty miles out to sea with a Status Eptilepticus (a patient suffering from uncontrollable and consistent seizures) on board. Coast Guard has the heelo and a crew of two, but no medics are assigned to their Air Station in Coney Island right now. They are doubling back to retrieve you and Jennifer and you are headed out with them."

"Lenny, you never cease to amaze me." I said smiling at Jennifer.

"Chris, you and Jen were in the perfect spot for this, and frankly I would rather you two take this one rather than anyone else. You two have trained with the military and you have trained military corpsmen, you two also have the tactical training equivalent to the crew on the Heelo. You will have a direct channel open to me on 800 channel 8-K, and whatever you need you got."

As Lenny spoke the last of his words, I could hear a chopper approaching. Jen opened the passenger side compartment and started grabbing equipment: Lifepak cardiac monitor/defibrillator, MEDS bag, Advanced Airway bag, while I grabbed the immobilization equipment, suction, Apcor telemetry monitor, and a trauma bag. I had a feeling that this was going to be one of "those" calls.

The heelo, a U.S. Coast Guard HH-65A Dolphin, red in color, shot past the Heliport and than made a swooping fishtail turn in mid-air, aiming for Heelo-Pad # 2. As they approached I picked up my EMS radio and informed Citywide that the Heelo was touching down. They knew within the next minute we would approach the chopper, board and lift off.

The Heelo was huge and the rotors remained in motion as Jen and I leaned down like the opening scene to M.A.S.H. when they approach the chopper, leaving our bodies in a ducking formation to walk to the heelo. You never want to approach a helicopter standing straight up, as you will get decapitated if the rotors drop. The coast guard airman took our equipment, one piece at a time as Jen and I hopped up inside.

Airman Griffin waved to us and pointed to our seat belts and headsets. We donned our headsets and seatbelts as we lifted off. As we went airborne towards the Statue of Liberty I kept thinking to myself, "Since we aren't officially employees of the U.S. Coast Guard, and we are no longer in a NYC EMS ambulance, if this thing crashes do we get hazard pay?"

Airman Griffin introduced himself and took a good look at Jennifer.

PARAMEDIC M.O.S.

Airman Griffin winked at Jennifer as he said to us, "Welcome aboard our bird."

The inside of the heelo was spacious enough for us to work a cardiac arrest somewhat uncomfortably, just the same as if we were in a studio apartment in midtown. There were several fire extinguishers above my head that weren't really instilling much trust in me. The cabin of the heelo was in the color of gunmetal gray, which would be appropriate since I am sure we were moving faster than a bullet. That speed of this particular craft was concerning me.

I spoke to Airman Griffin for us. "We are glad to be here, now what is the deal?"

"We've confirmed that an auto freighter has a male in his 50's on board having seizures, last report we could assess he has been seizing for two hours." Airman Griffin said to us reading from some type of print out.

I grabbed the mike to the headset to get a better voice inflection to Jennifer, "If this guy has been seizing for two hours, he may be in arrest when we get there." As we shot past the Verazzono Bridge in Staten Island, Jen nodded to me as we both began to look below us, to the empty darkness that was in the form of the Atlantic Ocean. We must have been at about one thousand feet, and I felt like we were in a bullet. There was a high pitch, heavy whining in the background, which were the rotors. I looked up at the cockpit and it was illuminated in numerous greens, oranges, and yellows.

Jennifer tapped my right leg and reaching for the microphone on her headset said, "I have a funky feeling about this."

"Me too." I replied. I looked at Airman Griffin and asked if he could switch my headset to my EMS 800 Channel so that I could speak with "my people."

Griffin reached above his head and pushed several buttons, and turned a dial. I heard an uplink signal and then I heard the EMS Citywide frequency.

"Airborne 10X to Citywide, K?" (The letter K is an acronym used on our frequencies to signify the end of a transmission).

"Airborne Ten X, proceed to Citywide, K." A deep male voice said.

"Ten X, eighty five successful, and we are now enroute to the location of the freighter. The subject onboard may have been seizing for up to two hours. If the patient is in extremis (critical condition) when we make contact, we are going to divert to Floyd Bennet Field for a ground transfer to Coney Island Hospital, instead of returning to the M2 for a drop at Bellevue. Give ESU (NYPD Emergency Services Unit) a heads-up that we may be utilizing Floyd Bennet as the landing zone. Also ensure that we have at least a BLS unit in both the M2 (Manhattan South) and in the K1 (Brooklyn South) ready to rock when we lift off from the freighter. Whichever LZ (Landing Zone) we use, we want ESU securing the zone."

As Citywide acknowledged my transmission, Griffin interrupted my thought process by saying that we were not going to be landing on the freighter.

"Well then how are we supposed to get down to it? It doesn't have a pad?" I said concerned.

Jen grabbed my right arm and pointed out the window. We began making a sweeping turn over this massive vessel that was stopped in the water. There were lights on below, but I didn't see anything signifying a landing pad for a helicopter.

Airman Griffin handed both of us what appeared to be harnesses and said to put them on. He also told us to put our gear in the stokes basket. I put the headset mike next to my head and said, "Are you thinking of lowering us down there via the hoist?" Airman Griffin smiled a smile so wide, that his dimples showed, "You learn quickly."

Jen looked at me and said, " You have got to be kidding me?"

I was shaking my head from side to side knowing that this was not a joke.

Pointing to Griffin's computer panel above his head I said, "I guess I'll go first, but first give me my 800 channel on my headset."

"Ten X-ray Citywide," I was yelling into the microphone now that the side door to the Heelo was open and I was looking straight down at nothing but cold ocean water.

"X-ray if you can hear me, we are being hoisted down to the vessel, Coast Guard will transmit our exact coordinates momentarily." If I got a response in my headset I couldn't hear it.

I was now looking at Jen, who was looking at me, who was being looked at by Griffin. I took a few immediate airway supplies out of my bag and put them in my back pocket, in case I made patient contact before our equipment landed on the vessel or worse, fell into the ocean.

Jen was looking at me as I began my descent, and I actually saw fear in her eyes. I am unsure though if it was for me or for her. We were about

PARAMEDIC M.O.S.

fifty feet off of sea level, and I was beginning to spin from the force of the rotors. Wind and water was splashing in my face and I was deathly afraid of the enema I would get if this hoist inverted me.

As I got closer to the vessel, I saw seven men scurrying around making room for my descent. When I landed on the vessel, I really wasn't any happier than I was on the heelo. Since we were in international waters, I wasn't even sure if Jen and I would speak the language of the crew. This vicinity is heavy for international trade vessels, so anything was possible. We also didn't even know what this vessel was transporting, and the Coast Guard crew would not be escorting us on this situation. They would be staying aboard the heelo and hovering.

Jen was next down followed by our equipment. Once our equipment landed, I disengaged it from the hoist and the heelo ascended. Griffin gave Jen one of the Coast Guard two-way portables so we could call them back down when we were packaged and ready. We hit the deck of the freighter and tried to imagine something so large standing in place in open water. I couldn't tell exactly how many stories we were in the air, but it seemed to go on forever. The Coast Guard heelo lifted way up above us to hover.

The ship was actually bound from Turkey, delivering export goods. The ships captain, a small yet very muscular man greeted us in a professional manner, and I was so happy to find out that most of the ships crew spoke English, and not a language that I didn't have a knowledge of. It seemed to Jennifer and I that they had done this before, as they greeted us and immediately led us below deck.

The deck hands picked up much of our equipment, as we were led to a vertical stairwell. I tossed my medic bag around my neck and my Lifepak around the other side as I started the descent. I made sure to keep a careful eye on Jen, as I could see that these guys appeared to have a visual lock on her. My assumption is that they had been out at sea for quite sometime.

We followed the Captain and a few crewmembers through cavernous tunnels within the ships hull, leading to another stairwell. This stairwell was very rusted and went to another deck below. I began to assume that we were headed for the propulsion room. Jen grabbed my sleeve, her sign that she was worried.

I looked back at her and gave her a comforting glance that we were fine, and to follow my lead. We entered a room that was covered in rust and sharp areas of metal. In the rear corner was our patient. A male around forty years of age, large but good shape, seizing violently. He was blue from the face down, which would be consistent if he had been in seizure for so long.

"You gotta help him, he's really bad," a voice said that belonged to a person leaning down next to him.

"Okay, we are going to help him, just don't go anywhere as we might need your hands." I said as I dropped all of my equipment to get a full visual on the patient. Without me having to call for it, Jen popped out an non-rebreather mask and an oxygen tank. Smart thinking on her part, since it would take us a few moments to deal with this type of patient. It would be dangerous to attempt tubing him if he continued to seize so violently, so even if he is flailing about, he will get better oxygen than without the mask.

As his seizure calmed a bit, I whipped the mask on his face while Jen broke out an AMBU bag and tube kit; and I was preparing to pop a line. If I could get the line started when the seizures were light, I had the best possibility of administering Valium or Versed to bring those seizures to a halt. The trick is to do it fast enough so that he doesn't wig out on me again, blowing the IV. I put tourniquets on both of his arms and waited for the bulges to occur, but they didn't. His circulature was shot from being in seizure for so long and his body had to be tired. It would be the same thing as if an asthmatic was suffering a bad attack. At some point the body gives to the wear and tear of the event. I decided that since time was of the essence, I'd forego the arm veins and chose a nice big, fat jugular vein that was bulging in his neck.

Without even a second thought and before any of the shipmates knew what I was about to do, I reached for an alcohol prep, and swabbed the area over the site. He began to seize a little more violently again and I watched for a moment and hoped it would end. Normally I would have to call Telemetry Unit for an approval on narcotics administration, but given that no radios would work this far into the ships hull, I had no choice but to forget the attempt and act as I have in so many other situation when radio or phone contact was interfered with: autonomously. When his seizure slowed to a minimum I went for his neck again.

"What the hell are you doing?" I heard from behind me from one of shipmates.

"Relax! We are going to help him, just let us work our magic and stay nearby in case I need you," I said to the deck hand to calm him down.

PARAMEDIC M.O.S.

I reached in my waist pack for an 18-gauge catheter and almost as soon as I removed it from its pouch checking for the beveled edge, I went straight for his jugular.

I got the flashback on the first attempt and removed the needle. I advanced the catheter as far as necessary to secure it in his neck, and Jen handed me the line of D5W. I placed the IV tubing into the catheter and secured the IV with a Veni-catch.

This is like a large clear band-aid made for the securement of IV's, so that you can also monitor the IV site. Again without even looking behind me, while I held the IV tubing in my left hand, I reached back over my shoulder and Jen handed me a syringe with 10 milligrams of Valium already drawn. As she placed the EKG electrodes on our patient's chest, I dropped 5 milligrams of the Valium down the IV tubing and then flushed the IV to get the meds in him quickly. The patient seemed to relax all of a sudden and his heart rate dropped a bit, something Jen and I expected.

The patient was bleeding from the back of his head a bit, and with such violent seizures I didn't want to take any chances. I showed one of the deckhands how I wanted him to hold our patients head absolutely still while I bagged him for a minute. Now that I was bagging him with 15 liters of oxygen per minute he began to get some good pink coloring to his skin, which was blue as a grape when we arrived.

Jen placed a no-neck cervical collar on the patient's neck while I got ready to go for the tube kit. His respirations were pretty shallow and between that and the Valium, his body was going to either need rest or take it on its own. Once Jen got the collar in place, she took over respirations and gave him about ten quick but full lung fills of air so that I could tube him. In the back of my mind I was hoping that the chopper we came in on had full tanks of fuel or we were completely screwed.

I got the patient tubed on the first attempt and noticed his pulse rate still dropping, at this point below fifty, not good. I looked at Jen who gave me the look we share in our non-verbal medical consultation. It only took a look and each knew exactly what the other was thinking. It was the kind of look that made me proud to be who I am and proud to be working with Jen. Our looks spoke novels.

When I explained exactly how I wanted another deckhand to breathe for our patient with the tube I just placed into his trachea, Jen performed a quick survey of the rest of his extremities and body to note any other injuries or signs. I reached behind me and grabbed a prefilled syringe of

Atropine and dropped one half milligram down his IV tubing, hoping it would adjust his rate. I flushed the tubing again by opening the titration device to the wide position, and then continued to package him on a backboard with a few other deckhands. His rate went up a notch, which I was unhappy with, so I dropped the remaining half-milligram of Atropine.

This brought his rate up to about eighty; a good enough number for us to work with. I explained concisely how we would get our patient, whose name was Clayton, upstairs quickly and safely. Jen and I both went over our backboard straps once each. This was not that we didn't trust each other, rather we knew the importance of this gentleman remaining on the backboard as he was about to be lifted vertically up stairwells. One wrong placement and he would take a header straight down, which is something we do not want. We also were never offended if we both rechecked something the other did. It was just our way of being comfortably thorough and we saw it as having each other's back.

The deckhands were great, and completely willing to help. They offered to do most of the lifting since they knew the corridors and we didn't. Each time we reached a landing Jen and I would recheck equipment and breath sounds to ensure the tube was still in place. It was extremely humid in these portions of the ship, which made it an even tougher challenge. As we began to reach the surface I tried the portable radio given to us by the chopper crew. The first two attempts failed, causing me to wonder if they left us out there. As we were about ten feet from the surface, I tried it again and received a response from Airman Griffin.

"We are directly above you, and will be dropping the hoist momentarily. The wind conditions are favorable, so this should go pretty smooth." Airman Griffin said with confidence.

My stomach issued a sigh of relief that they were still there and sounded so calm.

We made it to the mid-deck of the vessel as the grappling hook worked its way toward us. Our patient's vitals were looking good, and he seemed to respond well to treatment so far. Little did he know that he was about to be hoisted 100 feet in the air.

The hook swung in front of us several times before one of the deckhands caught it. We placed Clayton in the stokes stretcher, especially made for backboard rescues, and I bagged him a few times before they would hoist him. I instructed the hoist operator on the aircraft that after he secures the patient up there, he needs to begin bagging him right away, no

PARAMEDIC M.O.S.

exceptions – even if we have to wait a minute. Clayton went airborne and I just hoped nothing else happened until we were onboard the aircraft.

As Clayton lifted, Jen and I counted our equipment to make sure we had it, and shook hands with the crew of the vessel. The hook came down and was ready for Jen and I separately, as we were both still in our harnesses. I told Jen to go first and I would take the end run. I didn't want her stuck on this vessel by herself. She lifted off and in no time made it safely aboard the craft. I saw her look back down at me and move into the compartment.

Before the chopper returned the hoist, it seemed to jolt hard to the right, and then corrected its position. I felt my heart stop. The hoist came down and as I hooked on the Captain extended his hand again. I informed him that the U.S. Coast Guard will post him on the whereabouts of the patient once we get settled. With that, I was hoisted into mid air. I was so glad that it was summer out and that the seas were very calm. The rotors were pulling water up into my face, but I felt so invincible at the moment. It was an incredible feeling to be part of this entire rescue.

Once on board the craft, I moved over to Jennifer who was bagging Clayton. I reached for my headset so that we could all communicate.

"You okay," I asked Jen.

"I am not sure. He is stable, but this thing just shook really hard." Jen said with a look of absolute fear in her eyes.

"I saw that down below. Hold on," I said as I pointed to the pilot. "Griff what the hell was that before you hoisted me up?"

Without turning his head, he put the chopper in a slightly nose down position, rocketing us forward. The rotors picked up intensity as we took off.

"I don't know exactly, it wasn't normal but we should be fine to get back." Airman Griffin said as he turned a few knobs on his console. "Do me a favor, leave the shoulds back at your base and just get us back in one piece." I said as diplomatically as I could, not saying I was not up for crashing today.

While checking the EKG monitor, I placed the mike on my headset right next to my mouth, "Airborne 10X to Citywide K." A deep, male voice answered, "X-Ray, go."

"X-ray go," A deep male voice answered.

"X, we are currently 10-82 to Bellevue with a 40 year old male, status ep. Call telemetry and let them know we administered Valium due to patient condition and were unable to secure communications with them. We should be back in Manhattan in about ten minutes, please secure the LZ for us." I informed the Citywide dispatcher with a very calm voice.

Captain Lenny chimed in. "X-ray, no worries on the Valium, I had already spoken with Dr. Robinson and he cleared you for standing orders for your judgment given the circumstances." As Lenny was finishing up his sentence, I heard a pop followed by hissing.

"Griff, what the hell was that," I asked with absolute fear. Griff didn't answer and we seemed to be losing speed. I could have sworn I heard Griff start saying the recital of an "Our Father, who art in Heaven."

Jen looked at me and I turned around, slapping the pilot's helmet with the back of my hand.

"Hey, this is not the time for a fucking sermon, you just keep this thing airborne, you got me?" I said this firmly to Griff who began pushing buttons and turning knobs. I kept thinking to myself that Jen and I were about to become the unfortunate victims of a fiery helicopter crash. That was a thought that did not sit well at all.

"I got it, I got it," Griff said confidently. Our speed began to pick up.

I got back on my headset radio to speak with the Citywide Special Operations dispatcher again, "X-ray, priority message!"

The dispatcher didn't even wait for me to unkey my radio completely. "All units clear the Citywide channel, X-ray go!" Said Lenny.

"We have experienced mechanical problems with the heelo, not quite sure what is going on, we are about 7 minutes out of Manhattan I would guess, will get back to you in a moment." I made my words as clear as I could through my fear that we may not make it back.

As I was finishing my sentence, we appeared to be losing altitude, but at a controlled rate. Our speed stopped and we were in a vertical descent though I couldn't see where, since land was to the left and right of us but nowhere below us. I felt us touch down onto something as Jennifer grabbed my arm, digging her nails in. As I was about to ask where we were, the side door opened on the heelo and I realized that I was on a flight deck. About eight naval personnel greeted us and told us we would be switching choppers.

Putting two and two together, I realized that this was Fleet Week. The week where the USS John F. Kennedy and its support fleet sail into the Hudson for limited tours to the public. While I was calling Captain Lenny on my radio, Griff must have radioed the USS JFK for an immediate and emergency landing on the deck.

PARAMEDIC M.O.S.

As the rotors on our heelo began phasing down, Jen and I jumped out a bit startled. We brought Clayton off the heelo and placed him on an awaiting stretcher. I heard the sound of a heavy elevator behind me, and when I looked I saw a NAVY SH-60 Seahawk helicopter being brought up from down below. We were currently sailing into the Verrazano Narrows towards the Hudson, so we could essentially head right for Manhattan.

As we were getting prepped for the new chopper, I enjoyed the warm gentle breeze on the flight deck caused by the forward motion of the vessel. The naval personnel were great to us and one of the ships physicians met us on deck in case we needed any hands or assistance. The new heelo we would board was huge. It's engines started up as we were loading our patient onboard and I notified Captain Lenny that we were safe and of the changes.

We lifted off just a few minutes later as Jen gave me a look of relief. Our patient in the meantime began to seize again, so I reached for another five milligrams of Valium, which seemed to control the seizure.

We made it to the landing zone back at the East 34th Street Helipad, where it was lit up like a Christmas tree. Apparently after hearing of our situation, every available ambulance, support unit and senior ranking officer that was downtown showed up. We touched down to a sea of hands helping us off-load our patient. Jen and I were just happy to be on solid ground.

As I was stepping off of the Blackhawk, the pilot grabbed my arm and informed me that the issue with that previous chopper was a loose lug nut in the rotor. A few more revolutions and it might have separated from the craft altogether. That was a little too close for my tastes.

We transported the patient without further incident up to Bellevue, where another crew of hungry wolves was waiting for us. When Jen and I cleaned up from the assignment, I told her what the Seahawk pilot told me, and she just looked at me for a long moment. Jen put her hand in mine, "I am so glad that it was you up there with me. Thank you for maintaining your cool. Christian, that was way too close."

I looked at her with a smile, "I know, but we are always here for each other. You know that I would never let anything happen to you. You know that we will always come out of any situation we get into, no matter how deep or impossible."

Jen smiled a charming smile, "I know we will, I know. That is what makes me so happy to have you as my partner. You make life easy."

C.B. Garris

We worked ourselves into quasi-normal laughter knowing that we faced something pretty foul and potentially one of the deadliest situations of our lives. Having called telemetry to log the administration of narcotics, spoken to Lenny and one or two of my favorite dispatchers just say hello, Jen and I cleaned up to head in for the end of our tour. Arriving back at the station and not wanting to really discuss the close call we had too much, we picked up all of our equipment to turn it in for the night, hoping to miss the entourage of coworkers who wanted to hear all about it. It wasn't that we didn't want to share it, because we did want to in great detail. We needed a night to let the fear settle, at which time we would most likely tell the story for a week.

When we walked inside, Lt. Yobi greeted us. "Just another one of your exciting nights in the city for you two I hear." He said this with a smirk to end all smirks.

"Uh, yeah, you could say that. I think this one is going down in our history books." I said as I opened the cabinet for the Lifepak unit.

Jen handed me her radio and I turned both in to the charging unit on the wall behind the station Lieutenant.

"Are ya'll in for the change?" Lt. Yobi asked as he catalogued the return of our equipment. In for the change means have you completed your tour. As I reached for my radio, I smiled at Yobi.

"Tactical X, 10X-ray, IFTC - OTP (In for the Change-Overtime Personnel)." This means that we cannot be used again unless a Level-7 Emergency is declared citywide.

The dispatcher came back with, "Good night 10X, thanks for your help tonight." I re-keyed the radio, "No central, THANK YOU!"

PARAMEDIC M.O.S.

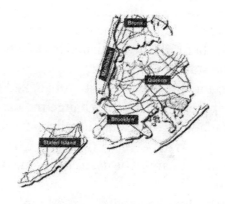

C.B. Garris

Chapter XI:

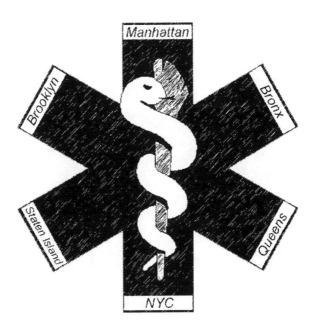

PARAMEDIC M.O.S.

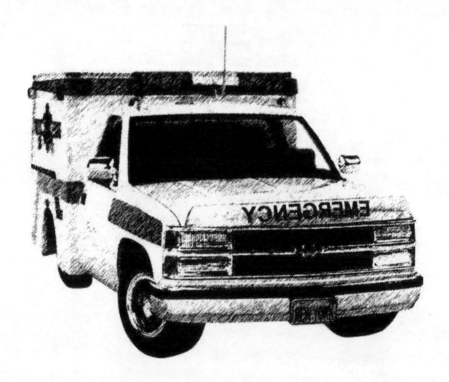

C.B. Garris

After signing in my narcs in the safe, I gave AMBU a long pet and walked upstairs. I told Jen that I was going to take a shower before I headed home to AJ's and she said she would wait downstairs. We always waited for each other when it came time to go home. It was just a habit we got into. If one of us was on the phone or taking care of paperwork, it didn't matter. We depended on each other every single day and night, and leaving the station before the other went home just didn't seem right. I always felt that if I let her drive off the grounds before me that she might get involved in some horrible car accident and die. I would be left blaming myself for years that I should have made her wait for me, and if I just gave her an extra long hug goodbye that she would have not been killed. It was a silent thing we developed over the seven years we knew each other and worked together.

We actually met at the academy and were in the same Paramedic class together. We ended up being assigned to the same station together and when our six-month probie time was up, we were assigned as regular partners. It was like going to your favorite party every day. We knew each other inside and out. We knew each other's habits, and how each other thought. I could not have ever had a better partner.

I was very fortunate to have her respect and care. Coming to work with Jennifer was like two kids at summer camp; we had an absolute ball. We watched out for each other in ways most never experience and we had an incredible bond. When Jen's apartment caught fire, I had her move into my place for four months until she got another place. Ours was a closeness built on mutual respect and care. When we met, aside from the fact that we worked together daily, we had both just exited really bad relationships; and knew that we were not ready for anything. Our friendship was everything. We had more fun together than I could ever remember in my past.

I peeked my head in the borough command to say goodnight to Erin, but it appeared that she was deeply involved in a phone conversation, so I let her be. I felt it was best to decontaminate myself by showering at the station before I even considered changing clothes. I would not think of leaving the station with all of the liquid pathogens from that last call all over me, and I was not going to go to AJ's like that. AJ, Jen and I were absolutely meticulous about our hygiene and presentation. We all felt exactly the same, that in order for a patient to trust us, they had to trust what they see since that will be the first judge for them.

PARAMEDIC M.O.S.

We knew our skills, but you have all of about ten seconds and eight words to gain a patient's trust, that is unless they are already unconscious when we arrive. In that case, we just assume that they will trust us. I finished showering and I was so glad that I kept all my bathroom stuff in my locker. Toothpaste, shaving gel, razors, towels, soap, shampoo, cologne, and of course, deck shoes (to avoid any fungal type stuff on the shower floors). Because our station was relatively new, we had a nice showering area with four large separated stalls.

Ready to go, I walked downstairs to an awaiting dog with a yellow ball in her mouth. AMBU must have heard my keys and footsteps. I would be off for three days now, and as I peeked in the office to say goodnight to the Tour 1 group, I let AMBU into the office. Tour 1 began at 22:00 or 10:00pm, and that crew was always shall we say, eclectic.

Lieutenant Alan Yobi looked at me as I walked in the door. "I gots overtime if you want, last minute vacancy?" I smiled quickly and said, "Sorry dude, I got somewhere I have to be!"

He gave me a nod and said, "So I guess I shouldn't bother paging you for OT over the next few days."

I picked the pager off of my belt and said, "Only page me if there is a citywide activation, but thanks for thinking of me." I let the steel door close behind me with a loud thud.

I put AJ's tape in my cassette player, and was immediately warmed to the sounds of *Sweet Love* by Anita Baker. I hopped on the FDR and began maneuvering the curves caused by the ongoing construction. This construction started years ago, and spans from 18th Street all the way to 96th Street. On a good day with little traffic, it reminds me of the races at Monaco. It was now just a little after 23:00 as I cruised past the United Nations. The city and the skyline were always beautiful on a warm summer night.

A little further up and off to my right would be the Tram to Roosevelt Island and the home of our employee health services at Goldwater Memorial Hospital. As I approached the exit to the 3rd Avenue Bridge that would take me into the Bronx, I was now listening to Michael Franks performing his song *Crayon Sun*. AJ and I picked up that CD titled *Blue Pacific* while we were in St. Thomas six months ago. It was amazing to sit on the beach, baking away and holding her hand.

There was something about AJ's touch that could stop a bullet train. When AJ reaches for my hand, it is as if my entire body is massaged. I drove past Yankee Stadium and saw the notice that they were playing the following night on the banner. I crossed the City line heading for the Hutchinson River Parkway, into Westchester. This meant that I had only about another 15 minutes to her home in New Rochelle. I passed through the Fleetwood section of Mount Vernon while little traffic followed. I exited off the Parkway at Exit 10, into the heart of a quaint section of Eastchester. I decided to get off there, as it made me reminisce about a great restaurant that used to be at the base of the exit called Sagano. This was a Teppan-style restaurant that I was introduced too as a child. It was where I established my love for Teriyaki.

I hooked a right and passed a great bakery and deli on the corner. You will not find better baked goods anywhere in Westchester than at that corner bakery. Just a few turns from there would lead me to a straightaway towards North Avenue. I pulled a right onto North Avenue, and then a quick left up the hill across from the Fire Station onto Route 125. A few blocks in and I was there.

AJ lived in a very nice home amongst a very upper middle class section of the city. After her parents died in the car accident, her uncle and aunt assumed custody of her. When she reached the age of twenty-three she was told that her parents left her a whopping amount of money. It was apparently very hard for AJ when the attorneys notified her, since it dredged up the past and brought on a wave of emotions that she thought she put behind her. AJ was smart about her parents' gift and bought a beautiful home, and then toured Europe for about six months after she graduated from college.

As I made the right into AJ's house I saw a few lights on upstairs. I exited my truck and walked up the lighted path to her front door. She owned this great three-bedroom home that she personally decorated and also worked with a few people to get the house just right. As I put my key in the door she opened it. At that exact moment, all time stopped. She was in a peach satin robe that covered all the way to her upper thighs in the front and covering just below her butt in the rear, exhibiting her fabulous legs. The peach color complimented her caramel complexion incredibly.

She had her hair wrapped up in a white terry-cloth towel and her skin glowed from the porch light. She had a gleaming smile that always welcomed me home.

There was clarity of purpose from her that never ceased to amaze me. "Hi," she said, almost bouncing in place like a kid in a sand box. When she welcomed me home it made me feel like I would never know what the

PARAMEDIC M.O.S.

word pain was. As I stepped in, she stepped forward and we locked on each other's eyes as we went for a kiss.

Her lips were unlike anything I ever knew. We made our kisses last hours. I remember the first night I cooked dinner for her in her professional kitchen. I was putting the final touches on the warm apple tart with homemade cinnamon ice cream dessert portion of the meal, when I couldn't stand it anymore. She was standing next to me, freshly showered and smelling incredibly fragrant. Just the sight and scent of her made me roll my eyes into the back of my head. Somehow while she laughed at one of my stories of the street, we ended up in a position facing each other.

Our eyes locked and I told myself it was time. I placed my hands around the small of her back, and her smile said to me that she knew that this was it too. As we closed in to lock our lips, what probably took a matter of seconds seemed like it took twenty minutes in slow motion. The feeling was so warm, tingly and encompassing. Our bodies sank into one another and when we finished that first kiss, it was two and a half hours later.

Any hunger we had prior to the preparation of the meal was completely fed by affection. When we realized it was so many hours later, we laughed for quite awhile. We did eventually eat that evening, and that was followed by an incredible night of affection. We have missed entire movies and documentaries as a result of our extended kisses. Our affections were like marathons that didn't end.

As I stood there appreciating her gentle body in the doorway, we kissed and she gently clenched on my lower lip with her teeth to lock me. Her lips were soft like the satin cloth she was wearing, and her body was gentle and inviting. AJ touched my face gently with her fingers as we kissed. I dropped my knapsack and placed my hands behind the small of her back, pulling her into me. About thirty minutes later, when we decided to take a break for some Gatorade and for me to actually step all the way into the house, we disengaged and she smiled at me.

There was no possession or claims to be made here; we were just very lucky to have established what most never experienced in a lifetime. I noticed that she had a Luther Vandross CD playing throughout the house. "How was your night?" She asked as she led me to the couch. I sat down as she mounted me, curling her legs under my thighs, still smiling. "It was a bit crazy. I assume you heard about the bank robbery in the M3?"

She said gently in my ear, "Thank you for the flowers," as I thanked her for mine. Focusing on my eyes, AJ brought her face closer to mine and rubbed her nose against mine gently in between kisses. AJ is the epitome of sensuality wrapped up in adorability. It all comes from her heart, a place that few ever connect too within themselves. I was having a difficult time with my current track of thought. Each time I went to speak and she acknowledged me, she would do so with a mischievous smile and another kiss.

After an intense hug she said to me, "I had a feeling you were on that one. I called Lenny, your buddy - Tour Commander extraordinaire to let me know that you were okay."

Knowing that I was a part of this network of people who I cared for and who really cared for and watched out for me made me smile internally.

"I hope that you don't mind that I got people out there watching out for you?" she remarked.

"AJ, I don't mind at all. You also know that I have eyes out there for you too."

She smiled and laid her full lips upon mine again "I know, that's only one of the many things that I love about you."

As AJ let her hair out of its towel, the CD in the player looped onto James Taylor's *Walking Man*. This girl was sexy au natural, and being held by AJ was warmer than a thousand suns.

I told her about the train incident and Jen's incident with the MTA rep, which had her laughing hysterically. AJ always loved how I told stories from the street calls we had. I told her I wanted to take another shower and she took me by the hand to the bathroom. AJ had her bathroom custom made and it was a fabulous set up. It was done in soft gray and tan marble, and had the his/hers sinks with a huge mirror, then she put in a bear claw shaped, spa whirlpool bath; certainly big enough for two. To top this off and my favorite, a large, glass enclosed waterfall shower with a built in steam unit and area for sitting, and a generously sized fireplace. The spa bath was always set up with scented candles and flowers. Tonight's flowers were the orchids that I sent for her. The aromatic candles were Pomegranate from Illuminations.

The steam/waterfall shower was huge, approximately 10 X 8. It had a waterfall where the showerhead is usually, and two shower heads on the sides so that you were immersed in water. The encased area had an area where two could sit and enjoy the steam generating at your feet. The ceil-

PARAMEDIC M.O.S.

ing had protected speakers built in. The CD now up was Herbie Hancock's *Maiden Voyage*. The CD that followed was Linda Ronstadts' *Skylark*.

While taking off my sneakers, AJ leaped on me, bringing with her an intense kiss.

She began taking off my shirt, "Would you like some company in that shower?"

I smiled under the kiss and said "Of course, but only if you let me brush your hair when we get out."

She disengaged the kiss with a smile and sneered a look at me, "I thought you would never ask."

As I slipped out of my clothing she stood about three feet from me and dropped her robe.

"WHOA!" I said to myself.

By the time I finished picking my jaw up off the floor, she walked slowly towards the bathroom, slipping one leg out "I think a bath will be in order first."

I stood up and made for the bathroom saying, "Works for me, besides, I get to be your loofah."

She ran a bath as I took out the spa treatment for the water, tonight's was a lavender/cucumber milk bath. I picked this up for her while we shopped a few months ago. Now I just have spa materials delivered on a monthly basis from her favorite spa in Los Angeles. Gotta take care of this woman, she is a keeper! She set the whirlpool on low and we both descended into the immense amount of bubbles together. The spa was all marble, and designed with several incremental levels. AJ rested her body next to mine, her head upon my chest. As we lay there in silence, I heard the beginning's of Pat Metheny's *Hermitage*.

As the room was skillfully and gently acousticized by Pats' guitar, we laid there in complete peace. There were no lights or sirens, no heavy weapons fire, no trains being lifted. There was just AJ and I. Somehow we managed to create something so different than either of us had ever experienced. She opened emotional doors to and for me that I never felt comfortable walking through before. It was as if someone appeared one night and pulled her out of my dreams. AJ didn't hesitate to speak her mind, but she did so without attacking me. Our appreciation of being in each others' lives was evident with each kiss, and in the gentle way we dealt with another. We could perform the tasks that our job called for, come home in one piece, and curl up together or take on the town.

I had never known what it was like to truly have someone who appreciated me before. My last relationship was with this female who was totally incapable of maintaining intimacy or trust. In fact I think the words will never be a part of her vocabulary. My fault in that was that I truly cared and wanted to make everything right. Some called her damaged goods. It took me years and a butt load of great counseling to get passed that, but I am better for it and without her. When I told AJ the story surrounding that situation from years past, I thought AJ was going to track this girl down.

Rather she just looked at me like she did as she reminded me tonight by saying, "It is obvious to me that you were severely hurt before, and by someone who didn't deserve an ounce of your time. She is probably one of those women who will bitch and moan about why she doesn't have a great guy who loves her and looks after her, while she is slamming down a beer with false friends. I have known since the first night we met how wonderful you are. Even if you hadn't jumped in and saved me from that piece of shit Eddie, I was immediately drawn to you. I do not normally cry in front of strangers, but it was the way you approached me and took the time. It seemed more automatic to be myself with you. Most guys just try to get into my pants, and none would have stepped in the way you did. Frankly, just by the way you calculated everything that happened that first night and how you leaped on Eddie, made me want to take you home with me and bang you silly. I also know that was the psycho-physiological and chemical combination of being saved by you and my attraction to you. I knew that if I had asked you out that night that you would have said no. You are so righteous."

AJ shifted her body so that she was now sitting on my lap rubbing my neck and shoulders. "You would have wanted to wait a few days so that I didn't get lost in my happiness of having an angel to come along and save me. I probably could have gotten Eddie off of me myself, but it was how you predicted the whole thing and how you were there in the nick of time; you cared for my safety. I didn't want to say it at the time but I was so glad that Chief Battieri decided to move me to Station 11 and pair me with you. I remember how she and I met about it before she made it official. She asked if I had any objections, and of course I said none. In fact I told her about how you stepped in when Eddie was fouling up patient care and how not only helped me do what I had to do, but you took the

PARAMEDIC M.O.S.

time to explain it. I told her you were extremely thorough and she smiled from ear to ear."

She said to me, "I have had a lot of people in my command, but none measure up to Christian. He is rational, caring, kind, completely professional and he treats his patients and co-workers like family. It is like he has this innate way of making you feel acknowledged and respected, and once you experience him you realize that he has a gift. I have seen good medics and bad ones. Then Christian was assigned to my command and there was something just different about him. I have never had a more conscientiously pragmatic individual under my command. If I had a hundred Christians, my job would be a breeze. Then we sat there in silence, almost like we were honoring you; it was very strange. I felt that she and I bonded in some way that morning too." She gave me a big kiss and then continued.

"I also knew by the way you treated me that you respected me completely and that you would not even think of dating until after my training was over. You truly did want to see if I had the right stuff."

AJ stopped long enough to allow me the chance to engage her lips again; this time I clenched for the lock. "And you do things to my body that I still can't describe."

I smiled, "You know if you are trying to build my ego, it's working." I paused for a moment in deep thought.

"I remember first seeing you," I continued, "I had to do everything to keep my composure. I didn't want to make you uncomfortable; but I could not keep my eyes off of you. There was this gentleness about you. I didn't know that I would be so lucky when I got the phone call from Davia informing me that I was being assigned to the detail as your training medic. I knew that she felt you might be more comfortable with me after what happened, and that with the two of us joined at the hip, you would not get any flack from anyone or there would be hell to pay. I was incredibly attracted to you, but the job is the job and I was not going to let anyone step in the way of you doing yours. I was also not going to be a part of the problem. Before you, it was my experience to have bad relationships. Before you I was always the sucker, always getting jammed up with some wacko. Being the caring types, we have to look real hard and be very cautious, as you already know."

We kissed and I continued, "Just how you listen to me when I want to talk, or how I have never allowed someone to protect me or just look out for me like you do. I enjoy how we can sit together quietly reading books, just touching hands and feet, and that is a world within itself. I love your laugh and how simple things are with us. You don't criticize me or chastise me for something I am not skilled in or have to get help on. You create a space in our relationship where I am accepted and it is okay to be me without hassle. I love how you let me shampoo your hair and brush it for you, as I will later. I must say that as you mentioned about what I do to your body, what you do to mine defies explanation. I love when you fall asleep to one of my massages or in my arms; that is the greatest compliment. I love shopping with you and watching you work a department store. I love how we secretly plan get away trips with another for each other."

AJ sat there motionless, as if held captive by my words. She took her head back and gave me this eye-squinting look, but it was more than that – it was intense and deep. She let her hair fall all around me as she kissed me deeply. We stayed suspended there for a few minutes and then turned the whirlpool up to medium. The froth from the milk bath was all around and the lavender and cucumber smelled great. We soon exited and stepped into the steam shower, sitting on the limestone seat. I admired her body as she reached over and ran her hand over my chest.

"So lover boy, I thought we would take these next three days and go up to a Bed and Breakfast in Burlington, Vermont."

I smiled and said, "Is that why you packed our bags before I got here?"

AJ began to laugh that joyous giggle that melts me every time, "Sure did. I didn't think you'd mind," she said in a very sexy fashion as she zeroed in for a kiss.

We rinsed off and stepped out of the shower. I heard a familiar cut from Sade's CD *Promise* now playing in the speakers above me. AJ had this way of wrapping herself in a towel that made me want to jump her every time. Her body was covered, yet her cleavage & butt were perfectly accented by the towel. Perhaps it was the way she carried herself that was so utterly sexy. She stepped into the bedroom as I brushed my teeth and shaved. While rinsing the foam out of my mouth I looked in the mirror and saw a leg creep into view. A brush followed the leg, tapping lightly against the wall to get my attention. AJ stuck her head in and said, "The sooner you finish my hair and the sooner you can have me." I spit out the foam and water, dropped my brush and made for my towel in one swift move.

AJ's bed was king size, done in either Oak or Maple, with posts that extended upward on a curve. She also had flowing drapes over the bed.

PARAMEDIC M.O.S.

AJ turned over on her stomach, so that I could begin her pampering with a long massage. I ordered this great citrus massage oil from her spa in Los Angeles when I was ordering her bath products, and tonight seemed like a great night to start using it.

When I was finished with her massage, it was time to work on AJ's hair. I sat back on the bed against the pillows as she was now back in her satin robe. She sat in front of me, resting her back against me as I reached for the brush. I began brushing, 100 strokes, fifty in front and fifty in back.

"I love how you are to me," AJ said to me softly.

I smiled and said, "Well I love being the person who is the focus of your affections. You are after all the smartest, sexiest and most insatiable woman I have ever known."

AJ said, "Okay that's it, now your mine!" AJ sat up, turned around and took off her robe, threw away my towel, and turned out the light.

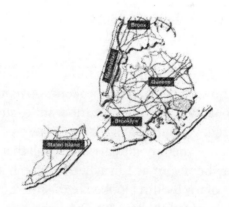

C.B. Garris

Chapter XII:

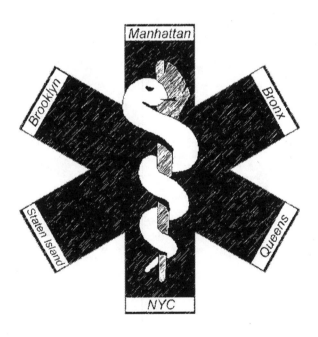

PARAMEDIC M.O.S.

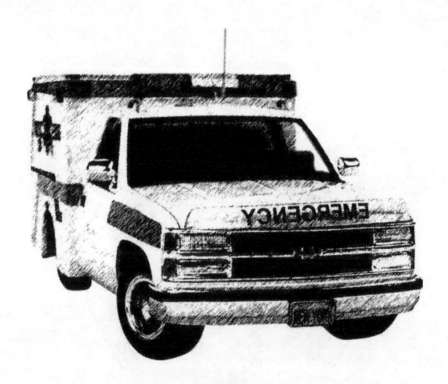

C.B. Garris

Our trip to Vermont was fabulous. Then again, going anywhere with AJ was a blast. She drove this trip, and although I like being in my truck high up off the ground, I was perfectly comfortable napping on the passenger side of her Mercedes. She had a great sound system in this thing and it drove beautifully; or perhaps it was the way she drove it. We drove very similarly, and I was always comfortable with her at the wheel. She decided to drive so I could relax after the week I had, and acrobatics that we put our bodies through the night prior. I offered to drive, but she mentioned something about that she wanted to ensure that I was well rested for round two.

The drive would take about six hours, so we stopped at the IHOP in Larchmont not far from her home. That way we could double back to Webster Avenue through Larchmont past the golf driving range, over towards the Hutchison River Parkway to get to the Merritt Parkway. We would take the Merritt up towards Hartford, and then pick up I-91 towards I-89. This was the scenic route through Connecticut and Massachusetts.

We would pass through Western Massachusetts, zipping by Springfield, stopping in Northampton before we trekked onto Vermont. This area is particularly beautiful and home to the Five-college area: Smith, Amherst, Hampshire, U-Mass @ Amherst, and Holyoke (a place that when I was a kid I pronounced "Ho-wee-oke"). We stopped on Main Street, at a great place called Elio's. An old friend of mine from culinary school happened to head the kitchen as the executive chef. I knew this area well as I went to culinary school in New England some years ago on educational leave from the service. I used to come down to this area every once in awhile. It is always great to go to a place where you know the chef.

AJ had a portabella mushroom sandwich on foccacia, with bean sprouts, avocado, and a great aged chevre (goat cheese). She skipped on the chips it came with and asked for cottage cheese on the side. I had the Copper River salmon sandwich with cucumber, a roasted red pepper hummus spread with shavings of Asiago cheese. We both decided on water; Pellegrino flat. AJ and I knew how to eat. We finished off lunch with a platter of homemade sorbets for two. Today's flavors were passion fruit, blood orange, pear and pineapple.

There was something passionate about the way AJ and I were together. When AJ got up to use the ladies room, the female part of a couple sitting next to us leaned over to me and said, "Is this your first date?"

I smiled softly and said, "Why do you ask?"

PARAMEDIC M.O.S.

She gave me that ATTA-Boy look and said, "You two cannot take your eyes off of each other and you are adorable together. You are just too sweet to each other."

I looked at her, then her counterpart and judging by the matching wedding bands, I was hoping they were married to each other.

He was ducking into his seat with a look in his eyes that said, "Why does she have too do this when we go out?"

I thanked her for her observation and informed her that we have been involved for a while and that I am the luckiest guy in the world. She smiled and said to me, "From where I am sitting, I think that she is lucky too."

As complimentary as that was, I was unsure how the hubby took that compliment, and I wondered if I was going to have to defend myself before the check came. AJ reappeared and even from across the room was able to grab my complete attention. When AJ looks at you, you listen. While we were waiting for our check, the aforementioned lady and hubby exited.

On her way out she leaned over to AJ and said, "I just want you to know that I had asked your friend here about the two of you, and he said he is the luckiest guy in the world."

AJ looked at me with her mischievous look and I could see her heart smile. I also knew that it was time for AJ to make a comment that would probably be questionable by some social standards.

She looked at the lady and said, "Thank you. Just so you know, he is not just my friend; he is my man and the only one that I would ever recommend. Unfortunately, he is signed to my camp and not a free agent. If you want to discuss lucky, perhaps I should share with you all the wonderful things he did to me last night."

AJ made these statements with a straight face and the most innocent smile you could ever imagine. I didn't know if the lady was going to choke on the mint that was left with her bill or ask me for my number.

The hubby just smiled and gave me this "YOU ARE DA MAN!" nod while raising his eyebrows. The lady said goodbye in absolute confusion. As they walked away AJ reached her hand out to mine, caressing it.

With a satiating sneer in her look she asked me, "So friend," her touch on my hand grew firmer, "would you like to hit the road so that we can perfect our frequent friendly extracurricular endeavors?"

I looked up in the direction of our wait staff person and said loudly, "CHECK PLEASE!"

AJ giggled gently. We continued our trip until we reached Vermont. We settled in that day with a walk in the woods near the Bed & Breakfast. We found this great Italian restaurant on Church Street in downtown Burlington. It was quiet and comfortably cozy.

After a sumptuous meal, we retreated to our lodging, repeating the events of the night before, this time we skipped the shower and hair brushing. The following days were spent canoeing on the lake facing the Adirondack Mountain range of northern New York State. I brought my guitar out with me and sang her favorite James Taylor songs. We even drove a few exits down I-89 and snuck in a day at Ben & Jerry's main production plant to watch all those famous concoctions get created.

Sometimes I was scared, not of AJ though. I was more fearful that something was going to come take her away from me. I was not concerned about her being interested in someone else, because I understood and trusted everything we had. I think it is a facet of working in such a violent profession, that I take the situation I have responded too and replace the face of the patient from some horrible traumatic incident, with the face of someone I love and care for.

I think those feelings would plague me forever; so my fear of losing AJ was to death itself. I think inherently she knew that from our long talks, and she always tried to make it better for me. I never took my fear out on her, but she knew that I worried more than most. She was reassigned to the academy on her first day back, as it was time for her re-certification upgrade class. This is something that all medics in the service are recalled back home once every three years. It lasts six weeks, and you return to your station and tour once completed. I haven't met one person yet who made it through the academy that failed refresher. That was comforting.

When AJ woke up at 4:00 am to get ready for the academy, I really wished she could have stayed. The comfort and warmth of cuddling with her always made me lose track of my thoughts. As I turned off the alarm, she stretched her arms around me and hugged me.

"You are the best snuggling partner." She said while my entire body smiled at her commentary.

"At your service." I said in return.

A gentle kiss and it was off to the shower for her. I wasn't due in until 15:00, so I stayed put. She came out of the shower and dressed. I sat up in the soft light admiring her. She stopped what she was doing and leaped on the bed kissing me. Her hair was wet still and smelled fragrant.

PARAMEDIC M.O.S.

"I would like it if you came back tonight." She said as cool drops of water fell from her hair onto my chest.

"I ain't no fool! I will see you after work."

I pulled her in for a kiss that she was already heading in to receive.

"I knew I could count on you," she said as she sat up to finish dressing.

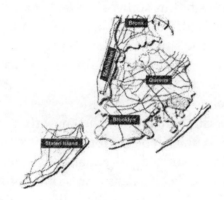

C.B. Garris

Chapter XIII:

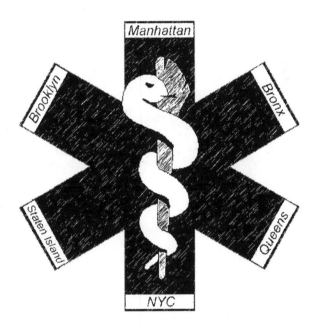

PARAMEDIC M.O.S.

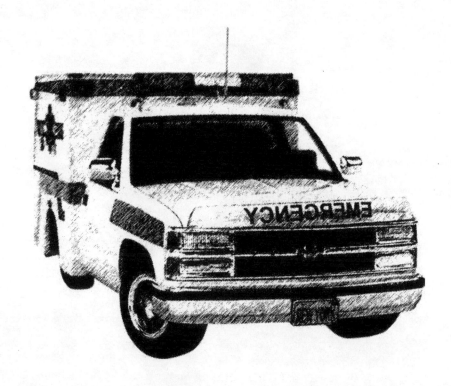

C.B. Garris

I awoke at 10:00am and made my usual breakfast. I picked up the New York Times from outside AJ's front door and caught up on news from the last few days. When I finished the Metropolitan section, I closed the paper and cut the lawn. It was now about 12:15 and time to get ready for work. I showered, shaved, threw on one of my white department t-shirts that said "NYC EMS-The Heartbeat of the City" in green and orange, jeans and a new pair of Nike's with a blue swoosh. I grabbed two Gatorades out of the fridge and hit the highway.

I arrived at the station around 14:00 and the place looked like a zoo. Fortunately, Mike Denieo beat me to the station to walk AMBU. In fact as I walked out of the office after checking in, she came running towards me. I grabbed the treats from my back pocket. As I made my way upstairs my alphanumeric pager went off. I was hoping it was AJ. I was lucky, it was. She was letting me know that she was heading home and to be careful out there tonight. I walked down for roll call ready to go. Keith Ribort was our Lieutenant for the day. It seems John's wife went into labor a tad bit early, so he wouldn't be coming in today.

I was working with Deklund McDonough today. He was a relatively new medic who they were a little unsure of. He is a hell of a nice guy, but he is lacking the aggressiveness that his patient care skills demand in the street. They asked if I would take him out to break him in and find out what the trouble was. He grew up in Oyster Bay, Long Island, and visited the city on school field trips when he was a youngster. This youngster was now 33 years old and about to have his ass kicked by the street and everyone in it if he didn't get with the program.

The streets are a difficult place. There are people of all denominations cohabitating in condensed areas, with all kinds of problems and issues. You have families, kids, lovers, loners, ex-cons, psychopathic predators, people with weapons, victims, and a host of different species. Our job was to keep them alive, no matter what horrible condition their bodies are in and no matter what mind-boggling trauma will be inflicted by or to them. Generally the people we get out here are great, but the city in a crisis situation can be a very intimidating thing. I had actually met Deklund weeks ago. He is always presentable, kind, and I can see it in his eyes that he has the stuff; he was just frightened.

Roll call was cancelled due to heavy call volume which means that we had no time to check our unit. I hoped that tour two restocked the vehicle. It was rare that you couldn't trust the previous tour, but every

PARAMEDIC M.O.S.

once in awhile someone gets scatter-brained. That isn't much of a big deal unless they forget something important: Lifepak batteries, refilling the drug box or replacing oxygen tanks. My bus was known as a floating restock vehicle. I found a way to triple up on just about everything, except for Lifepak Cardiac monitors since they cost about $10,000.00. I could only hide one extra in the truck. One of my tour two crews once sent me back out in the street with a broken one. Our agency Quartermaster's unit (supply division) knew I had the second one and why.

My bus was one that might get called into service if the President, Vice President or other dignitary came into the confines of New York City at the last minute, so we had to have a floating hospital ready. There were only thirty protection medics in an agency of 4000 strong, so we were on twenty-four hour call for that duty. Marcus the dispatcher was able to squeeze enough units around to give us ten minutes to go through our vehicle.

Somehow we slipped by the units that were being called into action, as a lull fell upon lower Manhattan. I decided to let Deklund drive for a number of reasons: one, it will immediately instill some confidence in him that someone believes in him, and it also gives me the chance to see how well he handles an ambulance on city streets. Lastly and if all else fails, it is one less time that I will have to answer to Internal Affairs as to why we drove right through one of those storefronts.

I was monitoring the NYPD Special Operations Frequency as we pulled onto South Street, and heard ESU Truck 1 get a call for a jumper up at the intersection of Pearl and Wall Streets. A "jumper up" is a person who is either threatening to jump or in position to leap, but has not yet decided to test the laws of gravity.

I picked up Deklund's EMS 800 MHZ which was resting on the center console and said to our dispatcher, "10X, Tactical X-ray, you got anything for a "jumper up" at Pearl and Wall?

A brief pause occurred and then Julie our dispatcher came back with, "X-Ray, 10-4, I just got it on my screen. I'll put you on it if you want it."

I hit the switches for our emergency lights and while popping the siren through traffic said, "X-Ray, 10-4, we are just coming out of eleven, you can show us in the wind (enroute)."

A few seconds later as we shot through the traffic light at Allen and South Street, our on-board MDT beeped twice with the call information. The call was categorized as a JUMPERUP, and since Julie entered a command into the CAD system on her dispatch console, my screen already showed us 10-63, so that I didn't have to depress the keyboard. NYPD ESU Truck 1, Truck 3 and R.E.P. (Radio ESU Patrol) Boy 1 hopped the call from 1 Police Plaza directly behind the intersection we just passed through. The ESU Trucks carry all of the rappelling gear if that is needed to gain access to the Wright brother's enthusiasts who attempt to jump and failing that, they also carry the inflatable rescue bags.

Since New York City is a city of endless skyscrapers, the fact that these bags are good until about 9 stories leaves a lot to be desired. But there is only so much protection that science and technology can provide against terminal velocity.

I told Deklund to take South Street past the firehouse. Just as he made a right, the NYPD Special Operations frequency now reported that the person may have jumped from the thirty-fifth floor. Pearl and Wall Streets are the heart of the financial district. All of the big and small brokerage houses are here; the main trading facility for the Stock Exchanges is here. We shot up to Water Street and then hooked a quick right onto Pearl Street, going the wrong way in traffic.

Deklund was frightened because he thought that he would get into trouble for doing this. Obviously Deklund and I needed to work together more often. We are emergency vehicles and we have carte blanche to do what we must for the betterment of the citizens. ESU Truck 1 pulled up from the opposite side of Pearl Street that we did, and we knew that this guy did jump due to the size of the crowd staring at the ground. There was a massive crowd in the street and on the sidewalk, and judging by the vomiting exercises in session, I knew this guy had to be dead if he did come from the 35th floor.

I leaped out of the truck telling Deklund to grab the trauma bag, airway kit and to just follow my lead. I started entering the crowd of suits and dresses firmly asking them to move to let us in.

Since that didn't seem to work I had to resort to language I preferred not to use in uniform, "You, get the fuck out of the way now!"

I did this while just pushing my way through the crowd, NYPD in tow. As I made access to the jumper, some guy in the crowd made a comment that my words were very unprofessional for a city employee. He was quickly issued a summons by the NYPD to appear in court for obstructing a governmental employee; and he also got his ass chewed out.

The jumper was about forty years old, in a very nice Brooks Brother's suit, which was now splattered with blood and bone fragments. He was

PARAMEDIC M.O.S.

very, very dead. He landed almost perfectly in the gutter – face down. As I adjusted my eyes from the sunlight that peeked through the area, I noticed that any attempts to save him would be futile. As I looked at his head I noticed that one thing was missing, his brain. He had a gaping hole in his temporal lobe, to the right just above his eyes.

Deklund came along side of me and said, "What's up?"

I looked at Deklund and said " Dude, just go grab a sheet, this guy's an eighty-three (our code for a DOA)."

I saw the look of disappointment in Deklund's eyes, as he wanted to work this guy, but he also realized that there was nothing else we could do. Further physical examination proved that his body was like jelly, and it appeared that he broke every bone in his body on impact. We found only broken segments of bones, some comminuted (closed fracture), and the rest compound (open fracture). A piece of his spine was sticking up out of the back of his suit.

We also had a BLS respond on this with us, and because the body was in public view, the BLS unit would end up removing the DOA to the morgue at Bellevue. Within the confines of New York City, if a body is inside an apartment or out of public view, it is the property of the Medical Examiner's Office, otherwise one of our units has to body bag it and take the body in after it has received its 95-tag, which is a paperwork for a DOA from the NYPD.

I tried to shield the body as best I could from the sight of others, but there were just too many people. It was obvious that several people knew this gentleman, as they were crying out a name that matched the identification NYPD found in the gentleman's wallet.

Deklund reappeared with a large white sheet, which we gently placed over the body while NYPD yellow taped a section of area including several cars right next to where he impacted. Before the body could be removed, we did have to await the Medical Examiners Office to send a pathologist to confirm everything. This is just a city protocol, kind of like red tape.

As the BLS watched over the body, Deklund and I corralled the friends of the victim. All three of the friends, two men and a female; were in business attire. All three were crying and trying to make sense of this. I had tried to console them as best I could, but it is difficult to console someone when the body that just went thirty-five floors or more is blood splattered in front of them. As we questioned them I noticed that the blood and various fluids were staining through the sheet. I told Deklund to take them behind our vehicle out of sight of the body while I went to retrieve another sheet to place on top of the original sheet.

I was trying to delay any more fluid leakage until the medical examiners arrival. I asked the co-workers if they had noticed any unusual behavior from the victim. I also asked if they knew of any enemies of the victim. While we talked and calmed them down, Detectives from the precinct arrived. I signaled to one that I knew, Andrew Billingsworth. He walked over and as we shook hands, I informed him of what we found when we arrived, and the fact that the brain was missing from the guy's head. While his partner looked under the sheets, I also informed him that we have three friends of the victim that he and his partner might like to speak to, as well as everything they told me. He thanked me and went on to interview the friends.

Deklund and I went back to the rig and started to do paperwork on the call, when a call came over for an address on Wall Street, almost adjacent to where we were sitting. Julie put the call out to 12X3 as an unconscious female. With all the confusion created by this particular call, she didn't realize that we were practically on top of the call, so I told her to cancel 12X3 since our patient was going to be a 10-83 left in the custody of 11(H)enry3, and we would go check out the unconscious.

We stepped back out of the vehicle and grabbed everything we would need for an unconscious victim, Airway bag, Lifepak Cardiac Monitor, Drug Kit, suction. Since the building had a working elevator, we brought the stretcher too. We entered into the building and approached the elevators, heading for the 15th floor.

An anxious female was waiting for us as we stepped out of the elevators. She mentioned that she had just called 911 back to see how long it would take us, and she then gracefully apologized for being impatient, as emergencies were not her forte. This female, a very attractive woman in her 50's was extremely professional and thankful towards our arrival. She introduced herself as Amy and said that our patient's name was Seema.

When we walked into the office, Seema was lying on the floor, being propped up and held up in the arms of a male counterpart. She was conscious but appeared woozy. Seema was about 27 years old, and appeared moderately overweight, but otherwise she looked healthy. She had no obvious skin disorders or discolorations (bruises, etc.); with her arms exposed I didn't see any track marks and her nostrils were not flared. She was well manicured and was wearing a nice perfume. The perfume didn't

PARAMEDIC M.O.S.

go well with the small waste can of vomit next to her though. I asked what happened and she was not speaking much at all. If I wasn't mistaken, she seemed upset.

I nodded to Deklund to put her on some oxygen while I sort the rest out. Her vitals were normal, as was her EKG. I looked around the room and searched for medication bottles, drug paraphernalia (scales, straws, rolled up dollar bills, needles, pipes, etc.) but found nothing. She seemed a tad bit altered in her mental status; and since no one had much information on her, I was going to go with the failsafe Altered Mental Status protocol. This consists of Narcan (generally known as Naloxone) which reverses the effects of most opiate based materials; Glucagon (an intense dose of sugar in case she is suffering from an acute lack of sugar (otherwise known as hypoglycemia, and finally Thiamine (a B vitamin). As I began opening the catheter I was going to use to initiate an IV on Seema with, she sat up, looked out the window and syncopized (passed out) in front of me.

I looked at her and the direction in which she looked when she sat up. There was a window there. I told Deklund to watch her for a second while I stood up. I walked over to the window and noticed there was an air conditioner attached to it on the outside. As I looked down I figured out what all this was about. Fifteen floors below this window was the perfect viewing point for a lot of emergency vehicles and one very large white sheet. As I focused in on the air conditioner, I figured out what made this all worse for Seema.

Perfectly perched on the air conditioner, minus a small chunk was the brain of our John Doe we left on the street. Grey and with a little blood and clear fluid all over it, the brain came to rest here. Considering that the air conditioner had a massive dent in it, we figured that on his way down from floor thirty five, John Doe slammed his head into the air conditioner with such force that his brain separated from his spinal cord and popped out of his skull. As I walked back over Seema and Deklund, I asked Deklund to give me his portable.

I called 11(H)enry3, "Paulie, have the Detectives meet us inside 2856 Pearl Street, Suite # 1524, and give them a red bio-hazard bag to bring with them. We found that missing item."

Paulie came back with a comical reply, "You're joking right?"

I informed him that I was quite serious.

We removed Seema from that office and talked to her for a while. It turns out that she was at the fax machine in her office, peeking out the window when John Doe slammed head first into the air conditioner. She thought that his body did a somersault on impact, but then she couldn't remember much after that moment.

When the Detectives arrived they told us that they found a suicide note on the guy's desk; but they were still leaving open the option that this might have been a homicide. I was able to talk Seema into letting us transport her to a hospital of her choice to be evaluated for emotional trauma. She wanted to go to St. Vincent's, and I told her that would be perfectly fine.

Now that we knew what caused her syncopy, and since she had no prior medical history or additional present symptoms, there was no need for anything more than oxygen and to transport. She was a very sweet person, and it sounded like she had led a very sheltered life up until now. Educated at Oxford, she moved to New York City a year ago for her new position. She has a double doctorate in business administration and investment banking; that just sounded painful. We wheeled her into Vinny's and helped her get settled in a quiet room.

Janice the charge nurse approached me with a clipboard saying, "Hey sexy, wadda ya got?"

I smiled and said, "By the smile on your face, either you ate a great bowl of cheerios, or you and Nancy hit an all new high last night."

She laughed and said "Yes and actually it was this morning not last night." Janice and I have worked with each other for about the last three years, and she is always in the ER when I bring in some strange and interesting call. I informed Janice about the events that brought Seema and us to Vinny's ER and she treated Seema with kid gloves.

As Janice took my paperwork back to her desk to sign, I peeked into Seema's room to say goodbye. As I approached her bed she looked totally distraught and vomited again. I went to the nurse's station and wet some towels so that she could wipe her face. When Seema was done wiping her face, she put her hand on my forearm as I leaned on the railing of her bed and she thanked Deklund and I for taking care of her. She looked at both Deklund and I, saying that she didn't know that people in our profession could be so nice after dealing with incidents such as the jumper. She said if it were her, she would have been unable to function. I smiled and told her if she ever needed us again that she should not hesitate calling 911; that is why we are here.

I nodded to Deklund who was looking at me for direction on when the right time is to leave the patient's bedside. I stopped at the sink to

PARAMEDIC M.O.S.

wash up and my pager vibrated. You always leave your pager on vibrate when working the street, reason being you never know when you are going to end up in a tactical situation where silence and the lack of anyone knowing that someone in a uniform is near will save your life.

It can be a deadly situation if someone's pager activates while we are fulfilling our role of Tactical EMS Medics with the NYPD ESU S.W.A.T. Unit or other law enforcement agency, when a door is being breeched (entered) during a search warrant operation. I have seen it happen and it is not pretty for anyone involved.

Deklund and I walked out to our bus, which was parked on the 7th Avenue side of the medical center where the ER entrance is. I put us 10-98(available on our MDT) and then we walked across the street to a little market to get something light to munch on. Deklund grabbed a Sprite and some mixed nuts, and I grabbed a bottle of orange juice, fresh squeezed, and a quart-sized container of mixed fresh fruit. Today's mix was Watermelon, Pineapple and Mango. These are foods that are great on the job, since they digest easy and they replace anything I might sweat off in my bulletproof vest.

I just finished my fourth fork-full of fruit when Marcus called us, "10X, I got a diff breather for you at 7808 West 18th Street. It's in a private financial office on its way to your screen."

Deklund started up the bus and since Vinny's was at the corner of 11th Street and 7th Avenue, we would be there in no time at all. I also grew up on the block where St. Vincent's sits, so I knew this area cold. I told Deklund to make a right on Greenwich (pronounced Grenich) and hook a right on 8th Avenue. Traffic wouldn't be that bad and once we made it across 14th, we'd be on scene in a matter of seconds. As Deklund hit the lights and blipped on the siren, I heard two familiar beeps from the on-board computer, and my MDT wouldn't transmit my signal to the dispatcher (not so uncommon).

As we passed 13th Street I called our dispatcher "Tactical X, our MDT isn't taking our 63 signal, Marcus can you please move us over (show us enroute)."

Marcus acknowledged and thanked me. We came up to 8th Avenue and scared some guy trying to wash windows. We jetted across 14th Street as if we were catapulted off of an aircraft carrier. I read the call out loud as we bounced down onto 8th Avenue.

"50 year old male, chest pain, difficulty breathing, history of fluid in his lungs. He is in suite 1535," I said nonchalantly.

I held on for dear life as Deklund made the right onto 18th street. We came through at a frightening speed, as those who were originally strutting across the street quickly leaped for life as we approached. They realized that we weren't stopping. Deklund double-parked the bus in front of the structure. We exited and when Deklund got to my side, I had already grabbed the monitor and drug bag. Dek grabbed the Airway bag with the portable oxygen cylinder in it and went into the back to get the suction unit in case this guy arrested and for this call the stretcher.

We entered the building, and I picked up my radio, "Tactical X, I forgot to hit the button, make us 88." Marcus acknowledged.

We approached the security desk and the guard looked up at me.

Raising my eyebrows as I spoke to the Security agent I asked, "Suite 1535?"

He pointed to a bank of elevators behind him to his right. We waited with the rest of the suits, and when the doors opened, everyone tried to get on before us. I looked at Deklund as he looked at me.

Our eyes said, "Can you believe these people. They know we are NYC EMS 911 Paramedics and that we are here for an emergency, yet they don't want to give us an elevator."

As the doors started to close without us on the elevator, I stuck my forearm right in between. The doors stopped abruptly and they re-opened.

"Hi everyone this is an emergency and we are commandeering this elevator. I need you all to exit now and fast." I said abruptly. Wow, did I get some funny looks.

Some guy in the back started to say something and was elbowed by his female counterpart. Everyone exited fast.

Deklund looked at the control panel and said "Oh man, they hit every button from here to fifteen. We'll be here forever trying to get up to the 15th floor."

I smiled, took out my kubaton key chain and placed a funny looking key into the Fire Department Emergency Access Slot. This cleared the panel and sent us right to the fifteenth floor.

Deklund shook his head and his eyes opened wide, "No fucking way!" I started to laugh as the doors started to close and said proudly, "Stick with me dude, I'll teach you some stuff today."

I thought to myself that all this guy needs is for someone to take their time with him, letting him know that they care about his career and enjoy working with him.

PARAMEDIC M.O.S.

We got off on floor fifteen, hoping that someone would be waiting for us. Ironically there wasn't a peep. We followed the signs to 1535 waiting for someone to come out screaming in agony, but it never happened. I looked through the slate of glass that accompanied suite 1535, and then opened the door. It was some kind of investment trading office, as people were everywhere. I found some guy who had a huge desk overlooking the room; the caption above his head said "Floor Manager," so we approached him.

As soon as he saw us he sprang off his seat, "Oh good, you're here. Come with me."

Something didn't feel good about this whole situation. Why wasn't there an escort waiting for us downstairs? Why wasn't there someone waiting for us off the elevator? Had Deklund and I not known that we were in the room for an emergency, by the activity in the room you would have never known something serious was going on. People in suits were yelling back and forth, throwing pieces of partially filled out paper back and forth. We were led to an office with its door closed.

The office manager opened the door and said, "OH MY GOD!" When I looked in I saw a mahogany desk, and two feet sticking up in mid-air behind it. I pushed through the office manager and leaped over the desk; there was our patient. No one was in the room with him to comfort him while he waited for EMS to arrive. Our patient was still awake but had that damn ashen gray look to him. I asked him if he could talk and he informed me that he had bad chest pain for the last hour and laid on the ground thinking he was going to die. He was sweating profusely. I knew that we had no time for leeway.

"Dek, give me the O2 and the monitor". A few people started to watch us work. I guess now that it was an event, business was less important, unlike when this guy was in pain by his lonesome.

Deklund threw me the Airway bag, and I explained the following to the patient while Deklund set up frantically, "Jim, my name is Chris and this is Deklund, we are going to help you. I need you to stay as calm as you can and we will get through this. We are going to do a few things to you here in the office and then we are going to transport you to the hospital."

Jim looked up at me with absolute doom in his eyes. I had a gut feeling that he was going to arrest. I placed a non-rebreathing mask at 15 liters of Oxygen on his face. This concentration of oxygen is the best way to administer large amounts of O2 without tubing the person. You don't want to tube someone conscious unless you have too; that can get real messy.

Deklund got a pressure of 170/100 on him, and he was tachy at about 120. I sat him straight up and his color improved immensely. While I set up to initiate his first IV and get 60 cc's of blood from him, he said that the oxygen made it easier to breathe. About two weeks prior, the service took part in a medication trial program of trans-dermal nitro-glycerin patches. Similar to the nicotine patch, we were testing the trans-dermal patch as a route for nitro administration. I got Jim's IV set in his left forearm on the first shot, drew 60 cc's of blood for cross, type and match (red, gray and jungle topped vaccutainer tubes), and locked his IV in place. I told Deklund to get a nitro patch out, but to make sure he put gloves on.

Once you touch the patch, if it is patch to skin, it will administer into you. I checked Jim's lung sounds and he had rales (pronounced rails, which are rice-krispie sounds during inspiration, expiration or both, which is indicative of Acute Pulmonary Edema or left sided heart failure).

Another form of this is called ronchi, pronounced ron-kigh. This is a more coarse sounding disorder, which is indicative of right-sided heart failure or congestive heart failure (CHF), a disorder that is gradual in its development. Both are deadly if not treated, but left sided failure is more acute, and sometimes more difficult to detect unless you know the sounds, symptoms, signs and general pathology of this cardiovascular disease.

As I opened a pre-filled syringe of 40 mg of Lasix (generically known as Furosimide, a diuretic), I heard Deklund behind me fumbling with the nitro-patch packaging. As I pushed the 40 mg of Lasix into Jim's IV tubing I heard a huge "THUD" behind me. I spun around and Deklund was unconscious on the ground.

"Fuck!" I said to myself.

I told Jim to sit still as I moved over to Deklund. Low and behold, there was Deklund, face down without gloves on and a nitro patch in his right hand. I didn't know whether to slap him, laugh or both. I pulled the patch off with my gloved hands and picked up my radio requesting an immediate back up with an MOS down for medical reasons. Deklund was on the shorter side at about 5'6" and all of about 150-lbs. wet, so he was a ripe conductor for the medication.

Where as AJ's partner Phil was as big as a Mack Truck, he might have become a tad bit woozy, Deklund had no body fat and his pressure

PARAMEDIC M.O.S.

bottomed out. Deklund moaned a bit and looked like he had a hangover so I laid him down and propped his feet up. He knew where he was, so that was a good sign.

I went back over to Jim, and just before I placed a new unused nitro patch on his shoulder, he went sheet white and displayed Ventricular Fibrillation on the Lifepak. VFib is an erratic and often deadly misfiring of the heart's electrical system. If it goes uncorrected, you will end up in cardiac arrest. I attempted a pre-cordial thump, a closed fist punch on the mid sternum to manually jolt the heart out of its irregular rhythm.

Unfortunately, that theory didn't work too well in this situation; so now it was on to plan B. While I looked back at Deklund who was still on the floor, I charged my paddles. I kept hoping my backup units would arrive, my partner would find his blood pressure, my patient would stand up and start doing jumping jacks, and most of all that I could be back in Vermont on a canoe with AJ.

Considering that the only fully conscious person in the room was me, and that my patient was entering clinical death and my partner was semi-conscious on the floor, I didn't think I had to say "CLEAR."

I shocked Jim twice at 200 wps (watts per second), with no change in the VFIB. As per protocol, my next was the big juice, 360 wps.

I placed the paddles on Jim's chest and jolted him; simultaneously I heard "Oh shit," from behind me.

Then I heard another THUD.

I looked down my left side and there was Deklund, upside down against another wall. It seems that in his altered mental state Deklund crawled over to Jim and me, and in his attempt to get my attention he grabbed onto Jim's foot at the moment I sent a huge charge through Jim's body, sending Deklund against the wall.

"Oh, you gotta be kidding me," I said to myself.

Jim stopped breathing, so after I checked Deklund quickly, I intubated Jim. Once I secured the tube and began bagging him, I helped Deklund get next to me so I could keep an eye on him. I was bagging Jim through the tube and apologizing to Deklund simultaneously. Just before the backup units arrived, Jim opened his eyes and began an attempt at pulling the tube out of his throat as I tried to calm him down and breathe for him with the AMBU bag.

Extubation, or the removal of the endotracheal tube gets very messy if done incorrectly or in a rush. A patient can be conscious while tubed, but they need to be coddled, assured and coached. With my other hand I reached over and checked Deklund's pulse, which was actually normal.

Deklund was now looking at me funny. Jim was looking at me funny. If there was a mirror in the room, I would have looked at me funny too. My back up crews began arriving and I didn't know if they were going to laugh or cry, since the office scene looked like a game of Twister gone bad.

William Vulant from 12X3 said, "Oh shit, what happened?" I explained as they set Deklund up on a monitor and treated him for acute electrocution. Two additional BLS units showed up and had a similar experience in the elevator that I did. Lieutenant Harry Jerti, 11-Patrol, showed up with so many units being assigned to one call and of course, with a medic down.

He looked and asked me, "Is he alright?"

I shook my head and said, "Lou, it depends on how much he remembers. They're taking my original patient to Beekman-Downtown, and I and 11(H)enry will take Dek to Bellevue since he is stable."

Henry asked, "Are you okay to transport him?" I nodded, "Sure, I just feel bad." Henry had an extra medic riding with him, so he joined us for the ride in case anything else happened.

As Deklund was admitted to the ER for observation, I called AJ.

She had pretty much the same reaction I had, "You have got to be kidding me." She asked how Deklund was doing and if I was going to remain on the tour, I told her that I just spoke with Davia and she authorized giving me the rest of the night off. I was going to remain at the Emergency Room with Deklund until they decided what they would do with him.

Aside from some occasional FLB's, he was fine and in good spirits. He still couldn't believe what happened. I felt like shit for shocking him, but at least Jim the patient was doing well. The ER decided to admit Deklund on general principles and I accompanied him upstairs. Deklund's girlfriend arrived at the hospital just before we took him upstairs. Jannelle, his girlfriend, was a pre-school teacher in Babylon, Long Island, and a very attractive one at that. She looked terminally frightened, and I was hoping this would go smoothly.

I was about to introduce myself to her when Deklund sat up in bed and said, "Hi honey, thanks for coming. This is my training partner Christian." As I extended my hand he said, "Jan, you gotta ride with this guy, it's an electrifying experience."

PARAMEDIC M.O.S.

He laughed hard, she looked confused and I just sank into myself. I explained to her what happened and she took it well. Deklund insisted that I go home and get some sleep. He said not to worry about anything and that he had "Seen the light."

I think the light he was referring to was when the 360 watts per second charged through his body. He had a great sense of humor. I felt horrible. These things do happen out here, and the good thing is that based on the early information, he will probably be in CCU (cardiac care unit) for a few observational days and then released back to work.

Since Deklund was in excellent hands, I decided it was time to let him be with Janelle. I was leaning over his bedside looking at him, thankful that he was okay. We joked about the elevator incident and I told him I would take off. He was going to be put through some tests and then sedated for sleep. He kept telling me that it wasn't my fault, and not to worry. I told him to page me if he needed anything and I would check on him during the night and in the morning. We shook hands, hugged our agency hug, and I said goodnight.

I took our bus back down to the station and parked it for the night. I walked into the Lieutenant's office and Andy was sitting there.

I looked at Andy with a small amount of frustration, "Yup, just a little pissed that it all happened."

I was putting equipment in the cabinet when Andy said, "You couldn't stop him from picking up the patch that way and there is no way you could have foreseen him grabbing onto the patient's foot. You know that shit happens out here. Don't sweat it dude. Go home and get some rest, come in tomorrow nice and fresh."

I patted Andy on the back thanking him. I paged AJ from the desk alphanumeric paging station letting her know I was heading home. About two minutes later as I walked towards my truck she paged me back saying that she was making dinner, the massage oil was warming and to be ready for a night of pampering. I love this woman!

This particular evening at the Spa de Anjoline began with a wonderfully long hug and delicious kiss when I walked into the house. She prepared a fabulous dinner of Linguini a la Pesto. This girl had a recipe for Pesto that was better than mine. She always put her love into the cooking; then again, she put her love into everything she does. The pesto was accompanied by a great salad of field greens, raspberries, tangerines, caramelized walnuts and a honey-balsamic reduction dressing. She prepared a special bath for me, followed by a massage, and ending with her retiring to bed with me afterwards.

Before I passed out I called the CCU to check on Deklund. I spoke to Dina the Charge Nurse for the ward; she said he was doing great, the tests all came back negative and he said not to worry. I thanked her, and rolled over into AJ's arms. AJ is the only person that I will completely fold up into. Even though I am bigger than her, she had this way of enveloping my body in her hug that was an experience each time. We complimented each other well. We kissed while lying there for quite some time and fell asleep gently. AJ's massage put me into a very deep sleep, as I didn't feel anything until she sat down on the bed next to me to say goodbye on her way to the academy.

PARAMEDIC M.O.S.

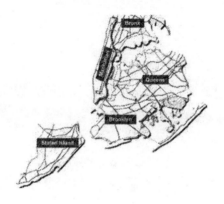

C.B. Garris

Chapter XIV:

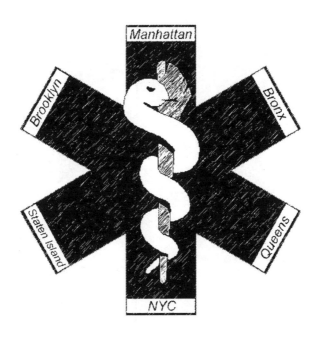

PARAMEDIC M.O.S.

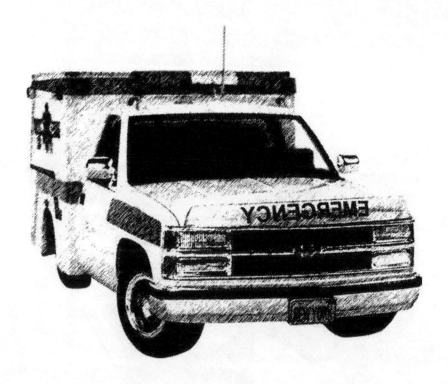

I woke up totally refreshed around 11:00 am. I called the hospital and it turns out that Deklund was discharged earlier in the morning. This meant I could go directly to the station instead of stopping off at Bellevue to see Deklund as I had planned. As I stepped out of the shower I heard my pager going off. I reached for it and it was a message from Chief Battieri. She asked me to call her in her car. I picked up the phone and dialed the number from memory.

"Chief Battieri," she said authoritatively when she answered.

"You rang?" I said with the distinctive voice Davia knew right away.

"How you doin?" She asked in a concerned manner.

"I'm good, getting ready to head down now. I checked with CCU and Deklund was released."

The phone signal appeared to skip like most cellular phone signals do.

"I picked him up from Bell," Davia said, "he was great and he got a good night's sleep too. He was totally excited at the prospect of working with you again. His eyes lit up when he began talking about someone having a Fire Department elevator key."

I could tell Davia was smiling when she said this.

"You wouldn't happen to know anyone fitting that description now, would you?" We laughed and I asked her how her fiancé was doing. Mike Vioreo, her fiancé, was a commanding officer for the NYPD. She said he was well, in fact he was down at Quantico (the FBI's training division), on a special dignitary protection logistics course and that he was returning in a few days. She told me to call Nora, our agency Medical Director, who was asking about me in lieu of yesterday.

She wanted to hear for herself that I was okay. She would have called but Davia said she would be speaking to me moments after they talked. I told her I would reach out to Nora (or as we professionally knew her as, Dr. Roberts).

I got stuck in enough traffic driving in to make me want to go mad. A bad accident on the George Washington Bridge (eloquently known as the GWB), had traffic backed all the way up to Yonkers. Once I broke through the traffic and headed east, it was already 14:10. The rest of the streets were open, so I made it down the FDR Drive in about twenty minutes. I hate rushing to work, because I like to get to the station, walk AMBU and feel the night out.

Rushing in means the rest of the tour will probably end up in disaster. I need a few unhurried moments to myself to think towards my higher

PARAMEDIC M.O.S.

power. There was someone or something keeping me alive while I worked these streets, so I needed to mentally prepare myself for anything at the beginning of a tour.

When Jen and I hit the street, it took no time to see that we viewed our work and life the same way. Jen grew up in the South Bronx near Lincoln Hospital, around 147th Street and the Grand Concourse. We both had great senses of humor and responsibility.

I walked in the office and said to Jen, "Hey you!" Jen turned around from signing out our radios and gave me a hug. "I hear you got a new way to break in the students," she said as she smiled from ear to ear as if to say, "I haven't given you any shit for about three days, so I am going to make up for it now."

I shook my head comically knowing how long of a night this was going to be. I am so glad that she was always in the mood to work, since 10X2 came in early due to overtime personnel. Jen spent the last hour and ten minutes going through the vehicle with a fine tooth comb. I trusted Jen implicitly because she was complete, thus I didn't have to wonder if she checked the vehicle out properly.

Nothing was worse than having a partner who you couldn't even trust to check out your equipment and bus. If he or she could not be trusted to perform such vital functions, then you should find a new partner. I went upstairs and did my super hero outfit change, while AMBU waited for me patiently at the door to the locker room. We walked downstairs together as she kept her head attached to my thigh.

As I walked into the apparatus room I heard someone yell, "Roll Call!" This is where we all line up in front of the station Lieutenant for inspection and to be notified of anything pertinent to the street that night. One or all of us usually got pulled from roll call for a 911 assignment, but it was an effective way to maintain our Para-military structure nonetheless.

We made it through roll call without getting called out. When all personnel were dismissed, I heard 10(A)dam3 get an injury on Mott St. in Chinatown, and 11(E)ddie3 got a sick call up on 11th St and Ave. B in Alphabet City. Jen and I headed for our bus and today was Jen's day to drive. She loved driving a five-ton emergency vehicle through city streets at top speed, since it was always a challenge. We deployed at our discretion today, so we decided to remain in the M1-M2 today. Each borough is divided into sectors, and it helps us as field medics as well as the dispatchers to assign calls and deploy units with these mnemonics. It gives everyone a general outline of what areas they are covering, even though most units are designated to sit at a particular street intersection when not on a call.

We decided to head up the east side for the beginning of the tour. 10(D)avid3 was sent to a PED-STRUCK (pedestrian struck by an auto) at 23rd. St and 1st Ave. Due to the high probability of someone getting pretty jacked up on this type of call, I radioed Tina and told her to put us on the back of 10D. I switched my NYPD portable to channel S2, which is the frequency for that sector. There was moderate radio traffic, some of it due to a felony foot pursuit currently under way on 21st street, unrelated to our call.

Because of this I could not get a perspective from any responding PD units. Jen was already heading up 1st Avenue past a bunch of school kids that must have stayed after today. We made so much noise that the bystanders in the vicinity turned around expecting a 60-foot truck to approach. The adults just held their ears. The kids stood at the base of the corner of 5th Street and 1st Avenue waving us on as if we were in a marathon.

In between the huffs and puffs of officers in foot pursuit of their robbery suspect, a very excited voice came over the PD frequency. "Central, rush the bus on two-three and one, confirmed ped-struck and he's not breathing central. Get me emergency services here forthwith!"

My day was just totally shot to shit.

"Step on it," I said to Jen in a calm voice. We were already approaching 18th Street and 1st Avenue right next to Beth Israel Hospital. I already knew the officer, Henry Dillinger. Henry is a former medic for NYC EMS and now with the NYPD, he was always good in the street, so I know we needed to haul. I picked up Jen's EMS portable and said "10X, Tactical X, PD confirming ped-struck traumatic arrest at 23 and 1, and they are calling for a forthwith on ESU. Do me a favor and give Bell a heads up and I'll get back to you in a moment. You can also show us "double up" (on scene)." As we approached it was evident that the body of this victim was in the middle of 1st Avenue. He was apparently hit on 1st Avenue before 23rd Street and according to eyewitnesses launched approximately 60 feet in the air, coming down on his head. 10(D)avid came screaming up behind us and completed the pattern to cut off all traffic attempting to get onto 1st Avenue. I have to say the officer was right, this guy was definitely not breathing.

PARAMEDIC M.O.S.

Much of his face came off when he landed, grating the blacktop for quite some distance. As we collared him and rolled him into position for ventilations, I noticed that part of his face literally stuck to the hot pavement. It wasn't so much that the pavement was hot, but the friction of his landing melted his skin onto the tar. When we rolled him into position, pieces of his flesh came right off, and unfortunately it was all we could do to ventilate him. You cannot ventilate someone properly face down.

I guessed by what was left of his features that he was in his 40's. He was wearing very raggedy clothing and he smelled really bad. Jen took over ventilations as I jumped in the back of 10(D)'s bus to set up for intubation. I also called communications, "10X, TAC X priority!" I waited for Marcus to answer, "C'mon Chris." Taking out a tube and watching them roll the backboard and stretcher towards the unit, "Marcus call Bell, 40 year old male traumatic arrest, ped-struck, multi-trauma, 2 minutes." Marcus heard me rushing so he knew that I had no time to say anything else. Jen, Bob and Juan wheeled our patient to the back of the bus, as I pulled the stretcher in.

All traffic was stopped at this major intersection and NYPD was diverting all cars away. NYPD never questioned us if we blocked traffic or did something that the general public frowned upon, because they knew we had good reason to do it. Juan put electrodes on the patient to help us see if there was any heart activity. I wanted to give him a try at a tube as we moved toward Bellevue.

Based on his injuries and the fact that he was not breathing, I had to get him tubed. Aside from the breathing issues or lack there of, judging by the amount of head trauma and pieces of his brain matter that were left on 1st Avenue, he was almost certain to have a large amount of inter-cranial bleeding. If we don't control the swelling in the field, his brain matter can and will literally herniate beyond his skull capacity and begin to creep out of his ears, nose and throat. I've seen this many times, and it is a horrible reality of inevitability.

With so much of his face and throat left on 1st Avenue, I didn't even need a laryngoscope to get the tube in place, since I could see all the way to his vocal cords without assistance so I performed what we call digital intubation.

I got the tube and secured it, as we made a slow roll towards Bellevue a few blocks away. His chest was partially crushed on his right side, which is where we believe he landed. We sometimes refer to this type of trauma as a flail chest, but in this case, it was totally crushed. I had a bad feeling that this guy was not going to make it and in fact I think he was dead on one of the two impacts.

Regardless, we were giving him every chance. Jen was having a hard time with getting IV access, so while she kept trying, I dropped 1 mg of Epi and 1 mg of Atropine down the tube as the 1st round meds of cardiac arrest. Since our endotracheal intubation method places the tube down the trachea where it splits into either lung at the carina (a wishbone like segment), we can use the lungs as a method of accessibility for drug administration. Between continued ventilations and cardio-pulmonary resuscitation, the medications are administered through the body.

We arrived to a well-rested pack of hungry wolves in scrubs at the ER Bay. One of the resident's said gaspingly, "My God, how did you get him tubed?" I just looked at her as we wheeled towards the Trauma Slot, "Didn't even need a scope." I had my feet rested on the bar of the stretcher that was not touching the ground. This was so I could reach across the stretcher and hold onto the stretcher with my right hand, while doing one-handed CPR compressions with my left.

As we headed for the slot, this nurse from behind the triage desk started yelling at all of us.

"Hey, what are you doing?" I told them that this hospital is on diversion and you should have taken that mess somewhere else!" I thought I was going to go over to her and throw her through the nearest window. We all looked at her strangely and then continued past. She yelled all the way down the hall, paying no attention to the blood droplets or pieces of flesh that we still emanating from this patient. The trauma surgeon's took over but didn't go to the OR, and I kind of felt that they were going to call this one. About three minutes into it, they did. The lead resident asked for the time on the clock to signify time of death.

I was covered in blood, as was Jen and Juan. Since Bob was driving, he was able to escape any blood splatterings. The three other medics and I stood there in the room as they pulled the sheet over his face. That is a feeling I cannot describe.

Even though I had a feeling that his trauma was too extensive, we all accepted that this might turn out bad. All you can do is go wash up, restock your equipment and hope that the next one isn't nearly as bad, so that there is something left to salvage. When someone is pronounced dead in the Slot, it is very business-like. There is generally no real sign

PARAMEDIC M.O.S.

of emotion except a quiet, somber meditation that we tried our best and wish that we could have done more.

The quiet, somber meditation is relieved by our combined experiences and acceptance that we can only do so much. We know that collectively, we make up the best team possible and will do everything we can. Thus, after a pronouncement of death the docs thank everyone for their efforts, and the nurses clean up for the next one. We just go get dinner.

When I walked out to the scrub sinks to clean up, that loud mouthed, insensitive nurse rounded the corner and leaped in my face. "I told your godammned dispatcher that we were on diversion and that you should have gone to another hospital!" She was directly in my face, antagonistically loud and so confrontational that Jen, who was in the restock room, was just waiting to hear the WHACK when my fist connected with her jaw.

I looked at her like she had horribly bad breath. She threw some paperwork in my face and pushed me away from the sink, "Did you hear me?" I had just lost a patient, by no fault of mine, but I just lost a patient and I was not about to be subjected to this tirade.

I got up in her face and said, "Look, I don't know who pissed in your Cheerios this morning, but you are way out of line! If you touch me again you will find your ass in jail for assaulting a governmental official!"

Jen, Juan, and members of the trauma team stepped into view.

"Exactly what the fuck is your problem," I said while awaiting her response.

She backed right down, "Uh, well, I didn't want you to come here with that mess of a patient."

It appeared that my look of absolute terror was beginning to take effect, "First of all," I started in on her, "Don't you EVER, and I mean ever walk up on me like that again. Second, don't you ever refer to one of my patient's as that mess! He had a name and if you were paying attention you'd know that he will not be answering to it anymore. Thirdly, if you read your citywide manual on 911 receiving hospitals, it states in relative paraphrasing that diversion is a courtesy status provided to a facility that meets the mandated requirements of the NYC EMS Office of Medical Affairs. Those requirements were created if a facility is unable to handle a certain criteria or all criteria's of patients that are transported by NYC EMS 911 ambulances, to allow said facility to return to a status of normal operation."

The charge nurse stood there in awe as I admonished her, and I was not quiet about it either.

I continued, "Knowing that YOU are the charge nurse tonight leads me to believe that you and your charming personality didn't follow the appropriate procedure for the aforementioned diversion request set forth by my agency; therefore your request is null and void."

The hospital administrator walked into view as our verbal altercation continued, "And lastly, last time I checked you are not only a 911 receiving hospital, you are also a Level 1 trauma center, which automatically disqualifies and negates you from being able to make a trauma diversion request. Any patient in cardiac or traumatic arrest by law has to be transported to the closest 911 receiving hospital, and since my last patient was hit by a truck three blocks from your front door, that also had a contributing factor in you being the recipient."

The nurse just looked at me like she wanted to take her broom out, hit me with it and then ride it off into the sunset.

The administrator took her aside and said something to her as I continued scrubbing. I dried off and went out to my bus to get a call report when the Administrator On Duty (AOD) walked up to me and said, "Do you want to press charges?"

I looked at her confused.

She informed me that another nurse called her down when she witnessed the nurse push me. I scratched my eyebrow as I sat in my bus to pull up the times of the call on the computer for my paperwork.

I looked at the AOD and simply said, "You know the beauty of this is that I know she is a miserable person, because it takes a miserable person to do what she did and say what she said. I am not going to waste the time of the NYPD to arrest her for assault or my personal time to testify in court. I just wanted her to back off because she was treading on thin ice." The AOD smiled appreciatively and thanked me.

"What also instills confidence in me," I continued, "is that she is going to do that to the wrong person one day, and when they haul off and hit her or worse, she will wish that she was nicer. It is called karma and I am a firm believer in it." The AOD nodded an approving nod as she adjusted her studious glasses.

After she began to walk back in the ER she turned around, "By the way," she paused and smiled, "Pissed in your cheerios?"

I smiled back and just shrugged.

After another approving smile, the AOD disappeared into the distance as Jen came out.

PARAMEDIC M.O.S.

Jen admired the beauty of the AOD and then asked what was all that about. She first thought that the AOD was out trying to get a dinner date. I reminded her that was an impossibility and we laughed about the fact that she thought I was going to slug the nurse. I informed her that the AOD was trying to ensure that I was not going to initiate litigation against the medical facility for damaged pride.

I told Jen that I had about four run-ins with this particular nurse, and she mentioned that I was not alone, as many medics had been complaining about her. In fact, when she went to get the signature from the nurse, she refused and Jen had to get the AOD to sign our paperwork. The nurse told Jen that the less she sends us back to the street, the fewer patients we bring in.

That was it for me. "Jen my dear, I think it is time we set her straight."

Jen knew that I had a good idea, but the look in her eyes was one that inquired as to how much paperwork this was going to cause her to have to write.

We cleared from the assignment and left the hospital. I always admired Bellevue Hospital and Medical Center, as it has one of the best trauma teams this side of the Hudson River. I know that if I was circling the drain, I'd want to go there. We drove over to a shelter for the homeless that was nearby.

The shelter is commonly a place that we get 911 calls from for patients with non-specific sick complaints, yet we do see a fair amount of legitimate medical calls from there as well. Some of the residents haven't had medical care or checkups for years. Many are now diabetics, riddled with lice and suffer from various topical disorders. Frequently they have severe hepatic (liver) disorders from years of alcohol and drug abuse with minimal or no intervention.

It was particularly cold this evening, so when we rounded the corner there were residents hanging around like there was a drive-in movie about to begin and they were waiting to get their popcorn. I had Jen stick the nose of the vehicle into the access way near the loading dock and front door, and I picked up the public address microphone attached to our siren saying, "Anyone want a warm meal?"

My announcement echoed in between the buildings and it looked like the worlds most diverse and hardened roadhouse bar emptied out. If it is cold out, the city hospitals are required to provide any patient who requests it and who is cleared for food by the physician, to have a nutritious meal. Jen knew exactly what I was doing, but that nurse had no idea what was coming.

Forward came eight of the skankiest, nastiest, most lice ridden, urine smelling, vomit ladened, shit-stained individuals I could have ever hoped to see. All wanted to go to the hospital for one reason or another. At first even I was worried that one of them would be truly sick. Luck came my way that night that all of the patients had no severe complaints.

My first patient looked like the cartoon character "Sam" from Bugs Bunny. He had a long, hairy beard, a long trench coat, underwear and a pair of cleats. He said he had chest pain. I asked him in a concerned manner when it started, and he told me five years ago when some girl broke his heart. That was the worst of the patients I had.

Since we were literally almost walking distance from the doors to the Emergency Room, I figured out how to get all eight patients in the back of the vehicle. Before we transported I put us out at the scene of a "Flag Down" (where we either come upon something or are waved down by a bystander); and Jen and I prepared eight perfectly prepared call reports. I didn't mention to Marcus how many patients we had for several reasons.

One is that if I said I had eight patients he would have felt compelled to send me back up. Secondly, I would have been required to receive a patrol supervisor and I didn't want to tie up any other units. I put us extended on scene for patient care reasons, and we finished all of our paperwork. I told all of my newly acquired ambulance mates that if any of them wanted a really good meal they had to demand it when they got into the emergency room.

All of my eight patients had either urinated, defecated or both on themselves before we arrived. The smell in the back of the ambulance was so foul that I was the one who was wearing an oxygen mask, giving myself high-concentration oxygen just to dilute the stench.

As Jen swung the vehicle around to the ER bay, I reminded everyone about the meal, and I also told them that if they didn't feel like wiping their own butts, that they were welcome to demand that the nurse with the blonde hair do it for them. I instructed each one of them to follow me in like Peter the Pied Piper in single formation. These guys were all just happy to be a part of something.

Jen opened the doors to the rear of the vehicle and I collected all of the paperwork. We began marching into the ER with all of my fledglings in

PARAMEDIC M.O.S.

tow. As we entered the actual ER area, a waft of horrid odor accompanied us as a few nurses turned around. I noticed the AOD and the EMS Station 13 supervisor were standing together chatting in the nurse's station. I stepped to the side so that my fledglings could strut in style or at least that is what I was hoping for.

What actually came out of it was three who dropped their pants as soon as they walked in, one kept walking in circles, one from the rear of the group who not only dropped his pants but decided to defecate right on the floor, and another who was trying to piss in the corner. I tried desperately not to laugh, but couldn't keep the smile from my face.

As I approached my favorite nurse she said to me, "What is this?"

I walked up to the triage desk and in front of the AOD I said to the nurse, "Here are eight patients, all who have individual names. I heard about your comment regarding not wanting to send us back out so that you wouldn't have to get patients."

Placing the eight perfectly and legibly prepared call reports on her desk I said to her, "Since you didn't want to send us back out that often, I thought I would round up as many as I could to brighten your day and save me multiple trips to see you. Read 'em, sign 'em, and we're outta here. Oh and by the way, don't you ever fuck with me again!" The nurse looked at the guy who defecated on the floor and realized that not only was he sitting in his own feces now, she also knew that she would have to be the one to clean him. As she looked me with complete disdain, she signed each form. As Jen and I walked past the AOD and the EMS Supervisor, they both just smiled big, cheesy grins and nodded approvingly.

C.B. Garris

Chapter XV:

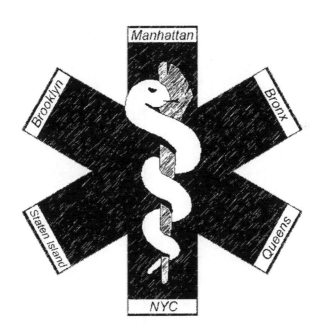

PARAMEDIC M.O.S.

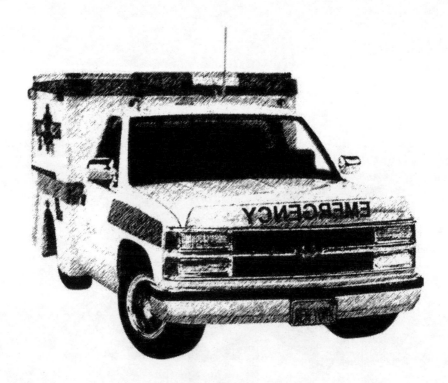

C.B. Garris

Since I had to testify in court tomorrow on a murder case I responded to over a year ago, I was given the following day off to keep my schedule on track. I arranged for Jen to work with Scott Beasley from Brooklyn's Station 36. Scott and I worked the West Indian Day Parade a few years ago on Labor Day and had a few very serious trauma calls from gunshots and stabbings. I liked the way he worked. Scott jumped at my request to take my spot for his overtime. Scott was born and raised in Brooklyn, but loved coming into Manhattan to play.

The cool thing is that I could take my day off and prepare a feast for AJ when she got home. One of the great things I love about what AJ and I have, is that although we work in an intense profession, we leave it at the office. We most certainly discuss things about work often, and we will stop on the highway if we see a bad accident, but we don't feel the need to let it take our lives over.

AJ and I have something unique and it is something that we both love to put our time into. We do our job and we do it well; we also manage to maintain a complete life outside the agency. Once we leave the station, we take care of each other. We made the decision to be with each other after a long process, realizing that it is very difficult to be without each other.

AJ said she would be home around 5:00 pm or so, after she dropped Nicole, one of the medics who carpooled with her to the Academy. AJ's feast for tonight, aside from hopefully being me at the end, would be a candle-lit dinner with special rose-scented candles I found at a place on Bleeker Street. They have the best-scented candles I have ever experienced.

I took out a few CD's to play while I prepared the feast, Charlie Byrd, Stan Getz/Astrud Gilberto & Antonio Carlos-Jobim. AJ's kitchen was custom designed, including a restaurant-professional chef stove with six burners. She also had a convection oven, an island in the center of the kitchen work area, and a ceiling pot rack. She had that put up for the numerous pots I would need handy when I turned her home into a restaurant if our friends stopped in; and I wanted to give them all the amenities of full-fledged cuisine. I would start early making the bread by hand, and preparing my mise en place (ingredients ready for service). Tonight's menu consisted of Bruschetta to start.

From the old country, Bruschetta is toast, which in this case would be my homemade hearth bread topped with my special mixture of tomato

PARAMEDIC M.O.S.

concasee (peeled, seeded & diced), finely chopped garlic and a lot of it, basil chiffonade (chiffonade is the same texture of the leaf as cole slaw), and extra virgin olive oil with a balsamic honey reduction. Bruschetta can be very tart, so the honey eases the sharpness. I started by boiling water in a medium saucepan to skin the tomatoes. I filled a moderate sized bowl with cold water and placed it on the side. I made a superficial X on the bottom of each tomato, going about one-third the way up the tomato. I dropped each tomato in the boiling water for about twenty seconds and removed each to the bowl of cold water. After about a minute the skin will come right off of the tomato.

Once all the skin was removed, I cut each tomato in half and removed the seeds. In the lengthwise position I made five long, thin slices through each section of tomato, turning the tomato one-quarter turn and slicing horizontally. I then placed each tomato under my fingers one at a time, slicing them into prepared chopped sections. Placing this in a bowl I then chopped about eight sections of garlic fine. I placed those in the bowl with the tomatoes and after chiffonading the basil from AJ's garden that I oversee, I added that with the olive oil reduction and let it sit in a covered container.

The entree tonight would be Coq Au Vin. I make mine with caramelized onions. I start sweating (slow sauté) very lean bacon in a large casserole or even a lobster pot. Once lightly caramelized (browned), the next step is to caramelize about 2 lbs of sectioned chicken get the fond.

Fond is the result of the caramelization of cooking. Thus that brown stuff left from cooking meat in a pan is fond. It contains great flavor, especially when you deglaze the pan with the appropriate wine. Adding a little salt and pepper, I threw in three-quarters of a cup of Cognac. I ignite the liquid, keeping my face away from the pot just in case.

After shaking the contents of the pan, I pour anywhere from half to three-quarters of a bottle of a fruity burgundy, bringing it to simmer. I toss in 5 cloves of minced garlic, 3 bay leafs, and 2 cups of demi-glace (brown stock). I cook this for about forty-five minutes, give or take a few. About fifteen minutes before the chicken is ready I place about a pound of bulb onions in a large iron skillet.

I add about a cup of sugar and 3/4 cup of water. On high heat I let the mixture boil, making sure to wipe down the sides with a pastry brush. If one segment of sugar goes undissolved, it can ruin everything. As the simple syrup of sugar and water begins to thicken I swirl the pan. As it begins to brown I pay careful attention, as I only want a medium brown.

If it gets to dark, the sugar will become bitter. Once the onions are at a rich, caramel color, I add them to the pot on top of the chicken.

For the finale of this evening, at least for the dinner portion, I will prepare a Drambuie Crème Caramel. In a large skillet I make a simple syrup of three to four cups of sugar and 1 1/2 cups of water. While I bring that to a boil, I bring 3 cups of cold milk to a boil over medium high heat in a separate saucepan, boiling it just before it scalds.

Add the zest of one and half lemons and let sit for 15 minutes. I strain that through a Chinois (pronounced Shin-wa, a funnel shaped strainer) and let it cool at room temp. I gently stir in two and a half cups of sugar and set that aside. Whisking the 6 egg yolks only until they are broken, I then add a cup of the hot milk creation to temper the eggs so they are not shocked.

Once mixed, I slowly pour the rest of the milk mix into the egg yolks. I strain the entire mixture through the Chinois again, and then add one cup of raspberries and three quarters of a cup of Drambouie. Once the boiling simple syrup becomes a thick, medium brown color, I pour the syrup into each ramekin, about half an inch thick. I immediately pour in two tablespoons of Drambouie on top of the sugar, letting it temper for a moment. I transfer the egg yolk mixture to the individual ramekins that are set in a deep baking pan.

I fill the baking pan about three-quarters up with water and place the baking pan with the ramekins in a preheated 300 degree oven for about an hour, or once a fork can be placed into the yolk mixture coming out clean. When the Crème Caramel's are baked, I remove them from the oven, allowing them to reach room temperature and then refrigerate them.

When it comes time to serve, I place the needed ramekins in a bowl of warm water to activate the caramel on the bottom. Using a knife to remove the custard mixture by working my way around the edges, I place each on a separate shining white plate. I allow the caramel to drizzle from the bottom over the dessert. I place raspberries around the plate and voila, ready to serve.

AJ had no idea that I had planned the feast, so when she opened the door her eyes lit up at the aroma. I was on to the Stan Getz CD when she walked in, and she came right over to me as I was checking the Coq Au Vin. She put her arms around me and kissed me deeply.

She stopped the kiss for a second and looked around the kitchen and dining area with her eyes wide open. "What have you done my love?"

I smiled an adoring smile, "I couldn't help the urge to cook for you."

PARAMEDIC M.O.S.

No matter how many times I cook for her, I always find a new theme or way to present everything. Even if she knows what I planned on cooking, she is always amazed at what I create. I thought she was going to jump up and down like kids do when they see the ice cream truck coming.

I said to her, "Oh, you might want to check the bathroom, I think there is an avocado milk bath in there awaiting you. I think she just saw another ice cream truck. She kissed me again and said, "You really do take care of me like no one else can or will. I love you sweetie, and I will always look for ways to show you that. O YOU ARE GREAT!"

AJ gave me an intense kiss and then disappeared into the bedroom to disrobe. I stopped my cooking long enough to catch a glimpse of her tantalizing body. She caught me and using her finger, she motioned for me to come to her. Being a gentleman I had to oblige. She rested her body against mine, and I felt my entire soul melt in her arms.

Now I think I saw the ice cream truck. I placed the robe around her body, as she made for the bath. I was already showered, shaved and dressed casually. I wanted to hop in the bath with her, but I didn't want to set the kitchen on fire. When she emerged from the bath, she looked as she always did – radiant and smelling like a bed of roses. She walked right up to me with the most sincere smile and looked at me for a moment.

I took the look as amazement that I would take the time to make sure everything was right for her and for us. She moved closer as the next CD played a very sensual piece from David Sanborn and we just held each other. It helps that AJ understands and creates a safe place for me with the horrible feelings of my past. We just fell into each other and life has been different since.

After a fabulous meal and several games of Scrabble in front of AJ's fireplace, we turned on NYPD BLUE. Watching this was always exciting for some reason; perhaps it just made some sense of all the stupidity we saw everyday. Jennifer paged me about 10:00pm, asking me if I wanted to work overtime with her out of Jacobi Hospital (the north Bronx) the following morning. As I sat there on the couch watching TV with AJ, I reached for the cordless phone and hit the autodial to Jennifer's house.

She answered on the first ring, "So are you up for some fun tomorrow?" AJ looked at me and motioned to let her speak when we were done.

"Hey you, of course. What time is roll call?"

Jen started to giggle, "Actually we are the vacation relief unit tomorrow, and since we are tactical we start whenever we want and go wherever we want. Lt. Robertson said to just give him a buzz back to let him know when we want to have our bus all fueled and ready for play."

I looked at AJ and knew that she was working tomorrow, so I knew she wouldn't mind. "How 'bout we go in service at 10:00 hours. Meet you there around 09:30?"

"Great," Jennifer said, "I will call Robertson to let him know. If we are lucky, we can get over to Vincenzo's for a corner slice like old times."

I smiled at the thought that Jennifer still remembers our early academy days when we would drop into Vincenzo's on the corner of Willamsbridge and Morris Park Avenue, for the best Sicilian in the Bronx.

"Hold on one second," as I handed the phone to AJ.

"Hey babe!" AJ said.

Jennifer replied excitedly through the phone "Hey girl!" These two could talk forever. I was very glad that AJ had all of her stuff intact. Jennifer and I go back about seven years and although we were never intimately involved, we went through a lot together. AJ never tried to damage that.

After AJ and Jennifer put the final touches on our dinner date we were all planning over the weekend, she hung up the phone and nestled her body into mine on the couch. When the episode was over, I got up to hit the bathroom and she turned off everything in the living room. As AJ walked by the bathroom she knocked on the door and said "Don't drown in there." I smiled at her joke and went to brush my teeth.

As I walked into the bedroom, AJ was sitting up in bed with a book in her hands and her studious glasses on. She was wearing a dangerous black negligee that always made me drool, and she had prepared cups of chamomile tea for us both. I scooted in next to her, kissing her left shoulder. I felt her inhale deeply as my lips moved closer to her neck.

"You are making me lose concentration in my book," she said affectionately.

"How could I possibly be doing that?" I said softly.

As I finished my words, the book fell to the floor and our lips met.

I stopped for a second, "Oh, do you mean this?"

AJ smiled and laid her body over me as I slid into the bed. We examined each other's lips for a while, long enough for the cups of tea to cool slightly.

"You are dangerous," she said to me, as she reached for her tea. I did the same and we clinked our cups. Warmed by the heat of AJ's eyes, I finished my cup of tea in a good place. We turned out the light as I set

PARAMEDIC M.O.S.

the time on the alarm for 8:00am. We adjusted our bodies to one of our favorite sleeping positions, me on my back with AJ laying her right arm over me, tucking her head into my neck.

Morning came way too soon, and I found myself stepping into AJ's shower. That was an experience, sort of like a human car wash. There were jets everywhere and great smelling soaps and solutions all over the place. Today I even tried her Blueberry facial scrub. I figured since I like blueberries it couldn't be bad. After I got out and shaved in a steamed bathroom (better for the face that way), I looked on the counter and saw a basket of yet another group of body solutions. One of them was a peppermint foot lotion. I looked down and decided that my feet did not need to smell like candy canes.

I hopped on the Hutchinson River Parkway, just up from AJ's house and had an easy ride in. I turned off the Hutch at the Pelham Pkwy exit, which will put me right at Jacobi Hospital. Because of the way I came in, I would have to go up to Eastchester Road and make a u-turn into the Service Road, which will land me right at Jacobi's main entrance. I drove through the S turns and went past the ER bay; there were no rigs sitting there. Since Jacobi was the main trauma center, burn center, and replant center for this area, I was surprised. They usually have a large amount of patients on a regular basis, we usually bring in the ones in the worst condition. I went past the ER and made a left down the hill to our EMS Station.

I pulled in at 09:30am, and as I parked my truck, a black Saab parked right next to me. In it was a beautiful woman with Auburn hair, green eyes, striking features, and she happened to be named Jennifer. I hit the button to descend my passenger side window as she put her car in park.

She rolled down her window and said, "What's up there sweet cheeks?"

This was a nickname that AJ and Jennifer came up with for me, while were all on a white-water rafting trip together on the St. Lawrence River in Maine. I dove into the water for a swim and my shorts came off completely. They thought it was hysterical. I was hoping that I got to my shorts before some ill-fated creature underwater decided to get curious.

I smiled and said, "So nice of you to make it, come here often?"

She looked at me sheepishly and said, "Are you trying to pick me up?"

I stepped out of my truck and walked around to hers, and reaching in the back of her car to retrieve her lavender knapsack I said, "I would never do such a thing."

She stepped towards me and we hugged.

As we walked the dirt path that led to the blacktop near the station entrance she said to me, "I didn't see anyone up at the ER. It can't be that quiet."

As we approached the station, the station Captain, Juan Ramirez, appeared. Smiling and advancing his hand to me he remarked, "What are you two doing here?"

We all shook hands, "Just using up some of your overtime budget," I said with a smile. He rolled his eyes, "You know, too many people are calling in sick."

I shook my head, "I think that everyone is worried that we might all lose our jobs soon. Everyone is a little pissed off."

Juan looked at a unit that was pulling up to the gas pumps and said, "At this point, we really don't know where all of this is going. It is very premature, but that merger is being optioned in front of us and there is little that can be done if it goes through. Damnit we are too large of an entity to dissolve and we have worked too hard to establish what we have; you two know that most of all."

Jennifer and I looked at each other with concern. Patting the Captain on the arm I remarked optimistically. "Cap, we will do our jobs just the way we always have." He smiled his very disarming smile and replied in kind, "You two are always making us proud, thanks. You make my job easy, and you are not even from my station."

Jen and I headed for the garage to check in with the station lieutenant and sign for our narcs. I opened the door and held it for Jennifer as she walked right in.

Lieutenant Eileen Fray smiled when she saw Jen open the Narcotics cabinet with her keys as I replaced our portable radios with fresh batteries.

"You probably won't be doing much today," Eileen said, "it has been dead quiet all tour. Even when it rained earlier, most of the station units were 98 (available)."

I looked at Eileen with a look like I knew that the peace and quiet would not last for long since Jen and I were in.

"Well if you wanted it to remain that way, you should have called us up and told us not come in. You know we work!"

PARAMEDIC M.O.S.

Eileen answered her desk phone when it rang and informed the Borough Command that she was putting us in service at 10:00 hours. I guess someone didn't call the Borough earlier this morning to clue them in.

"You are in vehicle 958, it's a brand new bus," Eileen said as she threw the keys at me. "Don't wreck it. I don't know if you heard, but I gave the keys to a real wonder boy about two weeks ago. It was a brand new bus, #847, and for its maiden voyage he made a right turn onto Pelham Parkway, hit four cars and totaled the unit. It had just arrived here brand new two days before."

As I pulled the Lifepak cardiac monitor/defibrillator out of the opaque colored cabinet next to the Lieutenant's desk and put it through its automatic test I said, "Lu, don't worry about it, we got ya covered."

Eileen looked back up from her desk, "Yeah, that's what I am afraid of."

Jennifer and I walked outside to find the unit parked next to the building. It was definitely brand new and shiny. I pulled the bus up to the gas pumps to fill both tanks, as Jennifer started checking the rear of the vehicle. After topping off the tanks, I told Jen to hold on as I pulled the bus out of the gas area. I left the vehicle on, activating the lights and blipping the siren to make sure it all worked. I walked around the vehicle to make sure all of the flashing lights worked and watched the front light bar to make sure each bulb worked. I checked the wigwags, which are the flashing headlights to make sure they worked. Everything was good, and it was 09:50am. I turned the MDT on and signed into the unit so that the dispatcher would receive signals from our system and radios. Once I received the text message informing me that my computer sign on was received, I hit the 99 button to notify communications that we were available at the station. As soon as I hit the button, Gina, one of my favorite dispatchers called our unit designation for this overtime shift, 20X2.

"Twenty-Ray, good morning and welcome aboard, I have you in B3 area today, and we are so glad you could make it."

Smiling with Jennifer simultaneously, I picked up my portable radio out of my back pocket (we rarely used the holsters), "20X-Ray, Tactical X, thank you Bronx, and it is wonderful to be here."

Gina sent a message to our MDT saying hello and that things were quiet. Jennifer and I checked out our drug bags and endotracheal intubation kits. In service by 10:00 and we didn't have to attend an official roll call, we were out of the station by 10:20. It was a beautiful day out. We drove out of the Jacobi campus and onto the Pelham Parkway. Jennifer needed to pick up a few things at CVS, so we drove up towards Westchester Avenue.

This area of the north Bronx was extremely residential, with lots of different communities and people just the same. Westchester Avenue was a long block with the elevated subway # 1,2,3,9 lines. Cars drove underneath the subway platforms, which really sucked if someone got hit.

Jennifer and I had a patient here three months ago who was hit by the # 2 train enroute for Manhattan. After surviving the fall from four stories from being struck by a train, the gentleman actually landed in the path of an oncoming truck on Westchester Avenue. It was a pretty gruesome scene, as the truck was going faster than he should have. There were parts for about three blocks. In fact, I passed one of the legs until we realized parts of this guy's body actual ended up in a garbage pile on the sidewalk. "Remember that guy we had here," and as the words left her mouth I made a grimacing face. Jennifer gave me her smart-alec face and said, "Maybe next time you could stop when you see a leg."

I looked in her direction, "Oh yeah, a lot of help you were co-pilot."

Then we heard it over our radio's, "23(D)avid, ten thirteen, ten thirteen, 2301 Coop City Blvd in front!"

The message was broken up, but this crew was definitely in trouble. A 10-13 is a life-threatening emergency, where the crew is about to be badly hurt or has already been. It is a last call for help and the one thing you hope never to have to hear or worse, to say. When Jennifer heard it she immediately pulled up the unit's information on our screen so she could see what kind of a job they were on. She also knew to hold on as I take 10-13's very seriously, we all do. In one full swoop I hit the switches for the lights, threw on the siren, real, real loud and pulled a no point U-turn in the middle of Westchester Avenue (which is considered virtually impossible by most), heading for Pelham Parkway.

Gina made an announcement on the air, "Units, 23David calling a 10-13, 2301 Coop City Blvd, off Pelham Parkway, first units onscene give a 12 (situation report).

Before I could even raise my radio to tell Gina that we were enroute, my computer showed us enroute. Gina knows how we work and she knew we were already supersonic. I took Westchester to Pelham and made a vicious right against a red light on two wheels, bringing all kinds of traffic to a halt. As I pulled the corner I saw four NYPD precinct units com-

PARAMEDIC M.O.S.

ing up fast behind me. I was bigger and I was going to blow a hole right through traffic. I think New Yorkers know when it's one of ours in trouble, we drive more aggressively and in a fashion where they knew that we are not going to stop. I must have been doing 75 MPH on Pelham Parkway as Jennifer was listening to the garbled radio traffic on the NYPD precinct frequency.

As I approached the entrance to Jacobi off to my right, at what must have been the speed of light, I saw three additional ambulances shoot off the ramp in response to the 10-13 radio call, followed by two 4X4 Jimmy's (Supervisor's vehicles) and even two Caprice Classics (Chief's). By the time all of the units got back on all four wheels and centered themselves in the middle of the Pelham Parkway Jen and I would be far ahead of them.

Jennifer and I shot over the Hutch overpass and we heard it again, "Central 10-13, 23 David , he's got a gun and we are getting our asses kicked!"

I clenched my teeth as I felt my heart sink.

"WE HAVE TO GET THERE," I thought to myself. I could picture these scenes having responded to many and having had to call a few myself. It has to be your worst fear. Here you are, 911 and you have to call an emergency. Traffic came to a halt, so without even blinking I shot the vehicle up onto the sidewalk and took out what I think were a few parking meters and then made a left into Coop City. I saw the crew's ambulance, and both members involved in a viscous fight.

Their original call at Coop City was for an EDP (Emotionally Disturbed Person), and from what I saw I guess they found their patient. I came to a screeching halt as a combination of about fifteen various NYPD precinct cars, ESU units and ambulances pulled up simultaneously. NYPD went for their weapons and I had a perfect body shot to take this guy out. He cold clocked one of the EMT's for the last time. As he turned around to meet me, he swung directly for my chest. Bad move since I had a bulletproof vest on with a metal shock plate in the middle of the sternum. I heard about three fingers break when his fist connected with my vest, and he grimaced in pain. I spun him around and forced him to the ground as sixteen pairs of handcuffs appeared in front of my face to lock him up, compliments of the wonderful officers of the NYPD.

In situations like this, whoever gets the person to the ground first, whether it is one of us or the NYPD, cuffs him or her. Since medics didn't carry handcuffs, NYPD never minded throwing theirs to us. Now that this guy was neutralized and screaming bloody murder, I did a quick check of his sides, underarms, and then right around his stomach I felt it. It felt small enough to be a revolver and I was guessing a 38 caliber. I said out loud "I gotta gun," and about eight officers piled on top with the orchestration of an NFL blitz and the impact of a WWF Smackdown.

While the officers were rolling around on the ground with the EDP/suspect, I slipped out with the gun and handed it to an ESU member. I informed Gina that the scene was secured, but the crew would be checked out, and a boss was assuming command of the scene.

The entire block was lit up with emergency vehicles everywhere. One BLS unit took the EDP with a police escort to Jacobi, while I walked over to the crew who were both sitting on the curb looking like they both just went two rounds with Tyson. Their faces had some marks and bruises, and their uniforms were torn to shreds. It actually reminded me of the aftermath of our union meetings. They said they were fine, just shaken up.

Apparently when they arrived here for the call, this guy who was actually the EDP flagged them down acting as if he was the person who phoned 911. He pulled the gun on the passenger, and then put it back in his waist. The crew engaged him in an effort to hold him there until PD arrived, but they didn't know that their MDT was malfunctioning when they punched the emergency button. The signal never notified the dispatcher that they were in trouble. They exited the vehicle and the slugging began. They tried to get him down and that was a bad move. One of the partners got smart and put out a radio call.

Since units were tending to the crew, I walked to Jennifer as she came towards me. With frightened confidence and a smile, she asked, "Are you okay?" I stepped up inside the truck to adjust my uniform, "Yeah, I am just glad that didn't go any further, he was pretty strong."

I stepped up in the unit and Jen closed the doors behind me; once I adjusted my uniform back to normal I stepped out. "You really knocked him down, where did you learn that move," Jennifer asked me.

I knocked on my bulletproof vest and said, "Grammar school, my dear!"

I saluted the patrol Supervisor that meant to him that we were going back into service. I hit the 97 key on the MDT and Gina thanked us for our quick response. It was now about 11:30am, perfect time for a slice at Vincenzo's. I drove back up the Pelham Parkway, and hooked a left onto Williamsbridge Road. Once I approached the second light, I made a U-

PARAMEDIC M.O.S.

turn as Vincenzo's was on our right. There was a space big enough to fit the rig in, which was rare.

We walked in together and there was Eddie, our pizza man.

"Well look what the cat dragged in," Eddie said to me.

He walked around the counter and approached Jennifer; the two of them hugged. Eddie secretly had a major thing for Jennifer, but the fact that he was married and not her type kind of discounted him from possible endeavors. Eddie and I shook hands and he returned to the counter.

"What'll it be today, two corner slices?" Jennifer smiled her electric smile as Eddie dropped an entire pizza dough he was spinning in the air. Like AJ, I have actually watched accidents occur while men have watched Jennifer. Eddie picked the dough up off the floor, tossed it out and washed his hands; and then took out a fresh Sicilian pie out of the oven. I never ate anything this heavy on duty, but this was a treat to be with my favorite partner on overtime on a beautiful day. We got our slices and sat down against the window. The glare from our shiny new vehicle was so intense that we had to move so I didn't have to put my sunglasses on.

"Tell me a story," Jennifer said to me as she took a bite of her Sicilian.

There was something strange in the way she said it. It was something that I hadn't seen in her before; as if she was asking me to explain the meaning of life and why life is so hard. It was the strangest thing.

I said to her with a smile but a concerned look, "What do you mean?" As I said the words, we heard 25C(harlie) get a difficulty breather not too far away. I was almost sure we would have to take the call with them, but as I began to reach for my radio, 23Willy came up and responded with the BLS.

I focused my eyes back on Jennifer as she said to me, "I mean, tell me a love story. How did AJ end up to be so lucky to have you in her life?"

Something about her question seemed like she was asking from a place where she was upset that she no longer had Billy, her former boyfriend.

"You know Jen-Jen, I don't really know. You know my past history with my ex-fiancé. That silly bitch would drive anyone crazy. In fact if she is following the same regimen when I found out she was cheating, guys are getting more mileage out of her then a Goodyear tire. As for AJ, I didn't even think I was ready, but I guess the combination of being who I am and who she is, and the fact that she wanted someone who was totally a stand up person had a lot to do with it. Are you okay?"

She kind of stopped chewing and had this glazed look in her eyes. I thought to myself, is this why she wanted to work together today? Was it because she wanted some time to chat? She wanted to feel comfortable?

"I'm okay, I am just pissed about Billy. Last night I lay in bed all alone and it just felt weird. I will never forgive him for sleeping with my sister months before my wedding, nor will I forgive my sister. I can't believe I didn't know that he was using again."

I sat there with this desire to reach out and hold Jennifer. Jennifer began seeing this idiot Billy several year's ago when he had just come off of drugs, and I guess that she wanted to save him. Here she is, warm, sensitive, loving, drop-dead gorgeous and dependable. He was a waste. I sensed something about him when they began dating, but I couldn't put my radar on it.

He was a financier for some large investment-banking firm, and they met while she was shopping. He treated her well at first, taking her everywhere on vacations, and he did buy her quite a bit of stuff. She never had much in her life, and both AJ & I became suspect of his generosity. When she told me she suspected he was sleeping with someone else, I had a foul sense that something was up too. I called a friend who works for a governmental agency to check him out. It appeared that Jennifer's friend Billy was arrested several times on possession, once with intent to sell, and once for assault in a domestic matter. He was never forthcoming about his past, even after she had asked him if was ever in trouble with the law.

I gave her a call one night and we met at my place. I broke the news to her slowly and presented her with the rap sheet. She was in absolute shock. She revealed to me that night that she had just found out that he was sleeping with her sister. I felt a wave of dread come over me when she shared that information with me. Jennifer wanted only to trust and love. I always had this funky feeling that some other bad stuff happened to her in her younger years, but I could never put my finger on it and she never mentioned it; it was more of a sixth sense. I could have literally beaten this guy to a state of unconsciousness when she called me for help the night that she told him it was over.

She had walked into her apartment, not even his but her own home, and he had her sister in her bed. I was just about to leave the station when I got her page. I remembered she was crying hysterically when I called, and it took me way too long to calm her down. I raced out of the station

PARAMEDIC M.O.S.

still in uniform to her place in Brooklyn. I called AJ and told her what happened; I thought she was going to pass out. When I got to Jennifer's apartment, she buzzed me in from downstairs. When I got to the door I heard her crying in the apartment and a male voice speaking. No one was coming to the door. I knocked again and a male voice said, "Go the fuck away, we are talking here."

I closed my fist and hit the door so hard, the entire hallway reverberated.

"Billy, open this fucking door or so help you God when I kick it in your ass belongs to me!"

I heard a smack and Jennifer whimper even louder and then I stepped back and kicked with all my might as the door came right off of its hinges. Billy had a very tight and what appeared to be a painful grip on Jennifer's arm. When the door fell in, Billy looked at me in amazement, as did Jen.

"Let go of her now," I said approaching Billy. He tried to swing at me with his right arm, since he was holding her with his left. His swing was way off base and I cold clocked him with a right hook. My connection was powerful enough to make him let go of Jennifer as his knees buckled. Jennifer backed up behind me as Billy approached and came back for more.

"Billy, stop while you are ahead; you are no match for me and you are about to lose teeth." Billy tried an upper cut and missed, leaving me in perfect striking position to lay him out, so I did. Since his body was already in a frozen motion as his upper cut completed, I came from up high and went bulls-eye across his jaw with my right fist. Three teeth flew out with blood spraying all over the floor. Billy was now on his knees. "You come at me again Billy and you'll be getting a cat-scan in about an hour."

Billy sat on his knees crying about his teeth while I picked up Jen's phone and called the NYPD. Telling them what took place and that it was a M.O.S., they were there before I even hung up the phone. Jennifer pressed charges against him for aggravated assault, assault and battery, and a few other things that the D.A. threw in the pot. Billy wanted to press charges against me for his newly acquired dental work, but the bruises he left on Jennifer's arm and the hand print on her face cleared me from any misgivings.

I went downstairs, woke up the superintendent and informed him that the door needed to be corrected immediately. He was a little wishy-washy, so I put Jennifer in my car and I gave him $100.00 to secure the door right there.

C.B. Garris

I called AJ to let her know that I was bringing Jennifer over and she said she would get the extra bedroom set up. Jennifer cried all the way to AJ's, looking out the window most of that time. At some point she reached out for my hand and squeezed it hard. Crying very hard she thanked me for being there for her. It took about an hour to get to AJ's from Brooklyn, and by then Jennifer's tears turned from sniffles to slumber. AJ was waiting up for us when we got home. She opened the front door and stepped out to greet us, and she saw that Jennifer was asleep on the passenger side.

As I went to exit my truck AJ commented to me, "You are such a gentleman."

As I started to round the corner of the truck I looked over at AJ, "I am a gentleman all right, and one that is apparently capable of removing teeth."

AJ knew from the sounds of that, she knew that I must have clocked Billy, and that I would tell her about it when we got to bed. I stuck my hand through the window of my truck, holding Jennifer's head up as I opened the door. I then scooped her entire body up, as she woke up briefly. She looked at me with her puppy eyes that were still puffy from crying. She was actually somewhat dazed, and just did what I wanted her to do, to relax and rest her head against my neck, wrapping her arms around me as I carried her inside.

AJ closed the door to my truck and we went in. AJ had already made a pot of Lemon Zinger tea, and sliced some cucumbers for Jennifer to put over her eyes when she was ready. The cold cucumber slices take down swelling. I called Chief Battieri and informed her what happened and she put her out of work on emergency leave for three days to rest. That is a day that I am sure the two of us will hold in our minds forever.

As I began to take a vulgar bite of my Sicilian slice, a dispatcher's voice called us, "Twenty X please, two zero X."

As Jen reached for her radio, I began wrapping our food up.

"Tac - Xray," Jennifer answered.

As I turned the vehicle on, the job hit our screen for an unknown medical condition on Morris Park Avenue. The call had almost no information in it, as we headed for the assignment just a few blocks away from Vincenzo's. As we pulled up the dispatcher notified us that he thinks this is now an elderly person with chest pain. We arrived at a typical two story wood frame dwelling for this neighborhood.

It appeared as though the house could have been a duplex. I radioed to our dispatcher to inquire if there was an apartment, and he informed

PARAMEDIC M.O.S.

me that the patient was supposed to be in the basement. Unless the person is home alone, generally right about now is when someone will come out of the house screaming that the person is upstairs and not breathing. This state of hysteria generally results in a patient who is relatively fine, but the family lost their heads. No one was coming outside.

Jennifer and I grabbed our gear for this call and approached the house. I took out my flashlight and stepped to the left of the door as Jennifer stepped to the right. I banged on the door and got no answer. I heard what sounded to be a television faintly in the background.

I looked at Jennifer and said, "I don't like this." Jennifer and I locked eyes knowing what each was thinking.

As I banged on the door again, Jennifer picked up her radio and called for a BLS back up (Basic Life Support assistance) and for NYPD to respond in case we found a crime scene. We were both thinking this was going to be a homicide. I turned the knob to the door and it opened, another bad sign. Although it was bright as the sun outside, this apartment was poorly lit, causing us both to use our flashlights. I could hear the television far in the rear of the apartment, which must have been at least thirty feet away from us. That may seem like a short distance, but when you are totally unaware of what you are facing in that dark room you are about to enter, thirty feet is three miles. I called into the room to see if anyone answered. A faint, raspy voice spoke from the area of the television.

"Sir, did you call 911 for an ambulance?" I said out loud.

The voice was vaguely discernible and said, "Yeah, I did." At least we know someone was in there. As I stepped into the apartment, there was garbage, boxes and newspapers everywhere. This crap was literally almost waist deep. I kept calling to the person thirty feet ahead as we walked in. Jen and I looked at each other like we just stumbled on a smelly landfill. As I stepped in I kicked something on the floor that I couldn't see, and it felt like a pipe. It caused me to lurch forward, but I kept my balance. Once Jennifer knew I was okay she laughed at me.

"Watch your step Cinderella," she said facetiously.

I got about five to six feet into the rubble and I could have sworn something on the floor moved. I stopped my motion to look at Jennifer to see if it matched up with her foot motions; it didn't.

I asked Jen, "Did you hear that?"

She looked at me and said, "Hear what?"

I raised my eyebrows and kept moving forward. I kept wondering where our back up was. I stepped about another three feet in and something on the floor moved and made a noise like moving newspaper. It wasn't my feet, and it definitely wasn't Jennifer. Jennifer was behind me the entire time, and this movement came from the perimeter of the wall. Jen stopped and grabbed my bicep, "What the fuck was that?" I was thinking quickly, mainly concerned with Jen's safety as well as mine. I was still at least ten to twelve feet from the patient.

"Sir, do you have any pets?" I asked loudly.

Sir replied back in a scratchy voice, "No!"

Once again, I heard that newspaper sound, and I felt something brush my feet. Just as I felt that movement on my feet, I flashed my light towards the far end of the room where I saw a very long and thin cage.

"O fuck!" I said loud enough for Jen to hear.

Jen felt my body stiffen up and she said, "What is it?"

I turned slowly and said to Jennifer, "I want you to turn around and on three run for that front door, I think there is a massive snake at our feet."

As I began to count to three, Jen's eyes lit up and when I hit three she B-lined for the front door with me in tow.

As we came scrambling out of the front door, our BLS pulled up along with two NYPD sector cars. They were exiting their vehicles casually at first until they saw us bolting out of the front door. The medics went into Tae Kwan Do stances, and four officers reached for their service weapons.

The officers ran over and said, "What's going on?"

I put down my drug bag and said "You better get ESU over here and put a forthwith on them. I think there is a mammoth snake loose in that basement apartment, and the patient is still in there."

One of the officers, who I knew from previous calls when I used to work this area training students, had a bug up his ass for medics. I think either he dated one and it didn't go well, or he wanted to date one and it still didn't go well. He was as big as an oak tree, standing 6'6" at about 285 lbs.

He walked over to me and said, "You EMS whimp, there ain't no snake in that apartment. You probably just kicked a cat. Let me show you how a real man deals with this."

I smiled and gestured as if I was rolling out the red carpet for him.

"Man, the apartment is all yours, but I would be real careful if I were you."

PARAMEDIC M.O.S.

The officer sucked his teeth and strutted towards the apartment like Vinny Barbarino. You know the strut: I have eighteen inches of penis and the attitude to go with it. Meanwhile, his partner called for a sergeant and ESU to respond for a loose reptile. Well, off our wonderful officer went, entering the structure and disappearing from sight.

About thirty seconds later we heard, "Oh Shit!"

A series of semi-automatic gunfire followed, I think I counted eleven shots discharged. Springing from the door was Officer Attitude, who ran right up to us saying, "Holy shit man, that thing is huge."

I looked at the officer and smiled. "Doesn't bother me," my smile now gleaming, "I'm already out here. I just hope that none of your eleven shots struck our patient who is or maybe was still alive in there."

Due to the weapons discharge, this scene was about to turn into a fiasco. It would be the Patrol Sergeant, the Precinct Lieutenant, maybe even a Captain and an Inspector too. I called for our patrol supervisor, just to make the gathering equal and complete.

When ESU pulled up a few minutes later, they suited up and went in with the shuffleboard sticks. About 6 minutes later they appeared with an eighteen-foot anaconda wrapped up in the sticks.

Turns out that the snake was property of the son, who went away on vacation for a few days, leaving the anaconda too little food. When the snake got hungry, he slithered out of the cage towards the father's room in the basement. ESU said that he was what I first kicked when I tripped originally and he was as I heard him, around the entire perimeter on the room. While ESU removed the reptile to the Bronx Zoo, Jennifer, myself, a BLS crew I never met before and six heavily armed NYPD ESU officers returned to the basement. We trudged back through all of the garbage, and I was hoping that there was only one snake. Luck came our way, there was only one.

Our patient, a seventy eight year old man was sitting uncomfortably in a large recliner. He must have no idea that he was about to become a feast for the snake, so said the handlers at the Bronx Zoo hours later. Our patient's name was George, and he said he wasn't feeling well. He had no specific complaint, except that he didn't feel right. He had an extensive medical history including congestive heart failure, diabetes and renal (kidney) dysfunction. These three disorders commonly go together. The diabetes breaks down the kidneys, the fluid from the failing kidneys back up into the blood stream with toxin; and the cells become over saturated unable to flush. The combination of extra fluid and toxins invade the heart's ability to pump causing systemic (multi-organ) failure.

With George's history and his asymptomatic (without symptoms) complaint, both Jennifer and I were convinced this was going to be a serious medical call. It was just a gut feeling. You hope that you are wrong, but you prioritize by ruling out the worst and working backwards. George was about 5'6, a tad bit overweight, with flaccid skin, that was flushed and temperate, and he seemed a tad bit slow in his responses. His lack of response seemed to be accompanied by an obvious stupor; perhaps it was a lack of sugar.

He was very agreeable to treatment as we set him up on the monitor and high concentration oxygen. As I set up to pop a line in his left arm, I looked at his EKG, which was not good. He had faint ronchi sounds (those rice krispie type sounds) in his lungs and he exhibited peaked T waves and widening of his QRS complex's on his EKG, which strongly suggested to us that he had an elevated potassium level.

Since George had so many issues going on, I called telemetry to cover our asses. Jennifer and I had already both decided on at least .5 mg of Atropine intravenous to raise his heart rate, and one amp of dextrose to get his sugar level up, hopefully correcting his mental status. If we could correct his sugars and pulse, we may have a whole new patient in a few minutes. He did also exhibit pedal edema (swelling at the feet and ankles), and that concerned us but let us know that we were probably dealing with right sided heart failure, the lesser of the two evils.

After speaking with Dr. Wimert at EMS headquarters, he concurred with our choice of treatment. Jennifer dropped the half-milligram of Atropine down first, and waiting for about a minute after flushing the IV, she followed with an amp of Dextrose, 40 mg of Lasix, and 2 mg of Morphine. Within a matter of minutes, George was like a spring chicken. He wanted to know why there were so many uniformed people in his house, and where was Tiny. I figured Tiny was his son.

Wrong! Tiny was the anaconda; I should have known. Now that George was awake and with it, he wanted to stay at home and wait for his dialysis (blood cleaning treatment for patients with kidney disease) two days following. Jennifer and I both explained that it was better if we transport him to find out what was going on, coupled by the fact that no one was there to watch him. NYPD was trying to track down the son's travel agent in the meantime.

PARAMEDIC M.O.S.

I asked George if he remembered his early morning routine, which he did. He informed us that aside from his dialysis treatments and normal visits to his physicians, he had not had any other medical care issues in twenty years. He denied ever being picked up by ambulance or going to an emergency room. I called communications and had them run a history on the address, and he was telling the truth; EMS had no other calls there at least in the last year. What caused George to deteriorate so rapidly was really puzzling both Jennifer and I, so we decided I would check George's bathroom and kitchen for anything out of the ordinary. Jen helped package George for transport with the help of the other crew, while I checked out the house.

I looked in the medicine cabinet and found nothing but the medicines he informed us he was taking. I looked at each one and calculated in my head how many of each should have been taken times the date the prescription was filled. Everything was a perfect match.

I walked to the kitchen and looked around, seeing nothing but kitchen stuff. I opened the refrigerator, moving things around the shelves I found the culprit. I took a huge ceramic bowl out of the fridge, and it contained what was left of the stems grapes come from. Grapes contain large amounts of potassium, and they can be the nemesis of a patient suffering from kidney disease. High amounts of potassium, particularly in acute doses can cause the kidneys to shut down and result in systemic multi-organ failure.

I walked back in the room as the last seat belts were strapped onto George as he sat on the stair chair (a chair like device we use to maneuver and carry patient's with in close quarters). Bowl in hand I looked at George and smiled. Jennifer looked at me with that "What are you grinning at" look, while the cops were lost.

I knelt down to George and said, "George, what exactly did you eat for breakfast this morning?"

George gave me a roll of the eyes and a smile. He knew he got busted.

George put his hand on my forearm, "I couldn't help myself, I love green grapes and I had to have them."

I nodded my head with a smile asking "George, exactly how much of this bowl did you eat?"

George looked at me slowly like a puppy that knew that he did something wrong and said, "All of it."

Jennifer's jaw dropped as did mine. That should have killed him. For whatever reason, perhaps rapid intervention, George was safe, but he definitely would need a cardiac workup and a serious dialysis at the hospital. As we wheeled George out, I threw the IV bags over my right shoulder so that I could lift the chair.

George had this huge grin on his face like he got to have his cake and eat it too, which in fact, because we got to him in time, he did. Jen and I sat in the back of the bus with him, and he had us laughing all the way to the hospital. He told us a story of his past and how when he was a kid, how he used to play jokes on the other kids, and his favorite pastime, stickball on Bathgate Avenue.

He was proud of his childhood, and he was proud of himself now. George was now 78, and a joy to be around. I was actually very pissed that his son was so irresponsible to leave him alone. As we wheeled him into the ER, Jennifer smiled and it was a smile that I had seen a thousand times before.

It was a sense of comfort and confidence. We loved working with each other, and now that I knew there was something going on internally in her, perhaps it was comfort that things are going to be okay. My internal alarm was sounding, but I had to figure out how to get whatever was concerning me out of Jennifer. She kept saying that everything was fine lately despite the fact that we had just lost more than eight members of the service to accidents, a heart attack, a bunch of suicides, and one of them in a climbing accident.

Andy was about two thousand feet up when he got hit by a really hard wind according to his climbing mates. He lost his grip and went straight down the mountain. Two days later, Francis Jurio was found hanging in his apartment by his children, when they came home from school. Last week Tony had his heart attack. Weeks earlier, Michael Runowski had a motorcycle accident which decapitated him. Another one of our medics committed suicide by overdosing on tranquilizers.

After awhile, all of these deaths of co-workers start to blend into one big mess. These incidents took place over a four-week period and really shook the agency. We were getting tired of heading into work to find Critical Incident Stress Debriefing counselors waiting for us. You know that when you pull up to your station and see the counselors standing outside, that it is going to be a real bad day. Since Francis and Tony were from our medic class, it hit home really hard. When we finished with our patient, we went down to the station to restock a few things.

PARAMEDIC M.O.S.

As we pulled up we saw the counselors outside waiting for the incoming tour. Jen and I looked at each other as my internal alarms went off again. I didn't even want to drive into the station. I knew someone else was dead, but I didn't know who, and for that matter I was glad that Jen was next to me. I pulled up and one of the counselors was standing by the side of the building smoking a cigarette. He looked in my direction and recognized me right away.

"Hello Christian." Victor Bifroet said to me.

I looked at him with anger and he knew it.

"Who now?" Victor reluctantly walked over to me. "Chris, why don't you just come inside," as I cut his words off.

"Damnit Victor, don't fucking patronize me, who is dead now?" I said keeping my distance from Victor.

"Chris & Jen I'm sorry, it's Tanya Dubouis, she was the victim of a homicide last night. According to the detectives, one of her ex-boyfriends, a construction worker who lived in Bridgeport, Connecticut showed up at her apartment with a weapon. She begged for him to leave and as neighbors were calling 911, he shot her in the head several times."

I looked at Victor for a long while and then slammed my closed fist on the hood of the bus. Jen just stood there and began to cry. I walked over to Jennifer and put my arms around her, enveloping her as she let her body sink into mine. Tanya was also from our medic class, and that would be nine dead in five weeks. I closed my arms tightly around Jennifer, and she placed her arms around me. Tears started to run down my face, as Victor asked us to walk inside.

I reached into the vehicle and hit the 99 button (available at the station) on the computer and we walked inside. All of Tour 3 was corralled and accounted for. No one except Jen and I heard the news. Danny Newfell saw Jen and me in tears. Now he knew that this was really bad. He looked at me questionably, his eyes asked me who was it that they were all about to hear about, and I just swung my head slowly from side to side. He knew that it had to come from the CISD counselors.

Victor and his team began with their deepest apologies to have to tell everyone this, and then they laid it on everyone. Four of the girls at the station started bawling, while two of the male medics walked out of the room. There was a huge crash, and I ran out with Jen. One of those medics picked up his locker and threw it through the station office window in frustration. CISD team members ran after him as he was now running as fast as he could toward the Pelham Parkway. Paulina Keritil, a medic who I trained years ago, walked to me crying hysterically and put her arms around me. I sat her down and placed my arms around both Jen and Paulina.

There was an angry silence about the room and it was a horrible silence I was getting too familiar with. We all see death and destruction every day, and we are now facing the ninth of our own going down. We know better than anyone how horrible it is to face death since we see it every day. Some days are more merciful about it than others, and some days just down right suck. It is one thing to get to the home of an elderly patient who has lived a full life, say 92 or 93 years old. We know that at some point the body wants to rest forever. We still hate to have to pronounce the patient or work them up knowing that this is probably not going to work.

It is another thing to be the first medic at the scene of a child murdered by one or both of its parents, beaten to death with absolute malice. It is even worse to be the medic who finds a baby near death from the parent who burned it in scalding hot water, or threw it across the room into a wall when the crying got too much.

We see these things everyday, some days we can beat death, and some days we can't. We know how explosive a situation can get in milliseconds and that horrible feeling that goes through our minds of, "is this the end?"

Another medic was outside pounding on the side of an ambulance.

"I'm getting tired of coming into this fucking place and finding my friends dead. Fuck this place."

He began to punch that ambulance until he broke two fingers and his wrist. He was a large fellow and CISD decided to let him get the anger out.

"John, JOHN," I yelled at him to snap him out of it. "I can see that your wrist is broken, STOP!"

John stopped and looked at me like he was going to leap in my direction. He took a deep breath as his eyes grew wide and then he collapsed to the ground. Three members of the CISD team, Jen and I ran over to him. He was awake, but completely traumatized. He used to date Tanya and although things did not work out, they remained best friends.

He was whisked away upstairs to the ER up the ramp.

Paulina went to the bathroom with Jessica Landy watching out for her, and I wrapped my arms around Jennifer. Again we stood there in silence,

PARAMEDIC M.O.S.

not really knowing how to be, except just being there for each other. Jen was crying extra hard now, and I wish there was some way I could stop her pain. Her mother committed suicide when she was seventeen, while Jennifer was in the house. Jennifer heard the shot while she was getting ready for school one morning. I know she never got over that.

"Do you want to go out of service for awhile?" I asked Jen quietly

"No," Jen said as she sniffled. "In fact, let's just get the hell get outta here, I need to get the hell outta here. CISD is here, they will take care of everyone."

"You got it," I said as we both wiped our faces and walked towards our bus.

The entire station was scattered, as people were crying in corners, some got in their units and went right into service. This was a really bad day.

What happened to those who died could have happened to any of us. We witnessed horrible encounters of death and destruction every day, and somewhere deep inside we hope it is not one of our own. It was wearing on all of us though, and we would all go through our own hell.

C.B. Garris

Chapter XVI:

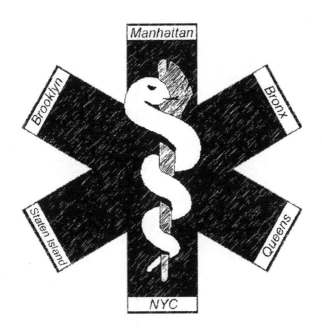

PARAMEDIC M.O.S.

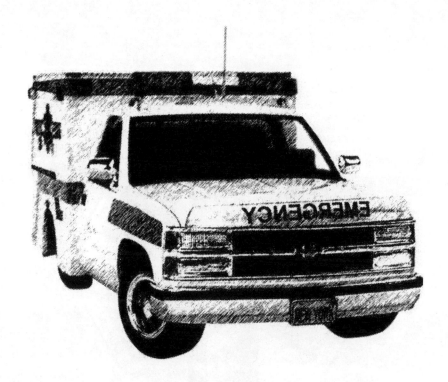

C.B. Garris

We were driving along Pelham Parkway when the assignment came over the radio. "Twenty X-ray for the trauma." Jen quietly answered, "20X go," almost as Jen let go of the button the dispatcher kicked in with, "20X-ray, I'm getting numerous for several children struck by a car, Radcliff and Morris Park Avenue. I'm also getting these peds are possibly crushed against a wall at the location, I'll get you a BLS."

As the information was being delivered to us over the radio we were already in supersonic mode, flying past Jacobi with our lights and sirens blaring. The area was full of people leaving the hospital at the change shift. I heard the familiar two beeps, which meant that all of the pertinent information on the assignment was now on the screen of our mobile data terminal. I heard another beep, which was Jen depressing the 63 key, confirming our response. We made so much noise that everyone turned around to see what type of emergency vehicle was passing by. "X-ray," the dispatcher chimed in, "ESU on scene requesting a forthwith, they are confirming two pediatric likely at the location."

I sped up even faster.

"Benny," I said to our dispatcher after picking up the radio microphone, "get us another ALS unit if you got it also."

Generally we do not call each other by name, but Benny has been our dispatcher for years and he knows our vocal inflections. Benny knew that if I was calling him for another ALS unit and by the tone in my voice, that there was no time to dilly-dally and that I was dead serious.

"23Eddie, 20Adam and 23William for the back at Radcliff and Morris Park along with 20X already 63. Units, PD confirming a large crowd condition at the location and some type of ambulance at the location, now you have three patients." While taking Brady Avenue on two wheels with my left hand on the wheel and making all types of sounds with the siren with my right hand, I grabbed the radio and said to the dispatcher "Tactical X-ray, Benny we are about 30 seconds out? Is the bus (ambulance) one of ours?" Benny came back in his strong Jamaican accent, "Chris, I don't know, let me know. I don't have any other units there yet."

We approached the scene to find complete mayhem. Several large fights were in progress, PD units already on scene were calling for backup and the Task Force (which is essentially riot control) and we are trying to find the children in all of this. As I lock in on the reason we were called to the scene, the crowds of bloody fistfights sway back and forth like baseball

PARAMEDIC M.O.S.

spectators doing the wave after a home run. Jen and I looked at each other as if they just dropped the H-Bomb on the Bronx. We grabbed our equipment and without even having to say it, we agreed silently that when we find the kids, we will get them into the rigs as quick as possible.

Our only means of getting to the critically injured children was to join the crowd. After all, these are all adults that know better anyway than to be fighting like this so my remorse for any wounds I was about to inflict was of no consequence to me; my only concern was the two children. After I literally picked up two guys by the seat of their pants and the scruff of the back of their clothing, tossing them into the swaying crowd, I then had to self-defensively back-fist the owner of a massive arm that wrapped around my neck, by what seemed to be the largest human being I ever came into contact with in my life. When I shook him off of me and got Jen away from these idiots, we arrived to find several EMT's from a private ambulance service tending to the driver of the vehicle who appeared to be unharmed. We looked around the car and saw no sign of the children, until I get up to the front of the vehicle, which is stuck against a wall. After processing the scene I screamed, "Jen get up here!"

Jen approached to render the same look I did. I reached down for my radio and keyed the hand mike to say amid the noise in the crowd, "20X, 20X, we got two peds, major trauma pinned against the wall. Call Jacobi and let them know we will be bringing them both in. We will give notifications when we are rolling!" I heard Benny's reply, "10-4 Chris, I'm on the landline now". I immediately checked the pulse on one, there was none. Jen told me that the female patient she found had a faint pulse.

I told one of the ESU cops to clear the area around the car and stabilize it. An NYPD Task Force of about forty combat-ready officers moved in and started clearing a path for us to work. Everyone scattered and it bought us some time. ESU stabilized the car while I set up to board and collar the child with the BLS crew from 20Adam.

My patient, the boy, was all of about six years old and he was in full traumatic arrest. Jen's patient, the girl, was about eight and she was barely clinging to life. Both were pinned against the wall at the abdomen, and we knew that when ESU moved the car, that would pretty much be it. The car was acting like a blood pressure cuff to them both. There was blood everywhere, and we could not tell who lost more.

Once we had the best cervical stabilization we could manage in that position, ESU moved the car simultaneously so as to move both children

C.B. Garris

together. I took mine down with the crew of 20(A)dam, while Jen worked on hers with the crew of 23(E)ddie. While the BLS crewmembers got both kids packaged, Jen and I intubated both children right there on the sidewalk. Both tubes were difficult, as much of their stomach contents came up just before intubation. We suctioned them and got patent (good) tubes in place.

At this point, ventilating them was the most important thing we could do for them. They would be headed right for trauma surgery as soon as we made it to Jacobi; at least I hope they would.

As we finished packaging our respective patients, there was screaming all around. I could not see Jennifer within the crowd as we split up to separate ambulances for transport. I was worried about her and her state of mind. We just left the station where all hell had broken loose, and now we were in this situation.

Jen boarded 23(E)ddie's bus, and there were no other ALS units on scene, so we transported. Enroute, Jen and I would follow our normal course of treatment. Because of the intensity of the trauma to both, we took 2 EMT's in the back of our rigs each. One would ventilate, one would do CPR compressions and Jen and I worked on initiating IV's and anything else our Prehospital Advanced Trauma Life Support protocols warranted. More units were pulling up as we were leaving. NYPD would be on scene getting that scene under control for some time, so the other units would take care of any other patients generated. I checked the pupils of my patient and they were open and fixed. As I established my third IV of Normal Saline to replace all the blood and fluid he lost, then inflating BP cuffs around two of the bags to get fluid in fast, I said silently "C'mon little man, come back to me."

While one EMT did compressions, I bagged and reached for my radio. "20X Priority," I said firmly as the dispatcher replied, "All units stand by. 20X go with it."

"20X enroute to Jacobi with an approximately 6 year old male, traumatic arrest secondary to being pinned by car against a wall. Major trauma to his chest and abdomen, he's tubed and three lines established; E.T.A. 3 minutes, my partner will have her notification next. "10-4 X," said Benny, our dispatcher. To ensure that no other unit stepped over her transmission, Benny continued right to Jennifer directly, "Jen C'mon with yours."

I knew Jennifer was monitoring and I heard Jennifer's voice as I was now pumping on the boy's chest feverishly.

PARAMEDIC M.O.S.

"Enroute to Jacobi with a 6 year old female, same mechanism of injury, unpalpable BP, a very faint pulse of 160, she's tubed, three lines, E.T.A. same!"

"X-ray, I got both notes. All units stand by," our beloved dispatcher replied instantly.

The wolves of Jacobi's Trauma team were waiting for us anxiously. Before the EMT's driving both units got the vehicle's to complete stops in the ER bay, the lead trauma surgeon jumped on the back step of the bus, opening the rear doors. There would be no talking other than what had to be said. There would be no "hello's", no "how ya doing's," nothing but the acknowledgement of this situation and the transference of information from one professional to another.

We moved both children out of our rigs as the trauma teams tried to assess where all our IV's were placed and exactly how bad the bodies were damaged. The doors to the ER were open and waiting as we hooked a quick right, bypassing the ER for the elevators to the Trauma Operating Rooms. The ER staff that was not tending to patients stood by the ER doors. They watched in silence, knowing how terrible this looked and may end up. The crowd that occupied the waiting room saw all of this commotion and heard all the sirens coming in. They watched, they stared; they covered their mouths.

Jen and I briefed the trauma teams on our respective patients, only to meet backing out of our trauma slots. I looked at Jen and she looked absolutely fragile. We knew that both children were in bad shape and their chances of survival were slim based on the extensive trauma their little bodies suffered. Jen looked at me as a tear rolled down her face, and even though we were both blood covered, I rested my back against the wall and let Jen fall into my arms. I tried to shield her face, but I know that would be impossible. This whole day had gone completely south. I knew that all of the recent deaths were getting to Jen, and Tanya's murder coupled with the trauma of these two fragile little children was getting too much. I eased her into the nurses lounge so that we could sit down.

"I'm fine," Jen said softly, as she wiped her tears with her upper shirt-sleeve and shoulder.

"This is nuts," she continued. "What the hell is going on? I don't even want to go back to the station."

I sat there for a moment and tried to collect my thoughts. "I know it seems like everything is getting out of hand. Everyone is tired and overworked, even though those that should won't admit it. I know that Tanya is a real whammy and this last call isn't great either." Jen let her head fall onto my shoulder.

"You guys alright?" I looked up and it was Charlene Turoe, one of our Captain's from the Bronx Command. "I just heard about Tanya."

Jen was whimpering on my shoulder as I just looked up at Charlene.

"You guys look a mess," Charlene said as she sat down opposite us.

"Don't tell me that you two just brought in those two kids?"

I looked at Charlene again out of the corner of my eyes.

"How much you got left on your tour?" Charlene asked concerned.

"We WERE OTP, so this is the last. I think we have both had enough for the night. When we get ourselves together in here, we are going to clean up, put that bus back together and call it a night." I said with complete firmness.

"I think that is a good idea," Charlene said in agreement. "You two take as much time as you need." With that she patted my knee as she stood up and made her exit.

Jen and I cleaned up as much as we could at the scrub sinks, mainly to get the blood off of us. We then re-gloved and went to the back of the bus to start putting our equipment back together. We were so drained that we didn't speak much, we just went about our duties.

PARAMEDIC M.O.S.

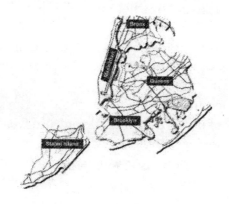

C.B. Garris

Chapter XVII:

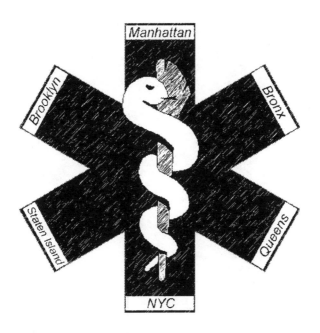

PARAMEDIC M.O.S.

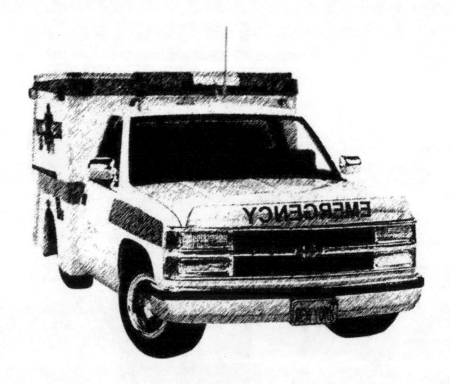

C.B. Garris

It was still the dark wee hours of the morning when my alphanumeric pager went off. Our agency pagers were programmed with two specific tones: a general page tone which let me know it was an agency notification, and then the other tone let me know that it was an internal agency emergency page only transmittable from the desk of the on-duty Watch Commander meaning something happened to someone, somehow connected to us.

Anytime I heard that page it always made my stomach sink; but nothing would prepare me for what I was about to hear. When I touched the button to illuminate the screen into its liquid crystal display green color, the message simply said 3611-TC Desk-911. I knew that 3611 was the shield number of Bob, the Tour One (midnight) Watch Commander, one of my best friends in the service. As the Tour 1 Watch Commander and one of my closest confidants, if he is waking me up with that page something horrible has just occurred.

I whipped up out of bed, putting my feet on the floor as I lifted the phone off the receiver without even looking at it. I immediately dialed the secured Watch Commander's 800 number, again without even looking at the phone. This number was imbedded in my skull early on in the service. Usually it was for me to make phone contact at the scene of a bomb job, where we cannot use our radios for fear of triggering an incendiary device. It was a scrambled-secured line that no one could breech. I would also use it only otherwise if a dignitary protection detail went south and I had bad news. AJ turned over as I whipped to the phone, observing me. Knowing that I moved that fast out of bed from her, something happened and it would be bad. AJ knew not to even bother asking me what was going on, as she would find out momentarily. She could see me breathing deep as the phone lines connected and it rang once. Bob picked up before the first ring even completed.

"Tour Commander." Bob said officially, though I knew he was expecting it to be me.

I heard the crackling of radios in the background and I noticed that the other background noise disappeared on Bob's end of the phone. This meant that he was closing his door for privacy. I took a deep breath and addressed Bob, "What happened?" I heard Bob inhale and I thought I was going to crawl out of my skin.

"Chris, I got to tell you something. I need you to hear me out and I need you awake."

PARAMEDIC M.O.S.

I was so scared now that I was dizzy. The light that AJ switched on next to her, lit the room up softly. Bob hadn't said that it was an emergency presidential detail, or that we had a major haz-mat job brewing. He didn't tell me that a major fire was underway somewhere with mayhem everywhere, and he didn't tell me that the city was in a riot. In fact, he still didn't say anything; somehow I knew this was personal. The thought of how personal this was about to get was making me choke.

"Chris," Bob said as I could hear he was fighting the need to tell me, "Is AJ there with you?"

"Bob, what the fuck is going on? And yes, she is." I snapped back in angered distress.

AJ reached over and put her hand on my right shoulder.

"Chris, I don't know how to tell you this, and there is no easy way to do this," Bob inhaled and I heard his voice crack. "Jennifer is dead."

I felt all kinds of doors in my mind shut. I didn't think I heard him right.

Speaking to Bob in an abrasive tone that I never had previously used with him, but for the matter at hand he was pretty much expecting from me, all that I could get out of my mouth in frustration was, "Bob, what the fuck are you talking about?"

AJ sat bolt upright and scooted across the bed right next to me onto my left side. She slipped her hand gently onto my right thigh to let me know she was there, without getting in my path of thought.

"Chris, it, it, it looks like a suicide." I know that Bob must have taken the phone away from his ear as soon as he said it.

In a distressful tone I said to Bob, "What do you mean suicide?"

"She uh," Bob began again, "NYPD Intel (NYPD Intelligence Division) says it appears as though she shot herself in the head." Bob took a deep breath, "and there was even a note." I sat there in silence and in an absolute state of shock.

"Babe," AJ said to me silently as she saw tears start to roll down my face.

I was breathing heavy now, hearing intervals of Bob's breathing and the radios crackling at his console.

"Chris, I am so sorry." Bob tried to say it as sincerely as he could, but he knew that I wasn't hearing anything else at the moment other than Jennifer is dead.

I dropped the phone slowly out of my hands. AJ looked at me slowly, her beautiful eyes were scanning me and she tried to figure out why I was crying. I was unable to move. Bob repeated my name a bunch of times as if we were losing our connection, while the phone just sat in my lap.

"Chris, I'm sorry dude. I am so, so sorry."

AJ pulled the phone from my lap to her ear and said "Bob, its AJ, what the hell is going on?"

AJ's inquiry to Bob came out swift and concerned. I heard the breath from AJ's chest gasp deeply, while tears were rolling faster down my face. The tears came on like a wave I had never experienced. AJ gasped in disbelief again as she etched her nails into my thigh. Bob just told her. I felt her body freeze in time and space. We were both lost, but together we were still connected. Her hand was now spread full across my thigh, squeezing it to let me know she was there. She knew that even though I was with her, I was lost somewhere. I was unable to hear anything or see anything around me. I just sat there deep inside myself. AJ told Bob that she wanted to take care of me and that I'd call him back in a bit. I looked up at her with my eyes full of tears, and I motioned with a few fingers for the phone.

Putting the phone to my ear I asked Bob, "Where is she, at her place?"

"Yes, she is." Davia and the crew are all on the way over there now," Bob said regretfully and softly.

"I'll be on the way in a bit." I said to Bob as I felt every ounce of my stomach wanting to empty violently. Bob and I said our good-byes.

AJ knelt down before me as I sat there crying harder and harder. She didn't speak; she didn't have too. She knew that this was too painful. She ran her fingers across my face to wipe the tears that just kept coming. AJ placed her arms around me trying to figure out how to hug me out of the pain that I was now enveloped by. She knew she couldn't, all she could do was exist near me. She knows how much I care for my friends and how important they are to me. She knew how special the friendship that I had with Jennifer was, and exactly how this was going to hit me.

We sat on the bed together, AJ just holding me. I was comforted by the feeling of her hair mixed in with my tears and the warmth of her body, but that was only a band-aid to the emotional evisceration I was about to undergo. I got up slowly and reached for my jeans. I went to the dresser to get my shield, department two-way radio and keys.

"Do you want me to go with you?" AJ asked gently.

PARAMEDIC M.O.S.

I looked at her and kissed her gently through my tears, "From what Bob told me I would guess it is a pretty gruesome sight. I don't want you to have to see her this way."

AJ looked at me, "Honey, we are together and I want to be there with you."

I thought long and hard, and didn't want to expose AJ to what I was about to see. I also know that I am unsure if I will be in any position to drive after I get there. Maybe I should have her come with me. AJ was her friend too and it would be wrong of me to decide for her what was appropriate or not.

"Um, uh, okay, but I am going to go inside before you. Oh HELL, I don't even know what I am saying." I said with complete frustration as I slammed my fist down onto the nightstand. My fist made a thunderous sound on the night table as the lamp fell off. AJ just sat there looking at me. She knew that I was going through enough of a metamorphosis in my mind to be able to withstand what I was about too. She also knew that I did not want to see this. I knew that she didn't want to either.

AJ reached for a pair of jeans, a t-shirt and a gray sweater that said "DUKE" on the front in blue writing.

"Hun," AJ said as she walked up to me and wrapped her body around me, "let's get over there." Her words were full of love and soft compassion, but sounded as if she was out of breath.

Jennifer was so sweet and kind, and she had the heart of anyone's best friend. After we graduated the academy together, I had just gone through a rough relationship situation, and she was a total friend to me. She was always there for me to cheer me up, to take me out to a movie, study or have dinner together. Whenever we went out everyone thought we were a married couple, as we were so close. We laughed at everything together and knew each other very well. Jennifer was family to me. We worked the street like no one else and always had a blast. Before I ever knew AJ, I experienced such a world of care from Jennifer that I had not received from anyone else. She taught me that it was okay to trust and love. Having experienced a number of bad relationships, she somehow always knew what I was thinking and how to help.

For reasons I will never know or so I thought, she took her life. As I walked about AJ's house, I could barely keep my thoughts straight, but I had to go to the scene. I kept walking in inconsistent circles, trying desperately to deny any of this was true. I kept seeing Jennifer in front of me, with her auburn hair, hazel eyes and her smile. She and AJ were the most attractive women I had ever known.

We preserved the value of friendship. We went on vacation together a bunch of times and it was just so nice to be with someone who cared. There was never any intimacy beyond hugs, and next to AJ, no one knew me as well. I adored the value of what we created together and when we were in the academy we always joked that later in life if our relationships ever fell apart, we would pack it up and take care of each other for life. That is what we thought best friends should do. It was a bit of a peculiar bond to most who never worked this closely in this line of work, but I was fortunate to have it with her.

I cried more and made for the door slowly. I was absolutely numb. As I opened AJ's door into the night air, I saw that a gentle amount of light was just starting to come up. I felt like a robot. I couldn't feel anything except that this was real and I just felt lost. As I sat with the driver's door open to my truck starting the engine, AJ locked the house behind her and walked up to me. I was staring at the ground aimlessly.

AJ hugged me. She looked at me and said, "Are you sure you want to do this?"

Without even looking at her I said, "Yes, I have too. It's Jen and she's dead." I said it in almost a struggled whisper. AJ shook her head up and down slowly and then made her way to the passenger's side of the vehicle. She was crying harder as well now. Although she knew that I was used to taking care of myself, she was trying to be as strong for me as I would let her be. Her nurturing instincts also told her that she wanted to provide me all the care I would need, being sure to give me enough room yet ensuring that I always knew that she was only a whisper away. After I put the truck in drive, I pulled onto the street, AJ just sat there looking at me. I was looking straight ahead, staring into blank space. I could navigate the streets and highways on autopilot, but she knew inside I was agonizing immensely. I barely looked at her, and she didn't mind; she knew not to take it personally.

She knew that I was silently looking in my mind for a sign that Jennifer was alive. She knew I was thinking about all the time we had spent together, hoping one of those enlightening moments would be able to revive her before I got there. AJ also knew that all I was really doing was reassembling my inner programming to accept all that I was about to see. She knew that I knew she was there and I would acknowledge that when I could.

PARAMEDIC M.O.S.

I flew down the Hutchinson River Parkway at what have must been eighty miles per hour; this was a fifty-five zone. Unlike most trips into the city limits, this excursion would be without music; just silence. I have seen patients who have shot themselves like this before, it was always a horrible sight; and it was even worse knowing that I was about to see Jennifer like this. I drove over the drawbridge that leads to Orchard Beach; the one that in my years of living in this area has never opened. I drove past Co-op City in the Bronx without even looking over at it, through the tolls at the Whitestone Bridge towards Bayside.

By the time we reached the tolls at the Whitestone, AJ must have touched my right hand about seventy times. We sniffled together as I reached mid-span on the bridge. If we would have had our faces together, our tears would have mixed together as our noses were now running too. I smelled AJ's shampoo and I was happy that she was with me. I made the left at the fork for the Cross Island Expressway and came off at the sharp exit for Bell Boulevard. Making a left at the light, I drove past Fort Totten (home to the EMS Academy) and further down Bell Boulevard. Trips to this area were usually for training updates, recertification exams and upgrades, haz-mat training, or some necessary educational reason to be back at the academy.

For all of us in the service, this is where life began. This is where we got our wings. Normally I would have stopped two blocks before the academy on Bell Blvd. stopping at a small mall of stores, which housed the 7-11, and a great pizza shop. Not today, not at all. As I drove down past The Blitz, our local academy watering hole after medic class, I approached Jennifer's block. I saw five NYPD unmarked detectives cars (or the equivalent of the entire night tour of the local precinct detectives squad, five EMS Ambulances with their lights off, numerous EMS patrol supervisor's and chief's vehicles. The one thing that I saw which drove my heart and stomach to the ground was the van from the NYC Medical Examiners Office (otherwise known as the morgue van) parked outside with its doors open.

I brought my truck to a stop in a space nearby one of the chief's vehicles. I exited and Davia walked over to me. Jennifer and I were actually known throughout the service, since she and I had a number of high-profile calls together, which ended up in commendations for us both. AJ exited the vehicle slowly as Davia raised her head in acknowledgment of her. Davia put her arm around me gently without saying anything as I just stood there.

The tears that just started flowing as Davia pulled me in for a hug and to shield me, ensuring that I could cry in as much privacy as possible. The press was already on the scene. Here I was, usually the pinnacle of strength for so many, the one that would walk into hell on any given day or night, and I am now crumpled to a pile of shattered tears and sniffles. AJ walked over and the two of them hugged. I looked at Davia and she began to cry.

There we were, no longer medic and chief, no longer commanding officer and subordinate, just nurturers and friends wiping tears from each others' faces with coat sleeves. Davia and I had been through a plethora of street combat before, and even the first terrorist attack on the World Trade Center, when they placed a bomb in the basement, but this took on a whole new pain.

I asked Davia, "Are we sure this is suicide?"

Davia tightened her grip around me while I felt tears run down her face onto mine. AJ was holding my right hand.

She quietly spoke into my ear, "Christian, we found a note."

She paused.

"It detailed some stuff and there is more." We hugged against her department vehicle, and I froze for a second and then pulled her away from me slowly.

I looked at her while my eyes went from crying to shock at the sound of her statement. "What do you mean more?" I asked.

Davia inhaled deeply looking away for a moment and then focusing back on me, "Christian there is a note addressed to you in there." She paused and inhaled again, "You don't have to see it, and you don't even have to go in there. It's pretty bad in there."

Before the words of her last sentence completed I had already detached myself from both AJ and Davia and was already in motion for the door. Davia and AJ both tried to grab my sleeves, but I had too much forward motion and they knew they couldn't stop me. They had both seen me jump to the rescue of partners and patients too many times before. They knew I was methodical, calculating, but most of all swift. I felt them behind me, just staring at my back in absolute heartbreak as I walked in. They knew this would be hell for me. Displaying my EMS Medic shield around my chest, attached to a minutely beaded silver necklace as we were required to wear under our clothing like dog tags off duty, the officer posted at the front door gave it a once over and gave me access.

PARAMEDIC M.O.S.

I walked to the front door of her apartment; a door I had been at many times before, always making sure Jen got home okay after we worked together or after we went to dinner, a movie or for ice cream. It was a doorstep where on many a night I thanked my luck for the benefit of a friendship so deep. As I stood outside the door I took a deep breath. I heard all kinds of commotion inside; I knew that would be the Crime Scene Unit & Detectives. I knew when I walked in there would be EMS personnel standing around in confusion, trying to keep their game faces to look professional; but I also knew that many people knew and loved Jennifer; so this would be a day without game faces. Right now this was a day without faces at all. I opened the door to find detectives taking pictures and logging evidence, as I heard the rattle of the Medical Examiner's stretcher coming down the hall. I was so dizzy that I wanted to puke.

All activity in the rooms stopped when they saw me, as an eerie silence fell over the room. All of the EMS personnel looked at me. Chief George Hujiker came up to me and placed his hand on my shoulder.

"I'm sorry, Chris," George said to me with complete compassion.

I could barely speak as I quickly recognized the smell of blood oxidizing.

"Where?" I said quietly and painfully to George.

He inhaled and nodded towards her bedroom, but I could tell he did not want to be the one to have to make that nod. I didn't know if I would scream or if I wanted to go in there. I inhaled. I felt the mucus in my throat well up into a ball choking me. I began walking towards her bedroom, my feet slowly touching the wooden floors that once knew her footsteps. The stench of exposed blood and death became more evident. Now I was wishing I brought AJ inside. Before I got to the bedroom door I stopped and took a few quick breaths, knowing that no matter how strong I attempted to be, no matter how loving of a person I am, nothing would prepare me or ready me for what I was about to see. I bowed my head and started to well up in tears again. I held the wall as I forced myself to turn the corner.

One of the medics from 40-Willy (a tactical medic unit from Queens) stood by the bedroom door like a makeshift honor guard. He had a look that I cannot describe other than angry denial. We locked eyes and we said it all without saying anything. I knew I had to go to Jennifer and be her friend. I looked in slowly, surveying everything in sight. I thought my life had ended. I slumped against the wall as the medic from 40-Willy caught me. I balanced myself against the wall and slid to the ground on to my butt.

There was blood and brain matter all over several walls, and I saw her legs exposed from the foot post of her favorite wicker bed. I tried not to look over the post, but I could not leave there without being her friend. I stood up telling myself to get it together, telling myself that I could do this. I walked around the foot post, and lying on her bed, there she was: lifeless and dead. I clenched my teeth as I tried to keep my footing. The bullet entered at her right temple and blew out most of her left skull. What once was one of the most beautiful women I ever knew and loved, was now a bloody mess of self-inflicted death. Jennifer's brain matter and skull fragments were splattered everywhere. Her auburn hair was matted to the bed with dried blood. I went for the garbage can closest to the bed as chunks of vomit began flying out of my mouth.

As I wiped away what I could with my sleeve, the medic at the door came down to help me.

"I'm okay," I said as I was now faced with this horrible taste in my mouth. I wiped my mouth with my coat sleeve again, and kept thinking to myself, "Damnit Jennifer, how could you do this? Why didn't you come to me?"

I was angry, sad, hurt, empty and full of rage. I got to my feet as everyone in the room looked away. With the wave of disbelief and sheer horror now upon me, I sat down on the bed next to Jennifer's corpse. I took her bloodstained hand in mine; it was cold.

There would be no more laughs, no more movies, no more smiles, no more hugs, no more of her nurturing care. There would be no more late night pages if we were working opposite tours to make sure I was okay. There would be no more. There would no longer be the comfort of showing up on some ridiculous mass casualty incident, only to find her there so that we could be each other's sanity through the incident. I remembered the time when I didn't have AJ, and I had gotten caught up in a large riot at the scene of a call. She heard me call a 10-13 in the Hunts Point section of the South Bronx, while she was working in Brooklyn. She made it to the scene from Brooklyn faster than units coming from Manhattan. It was like we were each other's lifeblood, closer than two could ever expect.

We had a friendship as if we were back in summer camp together as children. Our care, concern and love for each other was totally innocent, free of any outside force. I think we both missed out on that as children,

PARAMEDIC M.O.S.

so we really found something special in each other. It was as if we adopted one another.

As I sat there holding her lifeless hand, the detective in the room adjacent handed me an envelope and said, "I believe this is for you."

He handed me an envelope free of any blood or brain matter, which happened to be all around me at this point. Do I really want to open this? Do I need to know what she left for me? Of course I do. Jennifer is my friend, and I promised her that I would see her through until the end, until she rests in peace. I sat there, slumping forward on the bed, wiping the tears off of my face. Next, the Medical Examiners personnel walked in. I looked up and said to both of them abrasively, "Not now!"

They looked at me in confusion as a detective moved them out of the room. I opened the letter that was beautifully addressed to me.

Christian my dear, first I ask that you hear me through and please do not be angry with me. I love you with all of my heart, as you are the best friend I ever had. Though I am too far-gone, know that I will always be with you in spirit. I know this will hurt and that makes it so hard; but if you are reading this letter, then I pulled the trigger before I was able to get to you. You are strong and the best man that I know. No one ever watched out for me like you; and I wish I could have had a father who cared as much as you always have for me. Instead I got a rapist and molester for a father, and I have been having these visions lately of everything he used to do to me, and that his friends did too. Honey I want you to let AJ take care of you. She loves you as much as I, and she is fortunate enough to have the comfort of your arms at night. I know that if you are reading this in my apartment, she is outside at the moment, as you wouldn't bring her here first. You would want to survey the scene first and make sure it was safe for her to enter. Most of all you wouldn't want her to see me like this. You always bring out the best in people; don't let it stop now. I am honored to know you as I have and to love you as I have. I could not have a greater friend. You don't have to visit me if you don't want too, I will understand. You know of course that I would always love your company if you would stop by though. I love you.

Jen-Jen

The letter appeared to have been cried on, this apparent by the running ink. I slid off the bed holding her still and cold hand, crying hysterically. This time I vomited all over myself.

No matter how I tried I could not stop the tears from coming. Davia and AJ must have slipped in without me seeing or hearing them. I was curled up on the floor in a fetal position, not caring who saw me like this. AJ slid in next to me on the floor, right into a pool of fresh vomit and held me.

"Jennifer is dead." I said trying to focus on AJ.

Crying herself, she ran her hand across the back of my head and said to me, " I know Christian, I know. I am so sorry Hun." Davia leaned down and handed me some paper towels that were soaked in water to clean up with.

"If you want to stay, I can have the M.E. hold off awhile." I heard Davia's words but my response was slow in time. I picked my head up from the floor and said, "Just a few more minutes Chief, I cannot believe she is gone. I can't believe any of this." I cried out of control while AJ sat on the floor holding me. I know that she had no idea what to do, except be there.

Davia and AJ helped me lean up against the wall as the detectives peeked in. I looked at them and with swollen eyes and a swollen nose, I told them quietly, "Go ahead." I shook my head in disbelief and anger.

The M.E.'s personnel were very careful with her body. I stood there with eyes full of water that kept running down my face, while I became dizzier and dizzier.

Davia stood there as staunch as she could, though I know this sight was killing her. She loved Jennifer and she loved knowing that we were working the street together. AJ and I stood there for a while and I couldn't even speak. AJ knew how this was hitting me, and I knew how horrible she felt now too. Davia, AJ and I looked around the apartment saying nothing. I stepped out of the room while the M.E.'s personnel staged her body on the stretcher and I heard that horrible, but familiar sound of the body bag zipper closing. We all accompanied Jen-Jen's body out side, helping to lift it gingerly into the van.

PARAMEDIC M.O.S.

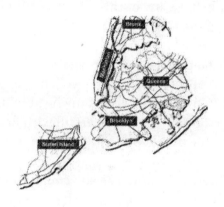

C.B. Garris

Chapter XVIII:

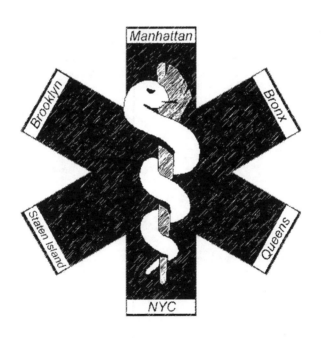

PARAMEDIC M.O.S.

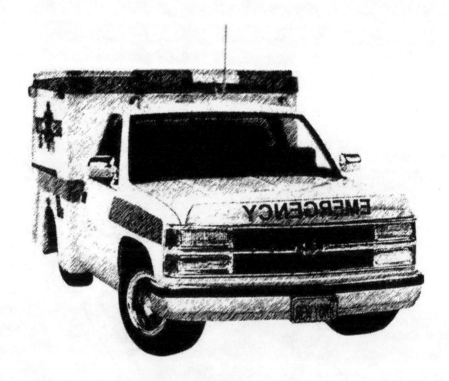

C.B. Garris

I walked in the door from the fourth session of Critical Incident Stress Debriefing, where I spoke to the counselor for two hours, reminiscing about Jennifer and crying. I felt as if someone hit me in my chest with a sledgehammer. I was completely winded and felt unsure about a lot of things. AJ was great to me the entire time. She told me to basically move in with her until I felt better. She knew I had my apartment up the road in Mt. Vernon, about ten to fifteen minutes from her house, but she felt there was no use in me spending much time there unless I wanted too. I already had the only other key to AJ's house and I had her heart. I didn't need anything else. AJ was sitting on her couch reading a book. She closed the book gently as she looked up at me slowly.

"Hey," she said softly.

I walked towards the couch, which was well lit by sunlight. "Hi," I said totally wiped from the counseling session.

Just saying the words made me feel winded. I knew that in AJ's presence I could just be me. Though normally full of life and smiles when with her, nothing could stop this constant pain. It felt like something that I couldn't shake. AJ was wearing a white cut-off gym shirt, which always complimented her body with her great lats, and a pair of jeans. Her toenails were painted a frosty light blue today. She opened her legs on the couch so that I could be wrapped up in them when I sat down. I just sat there, body poised forward off the couch. My head was down and I was clasping my hands.

AJ just sat there, running her soft but firm hand over my back, intermittently giving me back scratches with her perfectly manicured nails.

As AJ turned her body into mine, wrapping her arms around me, she asked softly, "Wanna talk about it?" AJ just held me, kissing me gently from time to time on my head and face. She let me be where I was. She didn't do what so many do, which is to tell you to snap out of it, or to just get over it. AJ knew that I would eventually come around, but I was adjusting to the reality of living without such a close friend and of seeing such a gruesome sight when I went to Jen's house.

The funeral had to be closed casket, since there was no way to cosmetically fix the damage to her head. Here was a girl who was absolutely stunning in every way. She was beautiful when she combed her hair; she was beautiful at 3:00 am if we were performing a rescue under a train together, or upside down in a car trying to extricate someone from of a wreck. She didn't need introductions when she walked into a room; she was one. My

PARAMEDIC M.O.S.

being partners with Jennifer never threatened AJ, and that made all the difference in the world. In fact the two became good friends. They could have been twins the way they thought. Just the same, AJ and Jennifer were mature enough to appreciate friendship and caring in its greatest forms. My life was so much easier when I told AJ I was going to work with Jennifer, since she was actually happy about it. AJ knew that we go way back and that we look out for each other. AJ knew that I would be well cared for on my tour and Jennifer would never let anything happen to me, nor I her. AJ knew that I would come home in a good mood and that I would have had a rewarding night on the street if I worked with Jennifer.

Before I met AJ, I was dating a woman who almost lost her mind when she saw Jennifer. Anytime I mentioned that I was going to work with Jennifer, she was so afraid of Jennifer's beauty that she swore Jennifer would steal me away from her. As you can see, that relationship had a very short life span. I was glad that I had some wonderful photographs of Jennifer both in uniform and from our vacations, but I had to put them all away for safekeeping. Maybe someday I would be able to look at them again.

Davia gave me a week off to get my head together. In fact, before I even arrived at Jennifer's house on the day she committed suicide, she had already notified Operations that I would be off for up to a week, on what we call release time. Release time is an administrative classification for time off for a job related situation. It could be given for any reason, whether we were being sent for specialized training such as our tactical law enforcement training, or perhaps when we are sent down to Jersey for HAZ-MAT training. Release time is also issued if you come in contact with a person who is either diagnosed with or has been exposed to a communicable disease. Very often we are released with pay for up to twenty-one days if it is exposure related. We are given that long to see if anything develops during the incubation period. It gives us the opportunity to be monitored by employee health services and it also keeps us from contaminating patients we would come in contact with in the field.

As I looked at AJ she asked me if I wanted anything for dinner. I told her that I really wasn't too hungry, but that I could pick a little. AJ prepared a platter of my favorite snacking foods while I was at the counselor's office; Kalamata olives, roasted red peppers, goat cheese, smokehouse almonds. She also informed me that she stocked up on protein powder in case I wanted to do a liquid diet for awhile. As I leaned forward to obtain a few of the items she prepared for me, she asked, "Do you want to watch TV or see a movie?" As I brought a roasted red pepper to her lips, she was already reaching for the remote to put on Great Chefs. I was happy to have her.

Sensing that she had something to say I asked, "Do you want to talk?" AJ lowered the volume on the TV, as the Chef was plating a special sea bass recipe. "Actually yes," she said touching my cheek gently.

I turned the TV off. "I am all ears for you," I said kissing her hands.

"This has been really hard on both of us, and I miss Jennifer too. I miss hearing her call here all excited knowing we would all be getting together. I loved to go shopping with her; we always devastated the stores. Did I ever tell you that I even let her pick out a few outfits for me that you absolutely loved? She loved you dearly and she said that you would love the outfits. Equally I remember how you and I would go Christmas shopping for her. You would always light up when you shopped for her. I always admire how you take care of me, and I love you for that. I also have always admired how you took care of Jennifer. I remember when you told me about the time you went late on a car payment so that you could get her what you knew she wanted but would have never asked you for.

That story of when the two of you did a call in a body and bath store that she had never been in. You went back to the store with her and you two window-shopped. You made a mental note of everything she said she liked but couldn't afford. It was December 23rd that year and you had one day to get down there to get her present. One of her brothers had just passed away a month before and she was upset. You went in and purchased something like $800.00 of bath & body products, showing up at her doorstep at exactly 12:00 midnight on Christmas morning in a Santa suit with a huge box just for her. She told me that story when we were away last year and how much just the thought of you doing that pulled her from a slump. She loved knowing that you cared and it meant the world to her, but I too sensed something was going on with her.

I asked her a few times about her past, but she was not interested in talking about it. She wasn't rude about it; it was almost like her past never existed. I realize from the contents from her letter that she was always in incredible pain, but it was not something we could see. I am angry at her for not coming to you or me, but I loved her and always will. She chose to take the route that she did, and it has left us all without her."

I sat there, tears running down my face again. I was frustrated. I shared AJ's thoughts and I was glad that she was sharing them with me.

PARAMEDIC M.O.S.

Part of me wanted to get up and scream, and AJ knew that. I think AJ wanted to scream with me; it was just not our character. I told AJ to sit tight and that I had to go to the bathroom. She swung her leg out and I walked up to her bedroom bath.

As I walked into her room I saw two very fat suitcases that were just about all packed. One had her clothes in them, and the other what looked to be mine. I was totally confused.

I turned right around and when I got back downstairs AJ said, "Hun, come here and sit down."

The last time I heard those words, it was from my ex-fiancé, and although my ex was not as pleasant about it, my stomach sank. AJ looked at me for a few seconds with the most loving eyes, and I thought I was going to short circuit. Is she telling me goodbye? What the hell is this? My eyes must have been wide with fear as AJ calmly said, "Christian," I gulped.

"Everything is fine, stop worrying," AJ said with a smile.

Before she continued she could see my legs shaking, and she started to laugh a laugh of relief.

She giggled gently, "Wait a minute, are you thinking we are having a problem?"

I was panting at this point and if I was a puppy, my ears would have been back and I would have laid my paws out in front of me in defensive mode.

"Honey, stop worrying, I packed the bags because you and I are going on a trip."

My eyes were still wide, my nerves frayed, and I must have looked pretty silly. AJ was totally amused at my body language in its defensive mode, and in fact I think it turned her on. She knew that if I was in that mode, whatever it involved was something or someone I was very passionate about. She had only heard about this particular look from a few partners I worked with, one being Jennifer, when their lives were in danger and I went into attack mode in the street. AJ never saw this before and was giggling herself silly at my look. I eventually broke out laughing and crying at the same time. It got funnier by the moment. AJ knew that I loved her and for the first time saw my vulnerability show in a form that was new to her. I could tell that she felt even more appreciated by what she witnessed.

AJ continued, "Christian, I am taking you away from here for some R&R."

I looked at her totally confused.

"Hun, I have to go to work tomorrow."

AJ smiled and reached behind the sofa to her answering machine, pressing the play button. The voice I heard was a very familiar one; it was Davia.

"Christian, hi it's Davia. I cleared it with the borough and operations, you are on release time for the next fourteen days and I know AJ will take great care of you. Go rest kiddo, and call me when you get back."

AJ had this huge smirk on her face like she was the mouse who snagged the cheese from under the cat's nose.

AJ dropped her smile for a serious look, "I called Davia to talk about how you are doing and we both agreed that you need some time away. I told her that I wanted to take you far away from here to a place where you can be guaranteed relaxation and a different view of things. She was all for it and took care of all the rest."

I sat there looking at AJ baffled that she would take the time, concern, and these measures for me. This is something I definitely was unaccustomed too. I knew that whatever she had in mind would be just what she said it would be, I just couldn't get over her actions.

She reached behind her again and pulled out two first-class tickets to Los Angeles International Airport in southern California. If I remembered correctly, the spa that I order her bath and body products is located near there.

AJ held my hand, "I want to take you to the spa that you always order all of my products from. I reserved us for a four-night stay on the spa property itself, and I have arranged for an abundance of spa treatments for you. We will have our own cottage with a fireplace and our meals will be brought to us at our beck and call. After we leave there, I thought we would drive to Los Angeles and stay by the beach for a week. I could show you LA from when I used to live there, and even introduce a few of my friends from there to you. When we get to LA, I put us at the Ritz-Carlton in Marina Del Rey, which is right on the water."

I sat there in absolute awe. I must have just looked at her for what seemed like forever, although it was only about a minute. I couldn't believe what she was telling me, nor that anyone would do this for me. I was always the one to provide the greatest present to someone. I didn't know how to even respond to such a generous gift.

"Are you sure?" I asked AJ.

PARAMEDIC M.O.S.

AJ said while she touched my face, "Christian, I love you, more than I can place in words. You are and have become such a force in my life and I appreciate every day with you. I love caring for you, and I know that you are hurting incredibly now. I will do anything to bring a smile back to your face. You have been treated like shit in all of your other relationships, and you are the most honorable man I know. It is time that you learn what it is like to be treated the way you treat others. I know this is going to be a difficult lesson, but I want to be the one to show you."

I sat there almost turning into myself, which AJ was expecting.

"Christian, I know this probably scares you, as anytime in your past when someone who you were close too was going to do something that seemed nice, it always came with a price. It was a price you have paid dearly for all of your life, always hoping that the next nice gesture from someone was not going to hurt you. It is my hope that you are able to find the place inside of you that will allow you to be loved and cared for, without the fear or guilt that you have walked around with for so long."

As these words left AJ's lips I was just rocking in place, crying. She knew I was with her, and she also knew that I was somewhere else. I was scared. Scared that someday she would lash out at me too.

"Babe," AJ said as she pulled me in for a kiss, "Don't worry, someday it will all seem natural, and when that day comes, I will be right here with you. We have been through so much together and we have also come a long way individually and together. I am going to take care of you the same way you do me."

We kissed deeply, and so many emotions and thoughts went through my head, I didn't know if I wanted to jump up for joy, scream in terror, or vomit.

AJ knew that this was where I was at, and she knew that we would be fine.

"AJ, I don't know how to say this, but I know this is going to cost you a bundle."

AJ placed two fingers over my lips.

"Don't you even worry about that," she winked at me, "this will not even phase my bank accounts, and besides I know you would do the same. So don't you worry at all about that. Let's just leave this place for awhile and go somewhere different."

I gave her the nod that she had waited for all night; the one that was my vulnerability giving in. Our flight was departing at 11:00 am, so AJ informed me that we would be picked up at 8:00am. AJ like me, preferred getting to the airport early, as you can always find something to do until it is time to depart. I slept off and on during the night, waiting for the other shoe to drop. Problem is, there was no other shoe. This is how AJ is and how she allowed me to exist in her life. AJ got up at what must have been 6:00am to start getting ready. She had to do her hair and makeup, although she never really needed any. Any makeup she wore just enhanced what was naturally there. I went down to her home gym and did a bunch of reps on my lats and on the chest press. I also worked on my abs a bit; just enough to get my blood moving. I was nervous, that this was the predecessor to the end of our relationship, when it was nowhere near that. In fact, my intellectual mind told me that it was an even greater step of how close AJ and I are. I went upstairs and hopped in the shower as AJ sashayed around her bedroom with her hair up in a towel. As I leaned over the sink to shave, she walked in and hugged me from behind. We smiled in the mirror, as I was increasingly more self-conscious. I realized that some bad experiences do remain with us for a long time. I asked her if I could brush her hair, to which she nodded excitedly. She sat in front of her vanity as I pulled up the hassock.

Sitting just off to her right I began using long strokes. Her hair was now down to her lower back and still beautiful.

"Thank you for being in my life," I said to AJ, as she turned to me with one of her heart stopping looks and spoke the same and ending it with a wet kiss.

We got dressed and made sure we had everything. I forgot that AJ packed, so I know we had everything. It was pretty cold out this time of year, as February was not my favorite month. AJ was totally decked out, and she looked fabulous. She was wearing a thick turtleneck sweater that was between beige and peach, with an iced tea colored suede jacket that was form fitting and stopped at her waist. Finishing off this outfit, she had on comfortable tight jeans and black knee-high platform boots with five inch chunky heels. AJ looked fabulous, and she knew that I thought so. At 7:59 there was a knock at the door, and our driver was there to take our bags.

"Good morning Sir, my name is Gerald and I will be taking you to JFK today. I'll take those bags and we can go as soon as your ready."

Man did this guy want a tip, I thought to myself. I extended my hand to Gerald and we shook. He had a solid handshake.

PARAMEDIC M.O.S.

I heard heels coming down the stairwell behind me and as AJ appeared in the doorway, Gerald looked up and dropped his bags in delight.

Almost as if he was a plebe fumbling to salute a major general Gerald said "Uh, you mmm, mmm, must be Ms. Sanchez."

AJ gleamed a thousand watt smile at Gerald, which I thought would make his knees buckle, "Yes I am."

She extended her hand to shake his and said there will be four bags, as she brought two more that I didn't see.

I looked at her and she said, "I had to bring a few extra things in case we decide to take on the town." She looked like a kid in a candy store. I could tell that she was excited about going to visit Los Angeles, and I think she was even happier to be taking me with her. Our car was in the form of a rather large limo, brand new from the looks of it. As I stood in the driveway, AJ was walking towards me.

When she reached me she knew why I stopped short. "Honey," she said, "When we ride, we ride in style."

She pinched my butt affectionately as I began to walk with her.

The ride down to JFK was smooth and even though there was traffic, the windows to our car were tinted and we were in fact, riding in style.

"It feels wonderful to be taking you away," AJ said to me while gently squeezing my hand.

I must have fallen asleep at some point on the drive, because the last thing I remember was placing my head on the window, sad about Jennifer; and then I woke up on AJ's shoulder as we were pulling off the Van Wyck Expressway to JFK.

"Wake up sleepy head," AJ said softly. I opened my eyes and worked on focusing. Opening the window for a quick wake up breath of fresh air, I was reminded of how cold it was outside. We were in a bit of a traffic snag when a small fender bender occurred in front of us between a taxi and civilian vehicle. The taxi driver exited his vehicle after he rear-ended the other car. He walked up to the driver of the vehicle and proceeded to pounce on him through his driver's side window.

Several patrol cars from the Port Authority PD pulled up as Gerald just shook his head. Gerald brought us right to our gate curbside. He exited the vehicle and quickly came around to my side opening the door. As I began to step out I placed my right hand into the car for AJ to use for leverage as she exited. Gerald popped the trunk and removed our bags.

He motioned for a skycap that was a little bit pre-occupied staring at AJ to notice he was being summoned.

"YO, redcap, take your eyes off the girl and get the bags; or do I have to do this by myself?"

Redcap, embarrassed that he got caught scurried to our bags. AJ saw that I had a very abrasive face showing, typical anytime I went to the airport. After my tactical training and experiences, I suspected just about everyone to be guilty of some crime.

AJ was determined to soften me up just enough to relax, though she loved my edge. We made it through security with over an hour to spare, so we went right to the Admirals Club. AJ and I both had chamomile tea, and we shared a large bowl of sliced fruit. We sat and watched the planes take off and land as several very famous celebrities snuck in and took up seating in the area below us.

AJ reached for my hand and nestled it against her face "This is really great. I have dreamed of taking you to Los Angeles. If there is anything you want to do when we get there, you just let me know and we'll do it."

I rested my hand against her cheek, "Really AJ, I am just happy to be here. I am kind at a loss for words and even a little jittery. I was up most of the night; but I was able to subside those wide awake hours tracing the curves of your luscious body with my hands."

AJ smiled, "Luscious, huh? It doesn't sound like you are at a loss for words at all."

As we enjoyed the moment, our flight was called for pre-boarding, so we made our way down to the gate.

I had never known the pleasure of first class before, though it appeared that AJ was able to ease right in. We both fell asleep somewhere after takeoff, and woke up for the last hour and a half of the trip. We woke up holding hands and I had this warm feeling all over. I was away from NYC. I was gone from all the pain that seemed to be surrounding me. Whether it was recent events of Jennifer's suicide or my demons of my younger years, I was away from it all. AJ went to the bathroom to freshen up as the flight attendant served mimosas throughout the cabin. I kicked my feet back in the seat, which reclined and was oh so comfortable. When AJ returned I just looked at her and wondered if I had died and met an angel. Perhaps part of me had died, the part of me that was used to being treated poorly. Could I have transcended and moved on? Our landing was the smoothest I've ever felt and walking through Los Angeles International

PARAMEDIC M.O.S.

was a breeze. As we stepped off of the aircraft, there was a rather large gentleman with blond hair, blue eyes and a solid tan waiting for us. This was evident to me because of his driver's black and white outfit and the sign that said *Mr. & Mrs. Sanchez.*

I looked at AJ with one of my comically puzzled looks and she looked at me smiling, "Hope you don't mind? Besides a girl can dream can't she?"

I was so pleasantly surprised by this. I am sure that most guys would have dropped a small land animal out of their ass since the sign was written as if we were married. More detrimental to most guys' egos was that it was advertised with HER last name. I on the other hand took it as the greatest compliment that I could ever receive. Even if for streamlining our trip, the fact that AJ would allow me the place in her heart to want to share her last name with me, and how much that meant to her was a priceless gift.

"I don't mind at all, in fact I am incredibly flattered!" Our driver led us to baggage claim and retrieved our baggage. Once outside he led us to a rather large stretch limousine. I stopped again like I did at the house and looked at AJ. "Just you wait," she said, "the fun is just beginning."

Before I stepped into the limo I noticed the California sun, and I was totally moved. It was hot and blanketing, but there was something in it that was far different than anything I had ever seen before. It was as if I could breathe for the first time. AJ walked up behind me in my stupor and said "Tantalizing, isn't it?"

She smiled as we entered the limo. It was about an hour and a half trip into the mountains, which I slept throughout on AJ's shoulder. This spa was at the base of a mountain, overlooking a gorgeous lake. The view was breathtaking and I felt as if I was I in a different world. When we arrived a representative walked out and reached her hands out for AJ. She was a tall, very healthy and striking woman. Her name was Leann. She was in her 40's, in amazing shape with long blonde hair, deep honey-colored, almond shaped eyes, an incredible tan, full lips and the body of a twenty-two year old. She was dressed in a gray business suit and black, platform chunky heels. The suit contoured her body in a very complimentary fashion. She was graceful, endearing and California beautiful. She extended her hand as did I.

"Christian I have heard so much about you. It is such a pleasure to meet the man who has been keeping this wonderful woman happy." Leeann said while AJ just raised her eyebrows and smiled. AJ and Leeann spoke as I dropped my jaw at the sprawling estate and facilities. The grounds were meticulously landscaped, and there were roman fountains everywhere. Something in the realm of delicious food permeated the air. As I was picking up the fennel and anise in the aroma, I heard a bunch of Terri-cloth robed women speaking softly. All were talking amongst themselves and giggling; but everyone around this place seemed relaxed. Leeann showed us to our cottage. Leann showed us the amenities; no expense was spared. I think I now figured out where AJ discovered the idea for her bathroom. We had a bathroom somewhat similar to AJ's, but even larger. As I looked around the bathroom, I tried to figure out why they put a phone next to the toilet. I assumed that most would be preoccupied when sitting there, but I guess some prefer to be interrupted. Leann said she'd be sending our treatment schedules up with our meal tonight. Both she and AJ hugged and then Leeann made her exit.

AJ and I settled into our cottage. We started by unpacking, and then took a long, hot shower together. Taking showers with AJ was always an event. To visualize her tantalizing body in all its splendor as the water ran through her hair was just an experience. I loved the tactile sensation of feeling her kissing me through the cascading water. My body always seemed to relax in her hands, as hers did in mine. We exited and put on our thick Terri cloth robes – emerald green for her and coral for me. Somewhere in the background I was hearing new age music, and it sounded like Kitaro. As we kicked our feet up relaxing on each other, there was a knock at the door. Leeann chose our meals tonight and sent them directly to us. The attendant brought the tray in and we said we would take care of setting it up.

Our starter tonight was Goat Cheese wrapped in baked phyllo dough, followed by a fabulous Maine lobster and corn gazpacho. We had entrees of roasted free-range chicken with a serious sage stuffing, chef's vegetables: a combination of daikon, carrots, eggplant and zucchini. The other entrée was salmon ravioli with a hoi son sauce. For dessert we had a fabulous flourless chocolate torte in an amaretto crème anglaise.. We ate up a storm, and my body was a little funky from the long flight, so we retired early.

Our schedule of treatments would begin in the Vespir Room for the his/hers two-hour shiatsu massage at 10am. We will be on tables next to each other so that we can remain close. Leeann said that she loved to hold hands with her mate while receiving a massage, and she thought this

PARAMEDIC M.O.S.

would be a nice bonding experience for us both. I was looking forward to the experience myself. Following that would be a soak in a private roman whirlpool for two, and then onto the wet room treatments. I believe that AJ wanted me to be detoxified, so I would get a eucalyptus wrap first, and then an hour body scrub. The eucalyptus wrap consisted of having specially harvested eucalyptus leaves placed all over my body, and then being wrapped in a hot, humidified towel for about forty-five minutes. This will open my pores and let them breathe.

The body scrub is performed by a technician who first uses a pineapple-mango enzyme body scrub to agitate your skin with massive mitts. Your body is welcomed into relaxation. You are then rinsed from a multitude of hot water jets above you. The next step in this process is that you are scrubbed with wheat stalks soaked in a cucumber solution, rinsed, and then massaged with citrus oil. I asked AJ how they do the entire body; obviously she knew I was asking if this is done naked. AJ explained that when you go in for the session in the wet room, you make a towel into a sort of diaper, covering your genitalia, which allows you to have both front and back done without anything slipping out. She thought my question was amusing. With the comfort of AJ's snuggling, I fell into a deep sleep.

All of a sudden I found myself in a strange place. She seemed so upset and angry with me, I just couldn't grasp why she was in her state of fury. Experiencing someone else's fury was second nature to me, but the beauty of adulthood now is that I could control it to some degree. All these years, I had just been re-living the same routine after routine. Women who are checked out, or are trying to check me out with their insanity. It should be no wonder that I ended up in weird relationships. All I wanted from Sylvia was her love. I came to her with no agenda, no angle to work from. Unlike so many men these days, I was truly interested in her, her feelings, desires, and dreams. I wanted to know her happiness, sadness, fears, troubles, and if there was a way to work it out.

I felt so adored by her when she would call and say hello, or that she was thinking of me. Receiving her letters and cards was like a deluge of water on a raging fire. She could douse my doubts and rage in an instant, and give me the promise of tomorrow; a tomorrow I never knew but so desperately wanted. I thought of where she would go after the phone call; was she sleeping with someone, was the lifeline I once knew as her name gone forever?

C.B. Garris

It all came to an end when she returned from her excursion away. She mentioned that she was going back to her family's home, and for the second time she mentioned that there would be no room for me there. In my experiences with the family, Sylvia's sister was always very considerate and kind to me, and every time I called to talk with Sylvia, her sister and I would have lengthy discussions on life and the pursuit of computer happiness. It was often that I would call at the height of a family computer disaster, only to save the day by playing Mr. Technical Support over the phone. Time had it that Sylvia was often unaware that the phone call was for her due to this friendly exchange.

When I met her mother and sister months before in New York, we hit it off from the beginning, as I escorted the family on a shopping spree and tour of New York City. I always felt uncomfortable around parents and family. I was always completely trusted, and known for my intense dependability and devotion to friend and intimate partner alike. When Sylvia made her comment that there would not be enough room for me at Thanksgiving, something about it just didn't sit right in my gut. Was my suspicion because her parents owned a house that could sleep sixteen comfortably? Was her deference something I could not see through? She seemed angry when she said it, as if I had no purpose in her life, or as if she didn't want me around.

I spent Christmas and New Year's alone, suffering terribly from intense loneliness. Five months earlier, I was basking in the delight that we both agreed it was time for me to move to that small mid-western town, after she accepted my proposal of marriage. A New York boy born and raised, picking up all of the belongings I had from years past, finally realizing that I found the most beautiful girl in the world. More so than that she adored me, or so I thought. I was sure that through it all, and no matter what situation came our way, that feeling of intense dedication to one another would stand firm, and we could conquer anything. All I wanted was to hear from her while she was away, and she didn't even make the attempt to say "hi" or "Happy New Year."

She left me, having asked me to watch her apartment, her fish and belongings; all the while, she was out doing the one thing she promised me she would never do, and the one thing that would turn my life in a direction I never ever hoped to experience. That was a rough time for me, each day performing in the kitchen as a chef. The last time I heard from her was that Thursday, when she arrived at her parent's house. She

PARAMEDIC M.O.S.

called me at my place about 10:30 pm, and it was much to my surprise. She opened up the conversation with a very warm hello, and she wanted to let me know she made it home safely. She said, "I knew you were there thinking of me, and I just wanted to say I love you."

When she left for home that morning, she took a shower without me (something very unusual, as we always bathed and showered together), and had I not awoken, I felt as if she would have just left. In her haste to leave, I so desperately hoped all was okay. Having slept naked, I grabbed the closest pair of shorts and a tee shirt, and putting them on made my way to the kitchen.

I looked at her and said, "Hey," lovingly, as she replied the same in a soft manner.

"Drive carefully please," I said as I opened my arms to embrace her.

We shared a long kiss, a quick hug, and she made for her suitcase. As she approached the door she turned to me with her beautiful brown eyes and full kissable lips, making a very disturbing, almost mischievous smile. The look and sinister feel from her eyes that I observed made my heart fall to the bottom of my feet. I knew at that moment that she was heading for trouble. I thought of our conversation in the bath the night before; and while she got to sit in the rear this time; I though of her comment that threw me into a different world.

As I lay there in her arms, while she sprinkled water over me and kissed my neck, she said "I don't know Christian, I just feel like I am going to hurt you."

I lay there motionless against her soft body; I could feel the droplets of water cool on the parts of my body that weren't submerged beneath the warm bath. It was not that my body was motionless but my mind went blank with pain. Our relationship was in a downward spiral and although I had been informed numerous times that I wasn't the cause, there was nothing I could do to stop it. I felt a sense of dread unlike I ever had before. I have had the experience of guns in my face, being pinned down by heavy weapons fire, and exploding buildings all around me, but nothing ever prepared me for what I was now headed for. How do you stop the world from crashing?

I told myself to stop thinking that way and almost believed my thoughts, but then she did something else inconsistent with her current demeanor. As she walked out of the front door, she took about six paces, spun around and said to me, "I love you."

C.B. Garris

When she said this, it was almost a loud whisper coupled with a look in her eyes that I thought was her laughing at me in some clandestine manner. She knew that she suckered me completely with her charms. My heart was now hers to break and destroy. Unbeknownst to me, she knew that I moved across the country to give us the opportunity to be together, she knew that my love was unconditional and perhaps she was intimidated by my free flowing emotion. I was consistent, something I'm unsure she ever knew the meaning of. With that frozen moment in time, she was gone. I felt as if I had just been told that the world was about to end. I couldn't explain it, but I felt as if I had met my demise. I closed the door slowly, thinking of how I was going to handle this.

There had been no discussion as to how we would contact each other. I knew the number to her parent's house by heart having called it all summer. I thought that maybe she just needed some time to collect herself. After all, school had been very rough on her, and she had turned into such a bitter person. That plus the fact that she gained about 35 pounds seemed to be some of the factors that added to her fury. "She will come to her senses and she must believe all the things she says I am to her," I thought to myself not knowing what emotional turmoil was looming on the horizon.

I showered and dressed, heading down the block to my pad. I slipped into the cold emptiness of that little mid-western town, looking around and reminding myself that all was going to work out. I decided to walk down the street to the local bagel establishment, get a little breakfast, and then perhaps pick up a movie. Work would not begin for another six hours, so there was time to think, and watch a movie, think, eat a meal, and think.

Sylvia was gone, and as I re-entered her condo to have breakfast, I noticed something that I had never felt with her in my life. All of a sudden as I closed the door, I felt as if I entered a parallel world. This was a world that was absent of me, one where I just didn't belong. It was -25 degrees outside, and it seemed colder in Sylvia's flat. As I made my way towards the dining room table, I couldn't help but feel as if I was a ghost and no longer welcome. It was as if I didn't belong where I was so often made welcome. Just a few hours before, I would lay with Sylvia, her arm draped over me in her slumber's silence, her lips pressed against my neck.

Now I felt like a stranger, an invader, and a ghost of the present. I guessed that feelings of hollowness were always uncomfortable, but this seemed to be something of a quantum leap that one might take walking

PARAMEDIC M.O.S.

through a black hole. You come out on the other end, but to a place so alien to where you have been, it is bone chilling. I walked into the living room, and placed the bagel on a plate on the floor, as its paper bag that held it made a light crumbling sound. I tried to bring myself to the present, but my fear was all around. I knew I would never be welcome in Sylvia's home again. Now there was nothing I could do. I made a cup of tea, Celestial Seasonings Wildflowers & Honey, our favorite.

With every movement I made in the kitchen, I quivered at the thought of our relationship coming to an end. Where would I go? What would I do? It was always so hard for me to find acceptance, love and after feeling this plethora of feelings for this past year, it is not only gone, but it is being deliberately vacuumed out. It was a feeling unlike anything I ever knew. It was a vast, festering hole that continued to bury deep within the walls of my soul. I did know that the days following would be complete with pain, suffering and confusion.

Once again, this situation was reeling out of control. I could save all those lives on the street as a medic, but this ship was sinking faster than I could respond to it. There would be no chance to start an IV, administer medication, intubate a patient, or defibrillate a heart that was temporarily out of control. The sentence I was about to undergo was a permanent one; one without chance, without understanding or mercy. It would be something I would have to deal with for years to come.

I sat alone in the room, eating my breakfast, watching a video, trying desperately to laugh at something the video store said was good enough to be in the comedy section. Breakfast eaten and the video now over, I decided to make my way home for a shower and to get ready for work.

The hot water in my apartment always fluctuated, but I was relieved by the fact that I was always welcome to use Sylvia's shower. I remember after one argument we had about six weeks prior. We had made plans to have breakfast together, watch a video and snuggle. I couldn't think of a better place to be. When we awoke on that Saturday morning, she seemed strange, even distant. Her mood swings were more frequent, so I felt it would pass like the others. She finally rolled over to me, kissed me deeply and said "Hey," in her soft morning voice.

That particular voice had enough adoration in it to light up a city. We agreed omelets and that we'd watch *Groundhog Day*. Almost as soon as we made these plans, the phone rang, it was Bill, her professor. They had a conversation full of her enlightenment, and her mention that "No, I don't have any plans today." My heart sank since I was the one lying beside her, considering what ingredients to place in our omelets minutes before. Her comment was full of my invisibility, and was followed by her acknowledging to get together with him within the next forty-five minutes to do some "house repairs," particularly the installation of an air conditioner. It was November. She then said she would drop me home, as she could only do this work with Bill.

I started to cry, and said, "I thought we just made plans to have breakfast together and cuddle with one another."

She replied, "Look, I really want to get this done, and Bill says he is great with household stuff.

You can't do this kind of stuff, so I'll drop you home."

I felt my insides jerk with her comments, since she never asked me about my ability to perform household repairs, which happened to be extremely efficient. I said, "How do you know what I can and cannot do?" With this, she thrusted out of bed and said that I was impossible. I was going home, whether she was taking me home or whether I was walking. Eyes full of tears and body full of anger, I started putting my clothes on unable to respond.

She said, "You know what? This is over!"

I began placing my clothes on in furious fashion, wanting to lash out verbally at her, but afraid that if I said anything it would crush her. Then again at this point, I didn't know that she was incapable of feeling. Nothing I said would have crushed her.

I remarked, "How can you say that? We just made plans minutes ago of a day of cuddling and snuggling, and then Bill calls and you are now getting together with him, throwing me out of your house?"

She looked as if she was the cat who was just caught with the mouse in her mouth, as if she had no idea of what she did. Could she be schizophrenic I thought to myself? Does the DSM-IV (Psychiatric Diagnosis Codes) even have a diagnosis for this load of shit she is handing me?

"You need to go, and I'll take you home," she said, and with that I made for the door.

As we pulled up at my apartment, my face was still full of tears, and she looked at me with that look of being sorry, but she said nothing. I exited and disappeared into the common area of my apartment building. I opened the refrigerator and poured a glass of juice. Still upset, I sat at my counter and thought. I tried to get the picture out of my head, but

PARAMEDIC M.O.S.

I kept thinking about Bill showing up at her place, and her welcoming him into her home. They would gracefully embrace and she would disrobe him, and he her. She would have sex with him in intense fashion, completely disregarding anything we ever shared together. While in this conscious nightmare, my phone rang. Sylvia said, "Hi, it's me. Look, I'm sorry at the way this whole thing happened, and we should be done with this air conditioner by about 1:00 pm. Let's get together then, and we can make omelets, and tea, and we can snuggle all day and night, we won't even have to go out at all. I really want to cuddle with you."

My sniffing came to a gentle whisp from my nose as I acknowledged her new plan. She sounded so sincere and genuine, and once again, I felt my heart beat.

There was a bright flash of light and I woke up in a cold sweat. I was breathing fast, having no idea where I was. I was holding a warm body in my hands, the face said it was AJ, but I was so disoriented I wasn't sure. I moved my head around, getting the cricks and cracks out of my neck, and I sat up. That warm body next to me was AJ, and I was totally freaked out. I was having trouble swallowing, as if my own phlegm was choking me. AJ sat right up realizing something was wrong as I looked at her as if she had several heads.

AJ focused her eyes on me and asked, "Christian, what's wrong?"

I was still panting, and after hearing AJ's voice I began to come back to the present slowly. AJ just sat there, trying to ease me back down to a pillow. She realized that my side of the bed was totally soaked.

"Hun, your soaked, what's wrong?"

I took several deep breaths and informed AJ, "I just had one hell of a nightmare and I didn't know where I was when I woke up. It was so powerful that I didn't recognize you."

AJ looked at me with puppy eyes, wishing she could have kept me from having the dream.

"Babe, this is going to be normal for awhile. I talked with Nora and she said to expect this type of thing. Your whole world just got fucked about two weeks ago, and it will be sometime before anything normalizes." AJ knew I was embarrassed, as I always was when I was deeply revealed.

AJ asked, "Will you tell me about the dream?"

I thought for a few seconds without answering, and now AJ knew this would be bad.

"Was it about Jennifer?" AJ asked softly.

"No." I said clenching my jaws tightly.

"Sylvia?" AJ asked inquisitively.

I nodded. "It took place back where I moved to live with her in the mid-west. It was just a repeat of some of that silly shit she used to do to me. What freaked me out was that it was so damn real. The frustration was real, my fear was real, as was my anger."

AJ was facing me now, with an approving smile. Her look said to me that she was quite comfortable hearing this bad stuff, and that I didn't need to be worried that she was going to fly off the handle or get psycho on me for having the dream.

"When we first met," AJ said while holding my hand, "You were so vehemently against dating or sharing yourself with anyone. You went years with either superficial, shitty dates or none at all. You were plagued by the demise of the love you thought you had from someone who was absolutely incapable of intimacy or love. The only thing she was absolutely capable of was hurting you, breaking your heart, trust and losing a man that would have loved her for who she is forever. Now I for one am glad that you got out and drew the line. I know it hurt you, but you took care of her as best you could until you realized that she was one psychotic bitch. If I see this waste of female flesh, I'll show her how we do things back in San Juan. You loved her enough to trust her and based on her promises and after all that you did for her, SHE FAILED YOU."

AJ eased me back down to a lying position, helping me loosen up my body's rigid demeanor. AJ took the covers away from our bodies and laid her body on top of mine. Now I was truly back in the present. Her warmth and presence is amazing.

She gave me a sweet smile, "And I want you to know that we are here and together. I will do whatever it takes to help you know that this is real and something that I want as much as you. Nora said that because of the recent traumas, especially Jennifer, you will have all sorts of things popping up in your mind of previous bad situations. It might be a relationship, or a traumatic work situation like getting shot at. The smallest thing or even the biggest thing that you think you may have settled in your mind may come up. I would suspect that one thing that might come up for you might be your part in the rescue efforts at the terrorist bombing of the World Trade Center in '93. I remember you sharing with me that you weren't allowed to make contact with the outside for about four days. You said it seemed like forever."

PARAMEDIC M.O.S.

I sat for a moment, shifting my head in the vivid but frightening feelings associated with that day.

"I remember you made the first call to your mom." AJ spoke softly in a clear verbal memory. "You told her that you love her, and that you were glad that she was not downtown the day this happened. You then went on to tell her that you were fine, at least physically. You walked down into the crater left by the truck bomb, and when you looked way up into the three-story hole left in the infrastructure of the Tower you mentioned that the only thing you could think about was what if the buildings collapsed?" I breathed deeply feeling that moment in time run through my system. I remembered the moment I stepped foot inside this cold, dark area of the Tower; I was stuck in a strange place of virtual realism. I could not believe that a massive bomb went off twenty-four hours before in the very place I was now standing in. I could still smell the acrid stain of smoke that was left in all of our nostrils. That smell would last for weeks.

"The other thing that really bothered you about that scene," AJ spoke as I visualized, "was that you were the only one to raise hell about where they situated you at the scene. Your command post was placed right under the Towers, and you kept mentioning that given the nature of what just took place, how were they so sure that there weren't other bombs set to go off later? You were vehemently against having your post set up anywhere near the bombing site, but no one would listen to you. You mentioned to me how you set up your own escape route if the structure started to fall on top of you. You knew that you stood little chance of getting out of there if the structure collapsed but that you wanted to at least feel prepared."

AJ slipped her hand into mine. "That my dear," she continued, "is an extremely traumatic event. Other things that might pop up or cause flashbacks are recurring thoughts of bad relationships or any situation where you were emotionally affected. Whatever it is, I will be here to help, and when you need time to be by yourself you have it. I am very glad that you let me take you away from everything, because I know that is a major step for you. Your trust in me is something I cherish completely, as I do the rest of you."

AJ took a second to look at the clock and it said 07:30 a.m. She looked at me with a very sensual look in her eyes, "And speaking of things popping up, we have a few hours before our services; care to indulge?"

I smiled a smile that AJ was used to seeing. It was the one that said I would always give in to her requests.

C.B. Garris

Chapter XIX:

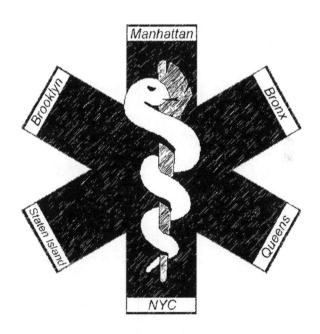

PARAMEDIC M.O.S.

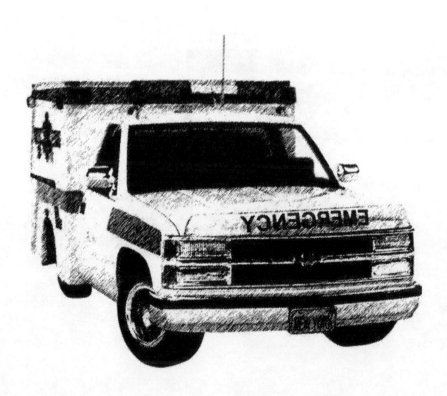

C.B. Garris

The his/hers massage was amazing. During the treatment we were able to hold hands as promised by Leeann, and they used heated stones as part of the treatment. They heat special stones in a warmer, and place them on certain affected areas of the back. The deep penetration of heat into the affected area causes an incredible release of tension and toxins. When the massage therapists were finished, they allowed us to stay there for a while. I had the immeasurable pleasure of lying prone (face down) on the massage table with AJ next to me. For about fifteen minutes after the massage, all she did was run her fingernails and fingertips up and down my right arm and back. Every couple should bond like this. I wish that everyone could be touched like AJ touches me; I think the world would be a different place, a better place.

The remaining treatments for that day left me strangely rejuvenated. When I arose from my massage, everything was clearer. I breathed easier and I was calm. AJ and I spent the following three days and nights in various treatments. These included more his/hers massages, oxygen facials, yoga lessons, reflexology, and incredible food by a fireplace. My mind now distracted and my body's chi (energy) balanced, or so said Master Yang, our Yoga guru, I felt somewhat displaced. AJ and I made love after a few of the Yoga sessions; now that was an experience.

When we completed our stay, AJ had a car brought to us that would shuttle us to Marina Del Rey. I stood by as AJ purchased a wholesale supply of products with a smile and gleam in her eye. I just smiled, as she looked like a kid in a candy store. Leeann was on hand to bid us adieu, and after she and AJ hugged deeply, I even received a hug from Leeann too with the instructions to come back and visit soon. We left the property and headed for the 101 Freeway. It would be about an hour and a half trip to Marina Del Rey.

We traveled south on the 101, opposite the direction of Santa Barbara. AJ and I stayed very close as I observed all of southern California passing my eyes. She was quiet, knowing I was soaking it in. As we got closer towards the Valley, AJ began sharing more information about where we were. We passed through an area called Calabasas, a very affluent and pretty section, which eventually gave way to Encino and Van Nuys. We turned off the 101 at the 405 and headed over the Mulholland Hill. It was about 2 p.m. and AJ said that traffic was lighter than usual. I'm glad because she had told me in the past of the ridiculous traffic jams that she

PARAMEDIC M.O.S.

sat in on various southern California freeways. We peaked the hill and it made several S curves as we approached Sunset Blvd.

"Isn't that where the Strip is?" I thought to myself.

As we passed the 10 Freeway, AJ asked me, "Different, isn't it?"

Studying how the 405 was looking much like the German Audubon at this point, I replied, "Quite. It is also kind of refreshing. I cannot quite explain how, but it is something more visceral than I have ever experienced."

AJ smiled wide, "I know exactly what you mean, I felt it too when I first moved here."

We pulled off the 405 at the 90 Freeway towards Marina Del Rey. Opting not to go to Slauson Avenue, our driver headed to the right. We drove into what appeared to have once been a marsh, but is now a well-developed community of two story condos, and homes called Mar Vista. We hooked a left on Mindanao and a right on Admiralty. We passed a park on the right hand side, several posh restaurants on the left and of course a fire station, LA County's Engine 110 and Truck 110. The station was perfectly perched against the backdrop of the Marina. Just up ahead of the firehouse, was an opening in the cement divider, and it gave way to a beautiful cobblestone entrance to the Ritz-Carlton hotel. I did a double take as AJ smiled once again. "I only take my baby out in style." She held my hand.

The driver took care of our baggage as we checked in. The expensive gallery artwork gave way to beautiful mahogany furniture throughout the structure in the lobby. We headed to our room or I should say more accurately, suite. The bellhop opened the wide doors to our suite and I witnessed an outstanding view of the largest man-made harbor in the United States. It was gorgeous and sunny. Boats and yachts were disentangling moorings and heading for sea. I noticed a bunch of Wave-runners making their way towards the Pacific. I opened the closet door to place my clothes in and I was greeted to a treat from AJ.

It seems that Ms. AJ decided to do a little clothes shopping for me and have the items perfectly placed for me in the closet. We enjoyed shopping for each other, and unlike most times, I was very comfortable with her shopping for me. Just the same I love that she let me shop for her. She had fabulous taste, and she thought the same of me.

We were both simple about the fact that when one shopped for the other, it was because we thought they would look great in something, rather than trying to make a statement that we didn't like their present wardrobe. I found what appeared to be California casual clothing in the closet. A great black sports coat by Gruppo, a silk Prada black knit shirt that complimented my physique nicely, black slacks, and shoes. I guess by the looks of things we had a few nice places to go.

AJ walked out onto the balcony as I walked out of the bathroom. I met her there and she faced me, kissing me very deeply. I felt as if I was being introduced to a different part of her. There were many depths to her soul, and even I was feeling the effects of being in California already. It was as if it blocked out all this bad stuff I have been carrying. It was bright and there was sunshine all around. They say that people who live in lots of sunlight generally are happier and lead fuller lives. It beats the hell out of living in Seattle, where although it is a beautiful city, it rains constantly.

A deep kiss. Another deep kiss, and I felt a freedom in AJ's body that was so alluring and appealing. Then again, she was always alluring and appealing. AJ picked up the phone and asked someone to bring up a fruit platter and several smoothies.

"Smoothies?" I asked.

"Great fruit concoctions that you will be hooked on when you try." AJ said as she pointed out a gorgeous 110-foot yacht as it pulled into the bay slowly.

"There is a fabulous restaurant just up ahead called Farma. I thought we would do dinner there, right on the water."

Trying to adjust to another wonderful evening in California I smiled, "You know that I trust your tastes!"

About fifteen minutes later, a knock at the door would just so happen to be our fruit platter and smoothies. The fruit platter looked sumptuous. She had picked out all of my favorites: mango's, passion fruit, papaya, incredibly sweet pineapple, strawberries, and some sharp cheddar to balance the palate. We sat on the balcony holding hands as I inhaled great Pacific air.

Every once in awhile I would have thoughts of Jennifer and New York, but they were very subdued. I was concentrating on the evening. We took a walk down to the Marina and even met a friend of hers who docked her yacht in one of the slips. After we made our first round of the boats, during our return trek to the hotel a female voice screamed out, "AJ?"

We both turned around and this stunning female of Asian descent in her 30's came rushing up to us. They hugged as I stepped back a few steps; apparently the friend of AJ's was ecstatic to see her. I could relate.

PARAMEDIC M.O.S.

As she hugged AJ, they disengaged and AJ said, "I want to you to meet Christian. Christian, this is Miko Irinokasa."

I stepped forward extending my hand as her friend opened her arms and pulled me in for a hug. I looked at AJ with this frightened look and she nodded approvingly. I gave her a gentle hug and she just stared at me for a second.

"AJ, how have you been? Where have you been?" Miko asked with a delicate hint of Japanese dialect in her voice.

As the two of them caught up briefly, I admired Miko's yacht. It must have been 100 feet long.

Actually, Miko looked vaguely familiar, though I could not figure from where. After the greetings were over, Miko invited us aboard. This was certainly the way to go. Not only was this yacht 100 feet long, but it was a home on the water. As we entered the aft portion of the craft, it looked like a living room sequence from a very expensive South Beach Miami penthouse.

Everything was pristine, but not overdone. It was obvious that Miko spared no expense. Miko disappeared below deck for a few minutes as a crewmember dressed in all white approached with selection of drinks for us both. I felt totally out of my element, but Miko's welcome made us feel very at home. AJ told me that Miko, who was originally from Kyoto, Japan, grew up in her father's import-export business.

What used to be mainly autos and clothing, gave way to tech support products and computers as well. Her father and brother were attempting to embezzle the funds from the generations owned family business so she figured out what they did and had them arrested. She in turn took over the company by unanimous decision of the board of directors, and now she does most of her business from Los Angeles, going back to Japan when she wants.

A crew member gave us a tour of the yacht and I thought I was going to faint. First, there is an eight-person crew that maintains the vessel at all times, and she even has another one for when this one goes into dry dock. They are identical with massive sleeping quarters, two navigational command centers above and below deck, a huge office with satellite video conferencing and an office for her personal assistant, Kathryn. Forget the galley kitchen, as she has a fully set up professional kitchen with a chef on board for her and any guests. This woman lives better than the president. She also has a small gym onboard, but she apparently goes to Diego, her personal trainer's studio for her workout in Santa Monica.

Miko reappeared wearing nothing but a bathing suit and deck shoes. She like Leeann was graceful and warm. We sat for a while as the two of them caught up. I enjoyed the view and this display of wealth.

"So Christian, you seem like a strong man and an honest one. Was it easy winning AJ? She is a tough cookie you know."

I smiled at Miko replying, "She does it for me."

Miko, who was expecting much more, seemed acutely pleased with my response. AJ filled her in on some of the recent events, and informed Miko that we came to get away from it all. AJ told her we would be heading down to Farma for dinner if Miko would like to join us. She accepted. We excused ourselves to get ready for dinner. We were to meet Miko at the slip in an hour; the restaurant was walking distance from her yacht.

"Wow!" I said as re-entered the Marina entrance to the hotel, "that was unbelievable."

"Welcome to LA honey," AJ said with a charismatic tone.

We approached the elevator in the lobby as AJ said, "Miko is great and she is a lot of fun. I am so glad that she has done so well for herself. She doesn't really have to work, just make sure that the company runs well. She is shrewd and very effective. She was married years ago, but she got rid of that dead beat. Good thing she had him sign a pre-nup first too, because not even I can imagine how much money her accounts hold."

"Let me guess," I said, "She is as sincere as you, but since she is a caring person with money, all the idiots try to score on her for her looks and money; no one is interested in her heart."

AJ put the credit card sized key in the electronic lock saying, "Honey, you never cease to amaze me. Like Davia said to me a long time ago, if they could clone you this world would be a better place."

The three of us had a great time at dinner. Though she grew up amid wealth, it appears that Miko had a good mother who kept her balanced. Our dinner lasted almost three and a half hours and I was getting many a look from both men and women. We were seated on a Marina side table, and the two of them looked absolutely stunning. AJ was wearing a mini dress and shoes that I bought for her a few months back. The dress was black, and very form fitting, with spaghetti straps from her shoulder blades to the top of her chest. The shoes were black platform, six inch spiked heel, with straps that went half way up her calves. I do believe that her

PARAMEDIC M.O.S.

outfit was responsible for a very loud kitchen accident when one of the chef's and an executive manager caught a glimpse.

Joining in similar fashion was Miko, who before shoes stood at 5'1", with long black hair down to her waist, beautiful almond colored and shaped eyes, and a very well toned body. Her outfit was devastating to most that caught a view of her. She wore gray & tan Anaconda Snake Hologram V-front pants made of Lycra, with a matching strapless, handkerchief top. She decided on black platforms as well, but with chunky heels that added six inches to her height, and accented her outfit perfectly.

AJ & Miko both looked like absolute royalty. Their presence was completely captivating as were their charms. Throughout the restaurant men were getting punched in the arm by their wives or dates for their staring. Admiring our fluid interaction, Miko admitted that she was quickly becoming insanely jealous of the connection AJ and I share. When we parted after the walk back to the boat, we promised to connect again before our return to NYC.

We retired back to our suite and enjoyed the warm breezes on the balcony. We sat sometimes in silence and sometimes we talked. AJ sat secure with me being who I am to her in her life, and I sat comfortable without having to make explanations for my thoughts. I desperately tried to step into the realm of comfort with the thought that AJ would be permanent in my life as long as we wanted to be with each other; but I was deathly afraid of getting hurt. It never stopped me from being loyal, faithful or completely crazy about her; nor did it affect my ability to love her with all of my soul. The only thing it did was keep me from a place of comfort, a place that she wanted me to experience in all its splendor. My fears run deep, perhaps too deep for even me to say; yet AJ understood my silence, and replaced my fears with affection and adoration that every man would wish for.

After an evening of keeping the neighbors awake, I awoke completely refreshed. When I opened my eyes, AJ was looking at me.

"Good morning lover." She said with a smile. "I want you to know that my body is still tingling."

I opened my eyes and focused, smiling at her comment.

"How about we order breakfast, and then take a walk on the beach? It is only a few blocks walking distance." AJ asked as she ran her fingers across my face.

"Considering we burned off a bundle of calories last night, I think breakfast is in order," I said as I stretched like a puppy, thrusting my arms all the way out, holding it and then wrapping them around AJ.

She slipped the menu from behind my pillow. I like a woman that is prepared. We both went with egg white omelets, both with spinach, avocado, and pepper, wheat toast, extra-crispy Peruvian blue home fries and large glasses of orange juice. After we showered, we dressed in summer attire and walked out of the hotel.

AJ was wearing her hair in a ponytail, with a dark blue NY Yankees baseball cap, a frosty blue tank top with the word "Taken" on the front, white shorts and a pair of white New Balance running shoes. I tossed on a great Hawaiian shirt that AJ bought for me, it was done in pastel blue with deep maroon and lime colored orchids, blue shorts/trunks, and also a pair of New Balance. We walked west on Admiralty, following the curve. When we reached Via Marina we walked right down to Washington Blvd.. We made a left on Washington Blvd. and I could see the beach from there. As we approached Pacific, I noticed a staple of our society on the corner, Starbucks.

"Up ahead is a great coffee meeting spot, it's called The Steaming Moose." AJ said like she hadn't seen an old friend in awhile. We approached this rather large outdoor cafe and the owner Bill Hynder looked up at AJ.

"Oh my God, could that be you?" He put his apron down and walked around the counter to AJ and I.

"Hi Bill." AJ said like she was being welcomed home. They hugged and I just observed. He was ecstatic to see her.

"What is his fucking story?" I thought to myself.

"Bill, I want you to meet Christian." AJ said with one of those thousand watt smiles.

Bill and I extended hands simultaneously, and he had a firm handshake. He looked like an okay guy. He stood about six feet tall, about 180-200 lbs., with a deep rich tan, brown eyes, short brown hair and he was well built.

It turns out that Bill is an ex-firefighter/paramedic for the Los Angeles County Fire Department. He fell through a roof fighting a fire a number of years back and was medically released from duty on 100 % of his salary for the rest of his life. He bought the cafe and has been running it ever since. We stood and talked for a while, and I became more at ease.

PARAMEDIC M.O.S.

In the back of my mind I found myself waiting for that other shoe to drop again. It was totally my issue and not my place to put it on AJ. I guess when you experience someone deliberately deceiving you in your past, it is difficult to break the habit of being suspicious. We picked up two great Iced Chai teas and headed for Venice Beach.

I stood at the base of the boardwalk near the Speedway looking west. There was sun, surf, and sand for as far as I could see. There were scores of people riding their bikes or roller blading on a special lane provided for them. There was a separate boardwalk lane for people to walk on, with enough distance and grass in between so if someone took a spill, they wouldn't take anyone else out. People seemed happy, as they were all smiling and laughing. Maybe it was the constant exposure to direct sunlight. I saw several males and females that must have had annual memberships to Gold's Gym, as they had more definition than a dictionary.

We walked for what seemed like miles. On our left was the beach, to our right one, two, or three story dwellings. Some of the dwellings were simply studio apartments on the ground level going for $2000.00 a month, although they provided a view of the beach out your front door. We walked north enough to where we walked past the gym at Muscle Beach, and then to the Boardwalk shopping and entertainment area. This was a mixture of fixed stores or private vendors selling their stuff. Clothes, music, food; it had everything. There were street performers, some guy in a turban with a guitar and a bulls-eye on it, who went by the name Dave. He performed this retro-60-renaissance music that sounded like Jethro Tull meets Godspell.

As I watched and held AJ's hand, she just smiled watching my reactions to everything around me. It was a far cry from being under a subway train.

Everyone seemed healthier than when I was in New York. Perhaps it was the sun, the sand, the surf or the food. Every establishment we passed had egg whites or avocado – very not the East Coast.

"I thought we would take a drive up the Pacific Coast Highway today and have dinner in Santa Monica tonight." AJ said to me as we slurped on the icees we bought from a stand on the boardwalk. I was so excited to experience California that I could barely stand still. AJ and I returned to the hotel where she had a convertible Beamer waiting for us. We hopped in and headed back in the direction we walked. She turned right on Pacific and took that straight across Ocean Park to Pico, and just before the

Santa Monica Boardwalk hooked a left onto the PCH. We drove north on a gorgeous day. It was about 87 degrees out and I was getting baked. Good thing we both put sunscreen on each other. AJ explained a little about the history of the area to me. We approached Zuma Beach and I was floored. It was like a beach paradise. We pulled into Zuma for a few minutes to watch the surfers. I felt like I was in a Beach Boy music video. I had heard so much about this place called L.A. and I was now in it, almost too quickly to realize it.

We continued on and after we passed through Malibu proper, we turned into a secluded place called Nicholas Beach. We parked and walked down the wooden stairs towards the beach. Once there we saw a couple of surfers gearing up and two scuba divers placing a buoy in the water. We walked towards a creek and joked about some of how some of our co-workers would not be able to handle this. We were going to have an early dinner tonight as it was Friday and she had other plans for us. We drove back down the PCH and I started thinking to myself, "I can deal with this!" If I wasn't mistaken I thought I saw a glimpse of "I'd like to move back here," in AJ's eyes.

We went to a place called the Promenade in Santa Monica to our restaurant. The Promenade was like a chic Venice boardwalk. It had all the hot, cosmopolitan stores, and a variety of indoor and outdoor restaurants. Tonight we would dine at Dente; a northern Italian restaurant. Anjoline loved raising my temperature, so tonight she was wearing an outfit that she picked. She was an absolute knockout; then again I was biased.

She was wearing black sheer flare stretch satin pants, the flare began about two inches below the kneecap and the knees had a lime green wavy design all the way around. Her top was a matching halter that was spaghetti stringed, and covered just to her cleavage. The area around her statuesque cleavage on the halter also exhibited a wavy lime green design, and it showed off her very impressively toned stomach, and was open all the way around her back. Anjoline's well-developed lat muscles gave the halter top extra depth. The satin pants were skin tight, and when she originally walked out of the bathroom at the hotel I thought I was going to faint. Her outfit was finished off with a pair of black platform six-inch chunky heels. She knew how to dress and how to make a statement. As we walked up the Promenade, most of the men who looked like Ken dolls, which was pretty common for Santa Monica,

PARAMEDIC M.O.S.

were in dead lock stare at AJ. She had that sexy New York girl flare that was completely insatiable. I even heard some guy behind me say, "Damn boy, you go!"

I smiled and so did AJ.

"You're popular tonight," AJ said to me squeezing my hand with a smile; knowing full well that the view of her just caused the maitre de to stumble over patrons at a Bistro next to our restaurant.

"No dear, I think it is you that is the popular one." With each day that I grew closer to AJ, she just became sexier.

The restaurant was owned by some of the boys from my old neighborhood. The place had serious New York flair. In fact, as we passed the demonstration kitchen, the executive chef sized me up and knew I was from the hood back in New York City. As we were led to the upstairs area for our reserved table, he and I locked eyes and I noticed that we even looked like brothers. The chef put skillet of pasta he had in his hands down, and motioned me over. "Good to see you papa," he said as we locked hands.

I smiled and said, "Great to see you as well." We were definitely from the same hood. AJ and I went upstairs and not long after we sat, the host returned with a platter of Amouse Bouch (the chef's complimentary gift). Tonight's Chef delights were house roasted sweet red peppers, house made mozzarella, stuffed mushrooms and topped off with lemon sorbet to clean the palate before the entree. Our meal was the best Italian meal I'd ever had. I had a Penne Saprori, which included seared chicken, house smoked mozzarella, and diced tomatoes. AJ had the Linguini Arabiatta, which consisted of homemade spicy tomato sauce with smoked mozzarella on top at her request. We finished with Panna Cotta (an eggless, whipped cream custard) with Strawberry Coulis, the best I have ever tasted.

After dinner we hopped in the Beemer and headed out of the parking structure onto 4th Street.

"We are going to have all kinds of fun tonight," AJ said as she made a left onto the 10 Freeway. It was wild to see a California freeway at night, probably since I was so used to seeing the sky around me in New York cut out by skyscrapers. Here in Santa Monica as we approached the 405 freeway, you could see for miles. When I looked into the southeastern sky, I could see a row of jumbo jets lining up for their final approach to LAX. We continued east until AJ came off at La Brea, making a sharp right to run down a nasty curve. Whoever designed these LA freeways needs assistance on how to build entrances and egresses; they all seem to mend together and I can only imagine the accidents that one can get into out here. We drove through an area that appeared to be somewhat run down after we came off the freeway. AJ explained that we would soon be approaching Miracle Mile, where La Brea and Wilshire meet.

As we cruised with the top down, AJ popped on the stereo and I immediately heard one of my most favorite artists, John Klemmer, on the local jazz station (94.7 KTWV "The Wave"). I was quickly becoming very comfortable in this Los Angeles lifestyle.

Next thing I knew, some guy in the car next to us rolled down his window and tried to get AJ's attention. He was driving a large black Mercedes, and looked to be in his early 40's, though I was quickly learning that out here you never really knew how young or old people were. It was a combination of either those who took damn good care of themselves, or those who decided to go the route of plastic surgery. He had a fair complexion with a good tan, broad shouldered, probably played football about ten years in the past, blonde hair, green eyes and a charming smile.

This putz rolls down his window and said to AJ, "Nice car."

AJ paid him no mind. "Hey babe," were the next words to come from his mouth. My dorsal fin went straight up as I was about to leap over AJ and show this guy what a Manhattan ass kicking was all about. Without even looking at the guy AJ just put the car in gear and we took off. When we reached Sunset we turned left and I suddenly realized I was on the Sunset Strip on a Friday night. There were people everywhere, and cars of all kinds. I could tell that a bunch of locals were cruising to show off their cars. L.A.P.D. was out in force, so I presume this area could go south if there was a drag race or an accident with one of these toy cars.

We drove a bit further and pulled off to the right at a valet spot. I looked up and we were at The Joke House, a famous comedy showcase spot. There was a long line going around the block, and when Anjoline stepped out of the beemer, all conversations in the first block of people ceased. I exited and after taking the parking sticker from the valet agent, she walked around putting her arm though mine with a proud smile. The bouncer at the door, a massive black male who was as big as a house at 6' 6", and he must have weighed in at 270, was all muscle. He had a shaved head, a goatee, and single loop earrings in both ears. He was an extremely handsome man, and I am sure that actresses and the like fell over this guy

PARAMEDIC M.O.S.

regularly. He had the aura of a pro football player without any attitude. He was talking with one of the staff of the establishment when his eyes caught a glimpse of AJ; he showed a huge tooth filled smile.

"AJ, baby, how are you?" He stepped off of his seat and leaned down to give her a genuine hug.

As they disembraced he extended his hand out to me with a warm smile.

"Anthony Watson, how you doing man," he said confidently. I followed by introducing myself. Anthony had a very warm presence, and one that I did not feel threatened by. AJ is easy to love and I was not surprised that she was greeted by so many the same way.

"Girl, where have you been? LA has not been the same without you." Anthony said as he checked off some paperwork he had on a clipboard.

"I went back to New York. I decided to become a Paramedic, and have been there for several years. This is Christian's first time out to LA, so naturally I had to bring him here." AJ spoke with affection towards Anthony. I got the impression that Anthony looked out for AJ when she lived here. An attractive female, who actually turned out to be the owner, stuck her head out to speak with Anthony for a brief second when she realized AJ was standing there. She was a very attractive black female, judging by her exotic features, I would say she was black, Latin and Japanese. Her heavy British accent was quite prevalent.

"Anthony, can you please make sure that..." realizing that AJ was there, "Oly shit, Anjoline 'ow are yuh?"

AJ opened her arms and hugged the statuesque and very well stacked black female with an intense, "Hey Julia." The two hugged intensely as they danced around in excitement.

"AJ, 'ow the bloudy 'ell ar' ya? Julia said looking in my direction. "Well by the looks of things, I 'ould say yu ar' doing yuh'self quite bloudy auright. Ooh 'is y'ur friend?"

"Christian, meet Julia. She owns this place." AJ said in complimentary fashion. I went to shake her hand and Julia thrusted onto me with a complimentary hug, making sure to outline the muscles in my back with her hands. She let go of me smiling back at AJ, "Eeee's purrrrfect." Now I know I was blushing.

Anthony interrupted for a moment, "Christian, AJ brought you to the right place. How are you enjoying LA so far?" It was nice of Anthony to ask.

"I gotta tell you, I'm feeling this something fierce." I said with a huge smile.

Anthony nodded his head approvingly, "You can get hooked real easy into the lifestyle out here. Some people from the East Coast have a hard time fitting in, but it looks like you've done it." Anthony summoned one of the hostesses.

"Are yuh comin' to see thah show tonight?" Julia asked.

AJ smiled and nodded, "We didn't make a reservation, and came in kind of last minute; but we'd love too. This is Christian's first trip to LA."

As the hostess opened the door for, Julia took me by the arm and said, "I 'ave uh special table just fuh' tha two oh ya." Julia scurried us in while Anthony stood back at the door. AJ walked in next to me and we were given a great table in the VIP section of the club. I was just glad that it was just far enough away from the stage. We were already seated with our drinks as the club started filling up.

"Y'uh ar gooing ta love t'is lineup!"

Looking at AJ I raised my glass to her, "I just want to say that this is really amazing, all of this. I am so relaxed and I feel as if my soul is being replenished. You my dear look absolutely beautiful!"

AJ rose her glass to me and thanked me. "Christian, I have not seen you this relaxed in a very long time. This trip is really working out like I hoped it would. I hope you are okay with meeting all these different people." I nodded very approvingly.

"L.A. was a huge part of your life and I am glad to see that you were as well received as I figured." AJ leaned forward and kissed me. She loves looking across a crowded room to find me, sending her that signal, the one that says, "when we get home, it's gonna be on!"

In between her laughing, I caught a number of very content and happy glances from AJ. She was glad to see me enjoying myself and laughing. She was glad that I, and actually we, were away from all that horrible stuff we left.

AJ knows I am a survivor, and have been through some pretty horrendous shit in my life. She knows that I have quite a road ahead of me, but through my laughter and my ability to remain who I have always been to her, she knew that I would be okay. It is a slow road to recovering from what I witnessed, since it wasn't the first time I'd dealt with suicide. When I was a teenager, a man by the name of Kevin Honnikcer who was

PARAMEDIC M.O.S.

like a second (and real) father to me, jumped off of the Verrazono Bridge in Staten Island. Weeks later a fellow student at my high school blew his head off with a shotgun. In college one of my neighboring hall mates hung himself in the bathroom, and I was the one to find him. With my own personal tragedies, AJ knew that I was never going to turn out like those that hurt me.

I was however very fragile in many ways as a result of my background. I would introvert myself, not knowing how to trust. Maybe AJ really is going to stick by me and not turn my world upside down.

It was about 10:30 when the last comedian finished his monologue. As AJ and I said goodbye to Julia and Anthony, we hopped back in the beamer and headed for The Samba Room. This is a fabulous salsa club in Beverly Hills. It is several levels high and when you walk in you have to go upstairs to get to the bar, which is neo art deco meets The Jetsons. To the left is the dance floor, and it looks kinda like a massive 50's soc hop. Men and women line the walls hoping that someone will ask them to dance and they are hoping even more that if someone does ask them to dance, that they know how. We walked up the stairs to find a restaurant and bar on our right and to our left the dance floor.

We chose right and both took a seat at the bar; AJ ordered an amaretto sour, and for me a virgin pina colada. As we sipped our drinks watching the atmosphere, we entertained our chosen silence with sensous touches of each others hands. AJ was stunning in the soft pastel-orange light that illuminated the room. The light bounced off of her tan warming all of my senses, and all of those around me. When we finished our drinks, AJ tapped my hand and then placed hers in mine, "C'mon babe, let's hit the floor."

C.B. Garris

Chapter XX:

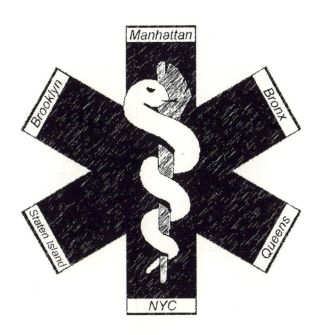

PARAMEDIC M.O.S.

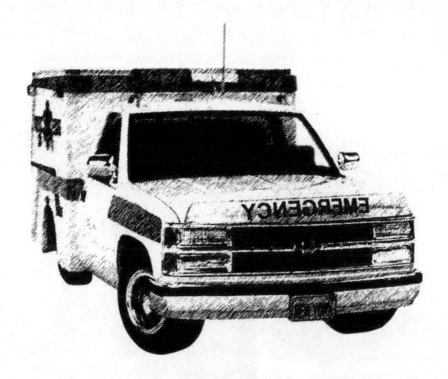

I awoke to the sound of glasses jingling in the room. When I sat up and rubbed my eyes, AJ was in a thick, white terrycloth robe and looking sexy as ever. She ordered breakfast for us and was bringing it over so that we could have it in bed.

"Well now, did you know that you amaze me every time we make love?" AJ said with a satiated smile.

"I like to think that I make you happy, and judging by the indentations in my back and shoulders from your fingernails, I hope I am correct."

AJ put her hand on my side and rolled me over slightly to see the pleasure wound she inflicted on me during the evening.

"Oops," AJ said with an innocent smile.

"I'm not complaining," I said with a grin. "I happen to love your body and being able to please you. I will always find ways or invent new ones to do that." I said this as AJ's eyes exhibited a look as if she was contemplating a list on a menu.

"Christian, Christian, Christian; how did I ever get so lucky?" AJ said as if she was contemplating a list of amenities of choices at the Spa.

"I think we are both very lucky," and feeding her a strawberry I said, "and I do love you."

AJ took a very sensual bite of the strawberry and fixed her eyes on me. After she chewed and swallowed the fruit, she leaned into me and we kissed. She smelled great, she looked great and I am in love with her. I would protect her at any cost, and am glad that I am the person that she confides in and that she likes to take care of.

"So what do you say about visiting a movie set today?" AJ said raising her eyebrows.

"Do they work on Saturdays?" I said pulling her close to me.

"Yes, silly. Movie making is a twenty four hour a day operation, just like EMS – except the pay is better." AJ said with a huge smile. "I thought we would take a drive up to Burbank and visit Warner Brothers to see Taylor Frentworth. She is filming a forthcoming blockbuster there now, and she told me to stop by the set if we came out."

"Taylor Frentworth? You know Taylor Frentworth?" I said in awe, as she is one of Hollywood's top leading ladies.

"Know her, we were neighbors when I lived in Marina Del Rey! We used to have barbecues on my porch all the time. We would just sit there and talk about non-entertainment type stuff, family, men and where our

PARAMEDIC M.O.S.

careers where headed. She is a real doll, and she actually expressed interest in me as a lover."

I sat bolt upright in my seat and imitating my best Buckwheat double take I said, "And?"

"Well, Schnookums," AJ continued, "I told her that I thought she was absolutely beautiful and if I was into women, I would be a lucky woman and the first to jump her bones; but that wasn't the way that I swing. She actually took it nicely and never gave me reason to feel uncomfortable after that. Although I could feel her undressing me with her eyes every chance she got. She became a great shopping partner and we developed a nice friendship. It was quite flattering."

I shook my head, "So let me get this straight, one of the worlds most famous and most sought after actresses tells you she wants to shack up with you and shag you, not necessarily in that order and you turned her down?"

"Yup!" AJ said with a confident smile.

"You are such a prude!" I said laughing.

AJ laughed and said, "Honey, I was saving myself for the man I always hoped to find."

I nodded my head thankfully, "Even I gotta say that was a long shot, don't get me wrong I am glad that we found each other, but what if we never met? You could have prohibited yourself from something that you might have enjoyed very much."

AJ gave me a mischievous smile "Who said I gave up on the prospect?" AJ laughed hard and began tickling me. We could take this kind of conversation in any number of directions, and I think the best part is that we could talk about it and not be frightened of what would be said.

"Are you serious?" I asked AJ.

"Gotcha!" AJ said as she tickled me some more. "Honey, you are all I want. It took us way to long to find each other, but no man or woman for that matter will ever take me away from you."

We were heading north on the 405 back over the Mulholland Hill when AJ turned right off to the 101. I could never figure out these California freeways. The sign would say west, but it was really south, and the same went for north and east. I am glad they identified what cities the exits headed towards, or I would have ended up in Vegas, which is not so bad of a thing. We went through Studio City and then hooked a left onto the 134.

C.B. Garris

I thought New York drivers were dangerous, but here I kept seeing people switching lanes without signals, and shooting across the highway four lanes at a time. We came off at Pass Avenue and made a few quick rights and lefts and all of a sudden we were pulling into the security gate at Warner Brothers. The lot was huge, with giant tan warehouse structures everywhere. If it weren't for all the giant billboards identifying the famous shows produced either by or at these studios, I would have thought I was entering a military base in the desert.

A very large security guard stuck his head out of the guard shack. "May I help you?"

AJ gave him one of her million watt smiles, lowering her sunglasses "Anjoline and Christian Sanchez to see Taylor Frenworth," she said thoughtfully.

"Oh yes Ms. Sanchez, Ms. Frentworth called down to the gatehouse this morning and told us to expect you." The guard, whose name tag said Tony, punched a few words into his computer and it spit out passes for us both and a map to the stage # 42.

"Maam, just make a right here through the gate, follow Denzel Blvd. until you reach Singleton Way. Follow the signs to stage 42, and the AD (Assistant Director) will be waiting for you. By the way ma'am, I do not mean to be intrusive but haven't I seen you somewhere before?"

AJ looked at me and raised her eyebrows up and down, "I have been here a few times." The guard pushed a button opening the gate and we drove through. The studios were a flurry of activity, with people in all kinds of dress walking around. There were men and women in suits, jeans, t-shirts, skin-tight dresses with all of there cleavage hanging out, women with huge diamond rings on everywhere, and a whole bunch of people with headsets on.

"What's up with all the security?" I asked AJ.

AJ laughed, "Those aren't security people, they are on the crews that are filming throughout the lot. They can talk to each other quietly even during filming if something is needed. The headsets also provide a method of privacy during the shoot for the crew." We pulled into stage 42, where a young, medium sized guy with a headset on put his hand out for us to stop.

"Ms. Sanchez!" He said with a charismatic voice. He was young, maybe twenty-eight, with dark hair and eyes, fuzzy beard from not shaving, slender build, and he was wearing dark sunglasses and a huge leather coat.

PARAMEDIC M.O.S.

"Hello," AJ said to the assistant director as he opened the door for her.

Hey, that's my job! I thought to myself.

As I was picking up a pack of mints I dropped, he ran around to my side of the vehicle and opened the door

"Mr. Sanchez, welcome to Hollywood." I thanked him and looked at AJ who got a kick out the look on my face when this guy opened the door for me.

"Thank you very much," I said, "It's great to be here."

"By the looks of who you just arrived with sir, I'd have to agree." He said with a serious tone. I didn't know whether to thank him again or deck him.

"Ms. Frentworth asked that you be brought right to set. Please follow me."

We did.

We walked through a maze of people, trucks, equipment and wardrobe. People in all kinds of odd-looking outfits were running around, and they had this pit in the corner called, "extra's holding." There must have been two hundred people in that pit: some looked to be talking to themselves, some were playing cards, a number of the women were on top of some of the men's laps. I couldn't tell if this was a movie, a social gathering or an orgy about to break out.

AJ took my hand as we were whisked into a "restricted filming area" of the studio. As the AD went to open the door quietly, I noticed that the red light above was illuminated; perhaps that meant they were actively filming. When we walked in, crewmembers saw the AD, and then saw AJ. The female members backed up to give her and the AD room, while a bunch of the male crew members were beginning to walk in AJ's direction. Then they saw me. Now the men were backing up. AJ pulled me along side of her and squeezed my hand.

Taylor was performing a scene of an upcoming spy thriller where she was an enlisted agent of the CIA, and as the routine goes she was out to save the world. When we walked in I didn't see her, and within a few minutes I realized the set was a replica of an office at the CIA. Taylor walked through with several other "agents" discussing how they would find who the double agent was. She was wearing an incredibly well tailored green suit, where the jacket came down just to her waist. The skirt came down to about mid-thigh, and then wardrobe decided to add a touch of sensual danger to the suit. They added a pair of black platform six-inch heeled boots that were laced up the front. She looked like a corporate dominatrix.

Taylor was a striking woman at 5'10", with hazel eyes, olive skin, and long straight blonde hair down to her shoulder blades. Her hair was so perfect that I was sure I had seen her in a Clairol or Pantene commercial. She had an amazingly large chest that if I learned anything over my years as a medic, judging by the dimensions of her waist, hip and chest, they had to be enhanced. She had a very small waist and perfect hips, but her breasts entered the room five minutes before she did.

"And CUT," said the director.

Taylor looked in our direction and screamed, "Girlfriend!"

Taylor dropped her props on set and ran over to AJ. I was trying to wonder how anyone who was 5'10" could run in six inch heeled platform boots without falling. It just looked painful. Taylor and AJ hugged for a few minutes, as the crew gathered around.

"This must be Christian!" Taylor said as she gave me an approving sizing up. She put her hand on my shoulder and rubbed it several times and then gave me a huge hug.

"AJ has told me so much about you, it is great to finally meet you. Come, let's go to my home away from home."

We were escorted out by the Assistant Director and several stragglers who I came to find out where called production assistants. We walked back out into the sunlight and were led to a massive Winnebago, known to the locals as a MOHO (motorhome). As we stepped up inside, I thought I was back at the Ritz. The entire vehicle looked like a hotel suite. There was fresh fruit and dips on platters everywhere. There was a wide screen TV, several comfortable couches, telephones, fax machines, a large king size bed in the rear, a stove, refrigerator and all the amenities. I must say the bathroom was ridiculously small. In fact when I went to use it I kept banging my knees and forehead trying to aim.

"Please help yourself to anything you would like Christian, I need help eating all this stuff. You know that a girl can't let her figure go in show business."

I smiled and thanked her. Picking a modest amount of fresh pineapple, strawberries and mangos off of the tray I heard AJ and Taylor catch up.

"I can't believe you became a Paramedic," Taylor said with a commendable tone. "It does totally speak of your nurturing side though."

PARAMEDIC M.O.S.

Taylor laughed. "Have you ever thought about coming back out here? You are still the talk in a lot of circles."

AJ smiled and said, "I hadn't really given it much thought. Though coming back here again has made me realize how much I miss all the sunshine. I lost track with how beautiful the weather is."

"Christian," Taylor called out, "how are you enjoying Los Angeles so far?"

"Taylor, I must say that it is amazing. I was just discussing with AJ about how there is something incredibly energetic about LA, and I can't figure out what it is. I feel like I have been reborn again."

Taylor put her hand on top of mine patting it, "L.A. is that way; have you ever thought about coming out here."

"I had always thought about visiting, as something about it always appealed to me. My work became so intense, I guess I lost track of the thought," I said with my hands up in the air.

"That's right," Taylor, remarked, "You are a paramedic also. AJ says you taught her everything she knows."

We sat for about an hour and a half while I listened to AJ and Taylor catch up and then a head popped in.

"Miss Frentworth, we are ready to put you through make-up and wardrobe again." Said the AD who escorted us around.

"Why don't you stay for awhile and watch." Taylor said as she rose from her chair.

We joined her back on set. After seeing her in another skimpy but well tailored outfit kicking the daylights out of her co-star we decided to say our goodbyes and walk around the lot a bit.

AJ stayed very close to me. I got the impression that her holding on close to me was not to say, "See, I have a man," but rather, "don't fuck with me or this man will rearrange your teeth." We walked out of the stage and onto the lot. We walked past a number of stages where all kinds of construction was in progress. AJ gave me the run down of who does what, the difference between a director and producer and what the difference is between a "Best Boy" and a "Gaffer."

As we approached the guard shack at the lot gate, the guard summoned us to stop.

"Ms. Sanchez, I have a message for you." The guard placed an envelope in her hands as she opened it.

"Taylor wants us to meet at her house for dinner in Malibu tonight."

"Cool," I said with a sun-baked smile.

AJ patted my thigh a few times and rubbed it saying, "It is really great to be here with you. L.A. can be a very lonely place, depending on your disposition. It can also be a fabulous place to share with someone. I am glad that we get to share it together."

Placing my hand in hers as she drove back towards the 134, I said, "I feel in some way that we were meant to be here. Thank you for making this possible. I haven't felt this relaxed and balanced ever."

AJ smiled and placing the *Eagles Greatest Hits Volume 1* in the CD player, she approached 70 mph on the 134 Freeway.

We arrived back at the hotel in time to shower and dress for dinner.

"Hun," I said, "what is the dress for tonight?"

AJ peeked out from the bathroom smiling and fixing her earrings, "Very casual. Taylor may strut herself in Versaci and Ralph Lauren when she is out and about, but she loves a good pair of sweat pants at the house."

I chose jeans, a gray v-neck, Club Room pull over (AJ calls it one of my muscle shirts), a black sports coat, and a pair of dark maroon Timberland dress walkers. AJ wore a fabulous black cotton sweater, with jeans and her black platform block shoes. It always amazes me how hot she can look even in dress downs. We left the hotel and drove back towards Pacific Ave. We were headed north up the PCH when we reached the light at Sunset Blvd.

"L.A. is a funny kind of place," I commented out loud.

"I had heard that this place can be hard to get to know people, yet at the same time everyone seems generally happy and polite."

AJ smiled, "It's the sun baby, it can do wonders for your demeanor."

We passed through Malibu proper once again and approached Serra Road. AJ made a hard right and followed the trail. From that trail was another trail, which led to a long driveway. We stopped at a gate, which had an armed guard, and I also noticed an unmarked police sector car sitting in the woods.

"Good evening madam. May I help you?" The guard said professionally. He was about 5'9", white, with brown eyes and hair, and very pronounced features.

"Anjoline and Christian Sanchez to see Ms. Frentworth." AJ looked over at me with a smile and touched my hand.

The guard walked back to the guardhouse and after speaking with someone on the phone, pressed a button to open the gate.

PARAMEDIC M.O.S.

"Just follow the lit path maam, and have a nice evening." The guard pointed towards a bevy of in ground dome lights that lit Taylor's driveway up like a runway.

Taylor's house was not a house, it was more like a facility. The grounds were spacious and perfectly landscaped. Her home, which was a giant Cape Cod style home, overlooked the Pacific Ocean. The facility as I call it must have had twenty-five rooms easy. When we approached the door, her personal assistant who apparently lives somewhere on the property greeted us. Out from nowhere came Miko. She decided to leave the boat for the day and come up to have dinner with all of us. Miko was very dressed down this time, but it did not in any way disguise her figure.

I kept thinking to myself, I could only imagine these three women on a shopping spree. They know what makes them look fabulous, and they have the money to back it up. Taylor came down from the long spiral stairwell. I heard a strange noise behind me and realized that Taylor had an elevator in her own home. I really didn't know what to do at this display of wealth, so I just thought I would appreciate it.

"I hope you don't mind, but I called up one of my chef friends and he is preparing us a meal tonight. Christian I heard you went to culinary school, so maybe you can give me a REAL critique on his food when he leaves." Taylor said smiling as she approached to hug me.

When she placed her arms around me, she squeezed my lats and made a sigh. AJ got a thorough kick out of it.

"AJ, he's a keeper!" All three women giggled and I stood there feeling like I had a little hat on my head with a propeller. Guess I am a little uncomfortable with compliments.

We were given the grand tour of the house, which took about forty minutes, and then sat down with Taylor and Miko in what I labeled the room with a view. Taylor had a sunroom specially designed with this massive bay window viewing the ocean. She had exotic plants of all kinds in perfect health throughout the house, and the sunroom led straight to the stairs of a gorgeous, professional kitchen. It blended nicely as I stood there staring at the sheer size of it all.

I have seen restaurants smaller than this place. The girls all had wine while I partook in a green magma-phyllo nutrient smoothie. Taylor heard I loved smoothies, so she had all the ingredients set up for me when we arrived telling me to help myself to anything I wanted.

C.B. Garris

Taylor was wearing very comfortable jeans, a pair of hot pink Pro-Keds and a gray blouse. She sat with her legs crossed, as if she was working on a collage. Taylor was very unpretentious and asked many questions of AJ and I. She wanted to know about what we do, but AJ made kind of a grimacing face when Taylor approached the topic, so she switched gears real quick. We decided to tell our most embarrassing stories, which I won the table on. Mine went back to an outward bounds trip in summer camp and a digestive disaster I suffered. Both Miko & Taylor laughed so hard I thought they were going to urinate on themselves. In fact at one point, wine came flying out of Taylor's nose; now that was funny. Our meal was served to us in the sunroom by a bunch of female hostesses. I got the impression that Taylor was more comfortable around women, which I could totally understand and relate too. I sensed that she had some foul situation with a male in her life, whether is was an intimate relationship gone foul or even issues with her father or brothers.

Her entire staff was female, and beautiful ones at that. They were all very presentable and kind. I guess she trusted women more than men. Miko and Taylor approached the subject of AJ and I possibly moving out to California, which I was totally unprepared for. Miko and AJ got up to go into the kitchen, leaving Taylor and I to talk.

Taylor leaned over to me and very softly said, "Christian, I don't want to harp on a sour topic, but I want to give you my deepest condolences on what just happened recently. I know it must be very tough, and we are all glad that you let AJ take you away from all of that. I don't want to put too many ideas in your head, but from what AJ's told me it's been a rough season for you. She has shared with me how bad it was and how it was very hard for you to smile. Since I met you earlier today, it appears to me that you have a marvelous smile and it looks to me like you have something for the Southland (southern California). I mentioned it to AJ already on the phone, but I just wanted to say that perhaps if you want too, you should consider moving out here. I have more pull than any actress in Hollywood, and I know that I can get you placed at any studio in charge of safety, dive rescue or emergency management. I don't want to offer this to take you away from what you do, because I have heard how close you are with everyone there. I just want you to know that AJ loves you dearly and she will do anything for you. I know she loved it here and it looks to me like it is doing you good too. Just from an observational point of view, you are a very fit individual and you obviously take excellent care of yourself. Just in that way, I think the southland lifestyle

PARAMEDIC M.O.S.

would fit your mind and your body better than New York. I know you grew up in Manhattan, but you know what Christian, so did I. There are times that I miss it, but nothing beats a southern California day or night."

Taylor sat there just staring at my eyes. "Think about it."

I looked at Taylor and smiled. "Let me begin by saying that I really appreciate you taking the time to talk with me about this and for even thinking of me before even meeting me. My head is really cluttered right now, and in fact I do love everything I have been learning about L.A.. I had never given thought to moving out here, but I do think I could get really used to it quickly. I too see how AJ looks at this place when she is here, and I can see her come to some inner peace just being in the sun. As I go through my options I will keep everything you have said in mind."

Taylor smiled and patted my hand, "We'd love to have you and AJ out here. If you decide to make a change, all you do is call me or have AJ let me know and I'll take care of the rest."

With that AJ and Miko walked back in and saw Taylor and I in a sort of huddle. I wondered if AJ knew that she would talk with me about this or if it was a surprise. From the look on AJ's face, I think she hadn't planned it, but she knew I was being briefed. Perhaps that is why she and Miko went to the kitchen. Maybe AJ knew I needed to hear a clear observation from someone totally unconnected to EMS. After hours of hearing about the mishaps that constantly took place when Anjoline attended Pepperdine, we decided to retire early. I received plentiful hugs from both Miko and from Taylor, as I was sent back out into the world. We were heading south on the PCH near the Ahi House when AJ said "You are very quiet, is everything okay?"

I thought for a second and looked over at AJ, "Everything is fine, I'm just soaking up the atmosphere. When you went to the kitchen Taylor gave me a little talking to."

AJ downshifted as we approached Santa Monica, "She told me, I hope that she didn't upset you. She means well, but she can be a tad bit overzealous at times."

I laughed and said, "Actually, she was very sincere and concerned."

I looked out at the Santa Monica Pier, watching the Ferris Wheel turn round and round when AJ tapped my hand.

"Look at the moon," which was low, full and the color of a blood orange.

"What did you think of what she told you?" AJ asked with a hint of excitement in her voice.

"I don't know. She made a very nice offer, but it is all too much to think about right now. I am thoroughly enjoying this place, and I can see the benefits to living here; it's just that I never thought of moving so far away from all I've ever known. The thought of it is a bit overwhelming. I guess I wasn't expecting to have a job offer handed to me. I am totally flattered. It is also obvious to me that everyone you come in contact with loves you. I watch you laugh and talk with your friends, and I know it must have been hard to have moved away from all of this."

"I am glad that I left when I did," said AJ, "things just got a little strange out here. But I sure do miss the life I created here."

We turned into the cobblestone driveway of the Ritz, as a concierge approached to open our doors.

"So many people have this weird view of life," AJ continued as I took her hand heading into the vestibule of the hotel.

"No one wants to take care of anything that means something. I have hoped and wished I'd find someone who would be interested in something more than himself or just getting over on me. It was hard to depart from California, very hard; but I felt that I had to go back to some familiar roots for a while. I promised myself that if I ever returned here, which I certainly could, I would only do so if I had someone special to share it with or minus that, after I adopted about five puppies."

I keyed into the room and turned on one little light. I pulled AJ into me and just looked at her for a while, appreciating her beauty, heart, words and soul. Every time I stood before her, I was amazed that I was the guy who shared her lips.

AJ leaped up, wrapping her legs around me, which was my cue to interlock my hands under her butt and hold her in the air. I walked us both over to the sofa and sat down with my back against it. AJ remained wrapped around me, but now folded her legs back, tucking her feet in the opposite direction.

Our balcony doors were open, allowing a gentle ocean breeze to flow through the room. The white flowing drapery swayed silently in the breeze.

"Christian, I know you have stuff you feel hinders you from having successful things, but our situation has been the total opposite of what you have routinely experienced. I want you in my life and I want to be in yours unconditionally. I know your past has been rough and nothing is solved in a day. I don't care what has transpired in your past, I want to be

PARAMEDIC M.O.S.

here when those things creep up and haunt you. I will always be here and I just need you to know how very much you mean to me."

We sat in silence holding one another.

"There are times when I get really scared, but your actions and consistency provide me something I never had or thought I would have." I picked up my end of the conversation.

"I have a pretty horrendous past, and it conflicts with my thoughts sometimes more than others. I remember being a sap as a kid, listening to "love songs" and the like. Loving you and being loved by you is a similar experience for me like hearing my most favorite music. It is that incredibly powerful, visceral feeling that takes control of my body. I can sink into it and savor it endlessly. It is as if you answer all the questions I have had and you make safe the places I would never dare to go, particularly after that whacko of my past. I have been ashamed for so many years of not only the feelings and fears that I have had, but also for the people I got involved with. I figured that I was just destined for emotional disaster. My world is very unstable lately, and I am really unsure of a lot of things. The one thing I do know is that I love you and I too want you in my life and I want to remain in yours unconditionally too." AJ knew her body well and she also treated it like a temple. Thus I knew when she chose to deliver something so special as a kiss to me, she meant it. I gather that when we kissed, not only did she feel safe, but she also felt understood, as did I.

We opted for a long hot bath together. I think one of the things we made real is that our love for each other was nutritious. It wasn't something we took lightly, and we made sure that every day was full of our concern and special moments. I know that she looked out for me in ways that I have never been looked after before; that takes a lot of getting used too.

C.B. Garris

Chapter XXI:

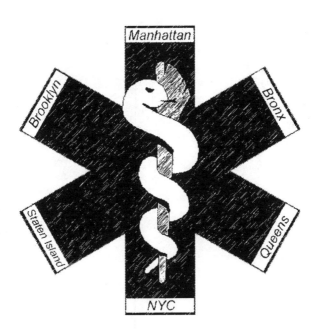

PARAMEDIC M.O.S.

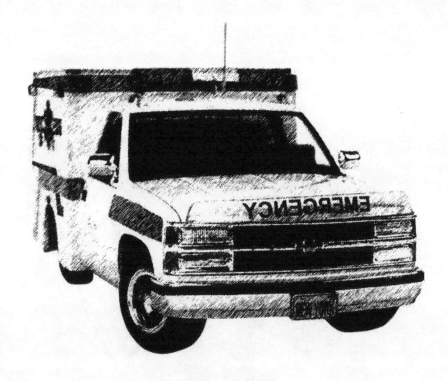

C.B. Garris

In the days to follow, AJ took me down the PCH to Veterans Park in Redondo Beach. We had lunch on the boardwalk, while we watched schools of dolphins toy with schools of scuba divers getting lessons. There was this very cool boardwalk that was just like the one on Venice Beach. People down here were also walking their dogs, roller blading and biking. We also drove down to Palos Verdes to get a great view of RAT beach. AJ mentioned that RAT stands for Right After Torrance. It looked a little smoggy, but it was quite a view from the windy roads that led to the beach.

AJ took me to this fabulous restaurant in Topanga the night before we left. It had a fitness-oriented menu of serious California fare and the establishment was situated in the Topanga mountain range. The road we took there, Topanga Canyon Boulevard, leads all the way from the valley right onto the Pacific Coast Highway in Malibu. It was a two-lane road, one lane in each direction, way up in the mountains. The restaurant was quaint and absolutely quiet. There was a long brook just off the left, and the natural cover of the area was the tree formations. Ironically there were no insects out, and they used these funny, mushroom shaped warmers to warm the outside dining area. I had actually seen these things when we were at Universal Citywalk, but I hadn't asked what they were. These people in California come up with some great inventions.

When it came time to leave L.A., I was actually kind of sad. AJ and I were back at our room as I walked onto the hotel balcony when AJ walked up and hugged me.

"You don't want to go back, do you?" AJ said as we watched a yacht power by.

"I am kind of torn," I said, "Lately everything is going to shit back there, and I know that when I return to work it will be without Jennifer. They appear real serious about disbanding the agency. If they do that, I don't know, but I am scared at that prospect. A lot of promises have been made, but it's all politics. If this thing goes through, it will never be the same. They are going to completely disband the Special Operations Division and everything that we have created. It has taken us years to get the training, the equipment and the right people in place to make what we do effective and what makes our agency world known. What we have all put our own blood, sweat and tears into is going to be whisked away. We are the place that the military comes to ride with when there are no wartime actions, so they can get skills in dealing with ballistic trauma. I can't tell you how many military corpsmen

PARAMEDIC M.O.S.

or just medics from other locales that I have taken out on the street. Each time they leave it is like they have been born for the first time. They had a blast, saw some incredible stuff on the street and always want to come back for more. Our own community of professionals has respected us for so long, and now we are about to lose the independent ground we created. It is really hard after putting all this time in. If the merger was going to be something of a positive nature than I would be all for it, but I just sense a lot of shit is going to go awry when it happens. So many promises, but something seems off kilter here. Jennifer is dead, nine other Members of the Service are dead, some from suicide and it feels like people are reacting on the fear that we really don't know what is going to become of us. I am really concerned that there will be more suicides when we get back."

Staring directly into my eyes, AJ commented with absolute affection in her voice. "I know that this has been unbelievably hard on you. I do also know that you are a survivor and you are strong. I know how very much this agency has meant to you over the years, and how the people you work with are like family to you, which is why you really dialed into NYC EMS so well. You needed them and they needed you. You needed to care for people, because for you it is a natural; it makes you feel alive. NYC EMS needed someone who defines the JOB the way you do. You make them look fabulous. You know from your past abuse how to treat people and what is right and wrong. You have developed ways to defuse situations that were by all means about to explode. You also developed the knowledge and skill to defend yourself at all costs if those situations reached critical mass. You have a reach and a presence that is very unusual, and when you hit the street in an ambulance, you are larger than life. I know that when you leave that arena, you often feel lost and unsure of what tomorrow will bring. That has got to be a very strange dichotomy to live with, but you do it with great style. You have this innate affect on every patient and partner you come into contact with, and when I have come across patients you have treated in the ERs, I cannot tell you how many times I heard them say they never knew that a person could be so caring."

AJ took in a deep breath. She continued, "If you decide that things are not what you want with the agency, and you feel that you need to make an adjustment in your life, I want you to know that I want to be with you when you do that and I will respect any choice you make. Sometimes change is good, and I will always support your decisions. You are a part of my life and you are my definition of love."

I didn't know what to say to such a subjective overview of my character or at the pledge of love and support AJ provided me. I did know one thing though: we are definitely permanent.

"I get the impression that you would like to come back here. Would you like to talk about that?" I said to AJ, as she seemed somewhat surprised.

As AJ took the look of surprise from her face she replied with, "Now that you ask, actually yes." AJ shifted herself in my lap and put her right elbow just below my left clavicle for support.

"I guess I am remembering how wonderful this place was to me; and I just feel kind of torn. I am glad that I left here since we ended up meeting each other. I enjoy being a medic too, but I think one of the differences between you and I is that when it comes to the job, I learned the job from my time at the academy and working with you.

As for you, my lover man, you are THE JOB! It's as if it begins and ends with you. You are fluid in it. You can do anything you want too, as you are incredibly intelligent about a lot of things; but you chose long ago to use yourself and your abilities to help people at their most desperate hour. I know that you have done this for a long time, and because of your absolute devotion to being the best Paramedic and caretaker that you are, to move out of it even if in a similar field would be really alien to you; I am unsure how uncomfortable that might be for you."

AJ breathed deeply for a moment.

"Given all that has happened recently and with the uncertainty of everyone's future in the agency, I guess, yes, I could really move back here. The trick about it is that I want us to be together and not separated for anymore time than we need to be. I am not going to put you or myself through a long-distance relationship if we can avoid it. I can do it with you, and in fact I would only do it with YOU; but I am addicted to you and your attentive pampering of me." AJ smiled immensely.

"I could leave the service; and actually I have given it some thought. The service seems so toxic, when so many young people in our agency are dying, whether it is from illness, trauma or suicide. It is an environment that I am very worried about you staying in. I would never get in between you and the job you love so very much, and I also know that you can handle yourself. I am more worried about the long term effects on your psyche."

I pressed my lips together firmly, resting my head on AJ's chest while she firmed her arms around me rubbing my neck.

PARAMEDIC M.O.S.

"This stuff that you deal with every day has got to have its effects on you, and perhaps your early traumas make it possible for you to properly compartmentalize situations quickly. You know when to zig and when to zag, without needing someone else's leadership. I think that is why your bosses love you so much. They know that you are steps ahead of everyone else and looking at the bigger picture. Granted I think your driving frightens the insurance carrier for the agency." We both burst out in laughter.

"So the thought of leaving the service and returning to Los Angeles presents a little dilemma. We are in no rush, so like we discussed before, I just want you to know that you and we have options."

I was so confused at the moment, yet I was crystal clear. She wasn't so surprised at the fact that I wanted to know her thoughts about her moving back to Los Angeles, rather she still was a little startled whenever I asked a question she was not used to hearing. Her previous gentleman callers were anything but gentlemen and her ex-fiancé never even asked her how her day went, let alone a serious question about what could be a difficult topic to talk about. AJ knew that I cared and that I didn't mind asking, nor would I mind the response. She knew I could see the thoughts that she kept hidden, which frightened her and also intrigued her greatly.

AJ knew that I always looked deep into her soul and with all good intent, as she did me. Her thoughts and feelings are paramount to me, and I sensed something different in her since we arrived. It was something that just was what it was. It was neither bad nor something I felt I needed to be frightened of, only something that I should be cognizant of. I could tell that there was a sense of clarity that New York didn't bring her. Perhaps it was being near the ocean and the solitude that comes with that. Maybe here she was a big fish and wants to be again. Maybe here there is enough distance between her and some bad memories where her mind is free to run amiss. If she loses track of the days here, it's no big deal. I can see how they all can just blend into each other. Hell, maybe it was just the ability to lay out on the beach or in the sun 365 days a year. There is solace in that as I am learning quickly.

We headed for LAX and its maze of terminals. I must have counted at least eleven movie celebrities walking past me. They were trying to be incognito, but if you have seen enough movies, it is pretty easy to figure who is who.

Our flight back was smooth, but as soon as the cabin door shut on the aircraft, I felt my neck tighten up. AJ leaned into my neck and kissed it.

"Don't worry. When we get back to New York, remember that you will get through all of this, that I love you and that you have options."

I turned to her and smiled as best I could. Thoughts of New York were beginning to creep up on me again. I kissed AJ before take off and then fell asleep on her shoulder before we even taxied down the tarmac.

PARAMEDIC M.O.S.

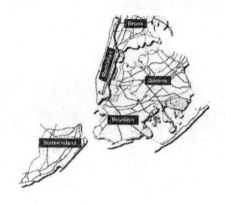

C.B. Garris

Chapter XXII:

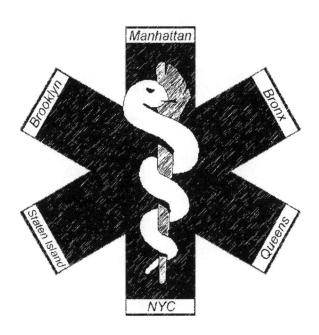

PARAMEDIC M.O.S.

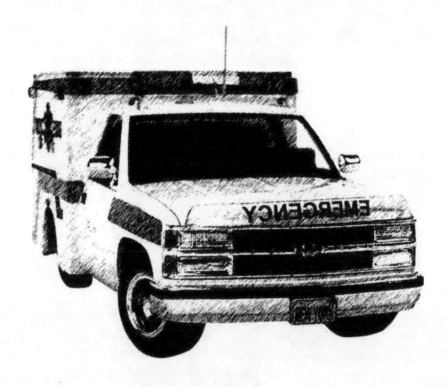

C.B. Garris

It was a relatively cold March day when Danny and I met up at the station for my first day back. It was bright and sunny, but the 38 degrees outside was able to penetrate my bones, making me dread nightfall. I hated those damn fake ties, and no one dared wearing a real one, since you could be strangled with it. My choice of official uniform today included the other option for upper torso wear, a department hunter green turtleneck.

We were deployed to the M2 (east side), stationed at the corner of St. Marks (8th Street) and 2nd Avenue. With an east side deployment, we would head up the FDR Drive after checking out our vehicle. Today was my first day back to work since Jennifer's death and Danny was taking one step at a time with me. He knew I was in shape to work, but he also knew that I had millions of thoughts running through my head, none of them too good. Today was also Jennifer's birthday.

Danny and I checked the vehicle out as usual, but this time with very little talking between us. Danny knew Jennifer too, and he knew how rocked my world was. Danny had asked if the previous crew replaced the extra Narcan in the supply cabinet. Without responding I hopped up inside the back of the rig and keyed into a small compartment on the passenger side of the wall.

"Those fuckers," I said surprised. "They actually left the station without even letting us know that they used up all the Narcan today. Damn, was there a street sale on heroin this week or what? How could they have used all of it?"

Danny stepped back inside the garage to hit the supply room to replace all that was now gone. Trying to make a small joke to lighten me up, when Danny saw me charging the Lifepak monitor paddles to ensure they charged properly Danny said, "Oh man, I think we forgot the nitro patches!"

I smirked as Danny howled, "Very funny. I'm sure Deklund would appreciate it."

Danny slapped me on the back as he laughed a few times, and I couldn't help but laugh with him.

"Ten X-ray, Tactical One Zero X," came from the radio on my hip.

Taking the radio out of my back pocket and placing it near my face, depressing the transmit button on the radio I replied, "Tactical X-ray,"

There was a one second pause and the on-board mobile data terminal (computer) beeped twice distinctively.

PARAMEDIC M.O.S.

The dispatcher read to us what I was reading from the yellow LCD readout, "Ten-X, unconfirmed P.O. (Police officer) shot, 98 Avenue D, 98 Avenue D with a cross of 12th Street, no further information."

We both hopped in with Danny driving, and I reached over and pushed the 10-63 (enroute) key, notifying communications that were rolling.

Ninety-Eight Avenue D had a long time history with our station and with the NYPD for that matter. Anywhere from two to six times a day someone (we assume children or some very bored adult) would call 911 saying that a police officer has been shot. We would come flying in with the NYPD, lights and sirens, lighting up the block. Kids always come to the windows, excited to see us but we never find anything. Generally aside from the caller saying that the officer is usually on the roof, we never get any additional information.

As we hooked a left onto Houston from the FDR Drive, Antonio our beloved PD dispatcher transmitted the same information over the NYPD precinct frequency. We have all heard Antonio transmit this call a thousand times. As we approached Avenue D, something in Antonio's voice alarmed me. He began transmitting very specific information that we had never heard before.

Antonio started by hitting the alert tones to get everyone's attention, "Okay, attention precinct sector units, 98 Avenue D, on a reported P.O. shot," there was a clicking of the computer keyboard he was typing on and he continued his transmission, "Units I'm now getting multiple officers shot, possible gold shields on the ground at location, report of multiple shots fired, six white officers in plain clothes."

I looked at Danny as he looked towards me knowing that this didn't sound right. Either someone has a great imagination or we may have a real problem on our hands.

"10-Xray, Manhattan South," I said to the EMS dispatcher on Danny's portable two-way radio.

"X-ray, C'mon," Wendy replied.

"Ten-X, PD is reporting multiple officers shot with more information than we usually get at this address, do me a favor and start me at least another unit and a boss this way until we figure this out."

Wendy didn't even waste time replying to me, "One-two Frank and Ten Patrol, along with Ten-X for the P.O shot, further information to follow."

I already knew that both units were monitoring and in the area as Willy who was aboard Twelve Frank(12F) whizzed past us smiling as they

C.B. Garris

headed eastbound toward the service road to the FDR Drive. A flurry of NYPD units began to canvas (search) the area and when the scooter unit who was in the 4th Avenue Walk area of the project pulled up all we heard was screaming.

"SP3 central, Forthwith on the buses, I got six officers shot here, repeat forthwith on the bus, Oh shit, 10-13 shots fired, I'm taking fire, ten-thirteen!" With that the radio went dead. What was about to happen was a first in my history with the agency. I had never seen so many police units mobilize so fast in a six-minute period.

Will confirmed the first officer he found was shot, DOA, as the dispatcher was redeploying units to our location as fast as she could.

"Chris," Willy called me on the EMS channel, "come up on the 7th street side of the FDR service road, I got at least six shot, one is an 83 (dead).

Willy's first patient, a police officer from whose jurisdiction we were unsure of, had been shot in the head, leaving most of his head gone. Although Will pronounced him, the arriving officers were unwilling to accept that he was already dead regardless of the amount of brain matter and skull fragments on the pavement so they frantically tried to help revive the officer with Willy and his partner.

Danny and I pulled up on the sidewalk and without having to say anything to each other, we both grabbed our trauma and airway bags (we each carried our own), and headed to a bunch of victims that were face down in the middle of the courtyard. We found two officers in plainclothes with their shields and weapons on the ground, both shot in the legs, chest and abdomen. Sirens were screaming everywhere, as the courtyard literally filled up with law enforcement agents from numerous federal, state, and local NYPD agencies in a matter of minutes. My first guess would be that there were at least hundreds of officers within minutes, all with their weapons drawn at the ready. I was glad I had my bulletproof vest on underneath my uniform.

Danny and I spoke to the two officers that we began to treat, both conscious and lying on their stomachs in pain. They had good skin color and were not sweating, which told us we had a little time. I went to remove my blood pressure cuff from my bag, and some officer ran over and snatched my trauma bag, along with my airway bag, backboards and c-spine immobilization equipment and took off.

"Hey, yo, what the hell are you doing?" I yelled out like someone just stole my last meal, as the officer disappeared into the crowd. There were

PARAMEDIC M.O.S.

so many emergency service personnel running in different directions that it looked like a swarm of locusts that just took off from a wheat field. I picked up my radio screaming for more equipment, units and to notify Bellevue and Vinny's that they would all be getting multiple gunshot wound patients who were police officers. The reason we inform the hospitals that the individuals shot are police officers is so that they can prepare for the onslaught of NYPD top brass, EMS Supervisors and media that will flood the hospital in a matter of minutes. Another team of medics appeared with equipment and assisted me in cutting clothes to expose the damage.

My first patient, George, was shot five times: once in the chest, twice in the abdomen, and once in each leg. As I went to cut his clothing off, shots were fired all around me. The officer who I was treating was lying next to a slatted iron fence supported by a cement foundation. The cement foundation came up about one and a half to two feet off of the ground. As several bullets either whizzed right by my head and pinged off of the fence. I laid down next to George, as flat as I could get.

As I heard another bullet ping off the fence I turned my head to the side as if I was trying to breath while swimming and quickly said, "George, stay absolutely still!"

The gunfire sounded like it might be coming from above, but there was just way too much chaos to be sure. Sirens, semi-automatic and automatic weapons gunfire, screaming, two way radios crackling, and all I kept thinking is that I am about to buy the farm and why could I not be back in a Los Angeles spa with AJ.

"George, GEORGE," I yelled to stop him. "I understand you are scared, but right now I need you to stay absolutely still and conserve your energy; we will take care of you."

George's eyes popped up, "I've been shot!"

I stopped cutting his pants long enough to say, "Yes George, you have been shot at least five times, just hang on."

I guess George didn't realize what was truly happening, which is to be expected. He immediately went from upset to thankful that we were there.

"Man, you gonna put me back together, right?" George asked liked he was asking me to save his cat from a tree.

"George, you are still intact, now just relax and let us work our magic." With this, George just laid back.

I wasn't going to move George until we had him fully immobilized. Any one or all of the five bullets that entered George could have lodged in his spine, lung or heart. If he is moved without being immobilized, it could be the only difference between life and death. Since one of New York's Finest ran off with my equipment at the sight of all this confusion, and for that matter he was probably headed west on 14th Street with it by now, I continued doing everything to prep him for transport with what I had left.

An officer ran over with a stretcher and literally tried to lift George from under my care as I was sticking him with an IV.

"Hey, what are you doin?" I said forcefully to the officer.

"We gotta get him to a hospital." The young officer said.

"No shit Einstein," I said with a very sarcastic tone, "but we are not moving until I say we are moving, got it?" The officer looked like I just pissed on his parade.

"Man, he's gotta get to a hospital!" the officer said to me.

Funny, I thought the patch on my left arm said Emergency Medical Service, City of New York, and the patch on my right arm said, EMS Paramedic, City of New York.

As I looked at both patches to be sure I had the right uniform on, George looked at me and said, "My back up weapon is on my ankle if you want to shoot him in the ass!"

One of my BLS partners, Reggie, pushed the officer aside and told him to stop trying to move him. As I got the second IV established in George's forearm, this pain-in-the-ass of an officer came back and tried to move George from under my care again. I told Reggie to secure the second IV that I just established and in one fell swoop turned around and I landed a full fisted punch in the center of the officer's bulletproof vest. I didn't want to hurt him officially, just knock him on his ass.

"I told you to stop!" I said abrasively, and then speaking as if I was scolding a child for something in pre-school I continued, "Now either get a grip on yourself or I will make you the next patient. You are going to hurt your own fellow officer if you move him too soon and if you've been paying attention, this situation out here has turned into the OK Corral, so I am getting my patient and my own ass outta here."

As the words left my mouth I thought the officer was going to strike me. I could see that the look in his eyes said he wanted to put me in cuffs. I turned back around and as I went to assist in rolling George onto a backboard, the officer leaned in and pulled me onto my butt with his handcuffs now showing. John Mcginty, a Detective Sergeant that I just testified with recently in court was right behind us when the officer forced me to the ground.

PARAMEDIC M.O.S.

"Reggie finish this, I gotta deal with this asshole now!" Reggie looked at me with a look asking if I wanted him to handle this, and I shook my head no.

I spun around and the officer had his handcuffs out and ready.

"What the fuck is your problem? We got work to do here." I said as my words were cut short by another round of rapid succession gunfire.

We both ducked, and returned to our previous stance.

"You punched me and I'm gonna lock you up." The officer said approaching me.

I kept thinking to myself, "Is this guy on drugs?"

With my arms spread and hands open in case I had to sock this fool, I said "I punched you because you're acting like an ass. What are we, in a sandbox here? Grow up and get a hold of yourself. You are having a stress reaction, and this is not the time for debriefing. I don't have time to play momma to you. If you can't help us, go find someplace to stay out of our way." I turned back to Reggie and paid the officer no mind. I felt a hand creep up on my right shoulder and I heard the officer's keys jingling behind me so I spun around and he went for me. He had very bad footing, so I just pushed him straight down to the ground. While he was flat on his face, Detective John stepped in to assist me. He lifted the officer to his feet and as the officer was about to swing, he realized that it was the sergeant in front of him, not me. John didn't even look over at me when he said," Christian, take care of your patient, I'll deal with this idiot."

Reggie, Danny, and some medic from another station I didn't recognize were just leaving with George. We were able to make it to my vehicle, which was still running while sitting on the sidewalk. There were police officers, FBI agents, Customs agents and ATF (Alcohol, Tobacco, & Firearms) agents everywhere. For as far as I could see, all I saw were law enforcement personnel everywhere. I kept wondering what the hell went down before we got here. We were about to take off with George when 10(Z)ebra informed me they had a serious patient, but that they could not even get to their vehicle that was close by, due to all of the hysteria. Since both were shot a total of ten times together, it is more ideal that you have one per vehicle; but in this type of situation you do what you have too.

I told Glenn on 10(Z)ebra to bring us his patient and we could take them both. As a medic from 13(V)ictor started to drive our ambulance away with Danny and I in the back, I yelled for him to stop since the crew of 10(Z)ebra was running down the street with their patient towards us.

C.B. Garris

This scene looked like a demilitarized zone. It seemed that no one had control of the situation and that was scaring the shit out of me. We didn't know who was shooting at us, whether it was coming from across the FDR from a sniper in the park, or if it was a sniper on a rooftop twenty-five floors up, or even a cop having a very bad day. Even the media was already out here running around with their cameras. How the hell did they get out here so fast? Our new patient, compliments of the medics from 10(Z)ebra, was the undercover officer that was next to George originally, by the name of Joaquin. I went to lean out of the vehicle and the guy driving my bus hit the gas and I almost went head first out of the vehicle. Catching myself on a handle, I extended my hand out of the bus for the backboard carrying 10(Z)ebra's patient. Police officers were all around our unit banging on the side of it telling us to just go. I was really in the mood to run a lot of these idiots over.

Generally we work perfectly with the NYPD, but something got into a few that were already present. In all my years, I have never known things to get all out of sync. Then again, six of theirs were down; it was very understandable.

There we were, in a very unstable street combat situation. I didn't begin to feel safe until we were blocks from the scene.

I yanked the second Lifepak cardiac monitor out of the cabinet I had stashed in my bus, and placed the electrodes from that unit onto Joaquin. Both George and our new addition, Joaquin were doing well considering. I established two more IV's on Joaquin, since previous attempts by 10(Z)ebra failed due to combat interference. The officers were so taken by the kinetic crisis in motion, that they didn't realize that there were about twelve ambulances parked all over the scene, with more on the way. They were literally trying to take Joaquin away from us while we worked on him in the courtyard. PD wanted to stuff him in a sector car despite the fact that on a backboard he wouldn't fit inside the car.

Once we got Joaquin into one of the ambulances that had its rear doors wide open, Danny got in with me, and began tending to George. Danny hooked George up to the onboard oxygen and gave me the portable for Joaquin. In their hysteria, the officers also managed to rip off Joaquin's oxygen mask, so I placed another non-rebreather mask at 15 LPM. In order to initiate an IV in an ambulance doing 30 mph, it takes the ability to perform acrobatics. Since Joaquin's right arm was exposed, it would be the easiest for access. I asked Joaquin about

PARAMEDIC M.O.S.

his family to keep him awake and talking, and hopefully to distract him from the screwdriver size catheter I was about to poke his arm with. I knew this was going to hurt. I took my handy mustard-colored tourniquet from around my belt and tied a shoelace knot around his mid bicep, placing one foot against the inside wall of the ambulance for balance. I could have knelt down, but being so close to the other stretcher would be uncomfortable.

I was already gloved up, so I found the vein and wiped it with alcohol prep. Always go for the veins you can feel, not see. The ones that you can see tend to roll and can be very deceptive. With my foot firmly against the wall of the bus, I took my left thumb and pressed down, pulling the vein towards me. This is what we call anchoring. Anchoring makes it nearly impossible for the vein to roll. If it rolls, you can say goodbye to your IV access. Every IV counts because you may not get a second chance, and I do not want to stick a person anymore than necessary. I was careful not to let Joaquin see the needle I was about to use. I pulled the catheter from it's packaging and told Joaquin to stay absolutely still. Danny in the meantime was already giving a notification to the dispatcher to pass on to Bellevue about our two patients.

"Joaquin, you are going to feel a bee sting in your forearm, DON"T MOVE!"

I pulled on the vein with my left thumb, and I swallowed quickly giving me that last millisecond to decide if I was happy with the vein.

I placed the 14-gauge catheter in between my right thumb and forefinger for maximum advantage, squeezing the tips of the fingers around the upper portion of the catheter – much like a baseball player "chokes up" on a bat before a swing. I landed the beveled side of the blade face up against his skin and with one swift motion entered his skin. Well that was a colorful moment.

"God-damnit," said Joaquin.

"Sorry dude," I said with a serious look, although the look on his face was priceless. "Just a few more seconds and the needle will be out." As soon as the needle entered his vein I received what we call a flashback of blood in the catheter, which means it was a good stick.

I tapped the catheter in with the nail of my index finger, removing the needle and leaving only the plastic sheathing still in Joaquin's vein.

"Sharp on the floor," I said out loud. This is what we say to each other after we establish an IV stick, so that we know there was no time to put the needle into the red container. It is safest to drop the needle and secure it until the vehicle stops. In this case, Danny knew exactly where it was; where I place all of my freshly used IV catheters, under my boot. My boots are thick and steel-toed, so I know that the needle will be safe there. You never attempt to put a used needle into a red container while the bus is moving. One short stop and you will be wondering if you contracted HIV for the rest of your life.

Before I connected the IV tubing, I drew 60 cc's of blood for cross, type and match; and then placed the tubing of Normal Saline into the injection port. I secured the IV and Joaquin was no longer angry with me; at least not until I started the next IV in his other arm.

"Sonovabitch." Joaquin squealed upon the second IV entry.

"Sorry, dude. It's either me or a med student in the ER. Trust me, I start IV's every day and night; most med students have only practiced on grapefruits."

Joaquin was not happy with either of his choices, but I knew he would forgive me. I thought at this point it was best not to mention exactly what would be one of the first things that will happen to him when we reached the Trauma Slot at Bellevue. If he thought my IV's made him uncomfortable, wait until he is the recipient the rigid plastic tube called a Foley catheter. This is where an ER nurse or physician rams a tube the size of a garden hose up his penis while he is still conscious, to measure urine output. This is the one medical procedure that brings me to my knees and rolls my eyes to the back of my skull every time I have to watch it.

We pulled into the ER bay at Bellevue and it looked like Graduation Day at the NYPD academy. There was a sea of blue as far you could visualize. There were officers in uniforms, plainclothes officers with their weapons and radio sticking out from out of their coats, sergeants, lieutenants, captains, one, two, and three star chiefs and Inspectors all talking on radios at the same time. I am sure NYPD Internal Affairs Bureau was lurking about in this crowd. My only concern was my favorite crew I called the Iditerods – that hungry pack of wolves known as trauma surgeons awaiting each ambulance. As our vehicle came to a stop at the ER bay, I opened the door to a flood of media cameras and camera lights to greet us. The media and the trauma teams made a beeline for the rear of my vehicle at the same time. It was apparent that the media was going to win. I slammed the rear doors shut and locked them. I stepped outside via the side compartment door.

PARAMEDIC M.O.S.

Captain Vonneger, who I have known for a while and never liked because of his miserable demeanor, ran over to me with a butt load of attitude.

"Do you have patients in there?" He said trying to look inside.

I am sure the look on my face said, "No you idiot, I just stopped by for a check-up!"

As he realized I locked the doors he said to me, "What are you doing?"

I looked at him with a stern look, "Both of my patients are stable and we have multiple IV's and Lifepak's hooked up. Except for the sheets covering them to keep them warm, they are also butt ass naked. Since their families haven't been notified yet, I am not going to have their bloody pictures strewn all over the evening news for their families and children to see. I want these cameras gone, NOW! "

"Just open the fucking door and let's go, your holding up patient care." The Chief said with a little more attitude.

I swung my head from side to side signifying no.

"Are you being insubordinate to me?" The Captain said to me as I was waiting for this comment.

"No, SIR, I am protecting my patients. Your priorities are all screwed up aren't they? You are not in a position nor qualified to question my patient care, and I'll address that issue with you once these guys are safely in the Operating Room. This is an unsafe environment out here. I know that you want YOUR face in the paper with the wounded officers, but I am not taking them out of our vehicle where they are safe, and putting them into this fucking melee you've allowed to form out here. YOU are the Captain, you deal with this!" With that I stepped back in the vehicle.

About thirty seconds later, all the noise diminished. I looked outside and the NYPD staged the press across the parking lot, so that if they wanted any Pulitzer shots, they would have to use their zoom lenses and fix their apertures. I swung the doors open and the trauma team brought out two black stretchers. We took each officer out as I heard the clicking of a few Nikons and Canons. I held Joaquin's IV's up as we wheeled them past the trauma slots and right to the Operating Area.

The EMS Captain who wanted his picture in the paper came round the corner.

"Just what did you mean that I wanted to get my picture in the paper. That was very inappropriate," he said attempting to admonish me in front of Doc Pete. Pete knew that this guy just made a mistake and since the trauma teams had to prep both patients for surgery, he had a few minutes to watch the verbal sparring that was about to take place.

I looked at the Captain and started right in on him, causing him to back up a few steps. "Let's get a few things straight here from the get go. You may be a Captain, but YOU don't ever tell me about patient care. First of all, my certifications supercede yours regarding patient care since you decided to take a promotion over your Paramedic upgrade. You became a basic EMT after I was already working the street as a Paramedic, and you were a shitty one at that. Your function in this agency is as an administrator. You have no, and I mean absolutely no foundation to make claims about my patient care. If you want to go down that road with me, not only must you be absolutely sure what you are saying, but also you need to be equally as qualified as I am, and the fact is you're not. You want to make any such accusations, you better be clear or I will not only have your Captain's bars revoked, but I will see to it that the State yanks your EMT certificate so that you don't even have a fucking job with this agency anymore." Captain Vonneger looked as though he had just seen a ghost.

Since I was on a roll, I decided to continue. I figure if I'm going to get written up for insubordination, I might as well make it good.

"If you think I am kidding, remember that not only am I a Field Evaluator, I also work closely with the Medical Investigations Division, and with the city Medical Advisory Committee." Captain Vonneger looked sheet white, and didn't even know how to respond; he knew I had him cornered.

I continued, "In order for me to treat you like a senior official, you need to start acting like one first. Now exactly where were you when we arrived?"

I thought Doc Pete was going to split his sides laughing at me chewing this Captain out. By this point, the Captain forgot that he had any rank at all.

"Well, I was right there in the bay." The Chief said defensively.

"Bullshit!" I corrected him, "You were sitting in your command car when we pulled up. Since the media didn't arrive until we got here, I saw you bolt from your car right to my bus when we backed up. You weren't going to help us lift the patients out, so that clearly suggests that you wanted a photo opportunity; and frankly, that disgusts me. Why didn't you secure the Emergency Room bay to preserve the integrity of the patients, facilitating a quick removal to the trauma slots, hmm? No, you felt it more

PARAMEDIC M.O.S.

appropriate to attempt to chew me out while the ONLY thing you should have done was get the ER bay secured. All you had to do was say one word to any top brass in the NYPD standing around and they would have gladly obliged. I am not going to take a patient out into a media storm if there is a way to protect his or her privacy. Oh and by the way you are welcome for all that we did out there. Perhaps if you weren't just concerned with your own ass, you would have responded to the scene and fulfilled your rank! Oh, I forgot, you just wanted your picture in the Times. "

The Captain just stood there with his jaw on the floor.

"You know what really gets me Captain," and I could tell he really didn't want to hear what I was going to say next, "we are busting our behinds out here, getting shot at. I just got back from release time after seeing my partner's head blown off from a self-inflicted gunshot wound, and I just buried eight other co-workers in the weeks prior. So if you really think that I give a rat's ass about your silly ego problem, you are grossly incorrect."

Captain Vonneger just stood there.

I think he felt I was about to lunge at him. Davia came around the corner. She was checking me out to see if I was about to clock this mope or if she should intervene. Davia never liked this Captain either and was just looking for a reason.

"Well, I'm glad to see we are all getting along." Davia said with a smirk. My eyes were fixed on this Captain. He was a miserable person who made his living attempting to make everyone else around him miserable.

"He has been very insubordinate to me." The Captain said to Davia like he was a kid saying "Nah nah ni nah nah."

I guess he thought Davia actually cared.

"Actually," Davia said as she looked directly at him, "From where I stood for the last, oh five minutes or so, it sounded to me like he said everything that you should have been told. Frankly, I'm just sorry that he beat me too it."

The Captain just stood there with his jaw on the floor again.

Davia looked at Captain Vonneger and said with a nonchalant tone, "So now I want you out of my face, back in your department vehicle and doing something useful like patrol. Be in my office in exactly two hours, as you and I have some things to discuss." Davia said very sternly towards the Captain.

"But Davia this guy got up in my face," the Captain started and was quickly cut off by Davia who pointed her finger at him.

"HOLD ON RIGHT THERE. I never gave you permission to call me by anything other than CHIEF, so let's get that straight right now. You don't have what it takes to call me by my first name. Although I really don't even like having you as a supervisor in the street, right now I need you out of my face before I start screaming. I want you on patrol, now!" Even I swallowed at how sharply Davia directed those words at him.

The Captain cleared his throat, putting together what little of his ass Davia didn't chew off as he made his exit.

As the Captain turned to walk away I said with a smile, "Thank you, DAVIA."

Patting me on my shoulder, Davia looked at me, "No problem Sir CHRISTIAN."

The Captain walked out very confused.

Pete knew it was time for him to get into the scrub sinks.

"You okay?" Davia asked as I walked to the scrub sinks.

"What an asshole he is." I said as I placed my hands under the water.

As I washed my hands, Davia leaned her back up against the wall.

I looked over towards her out of the corner of my left eye, "Was I loud?"

Davia smiled and shifted her body to turn towards me, "Uh, that would be an understatement. You didn't need a microphone, that's for sure."

Shaking my head, "Dav, I'm sorry."

Tugging on her ear Davia cut me off, "No need to apologize, you know he deserved it."

"I'll be fine, it is just that with all the shit recently with our jobs being in major jeopardy because of this merger, the other recent deaths and of all things, today is Jennifer's birthday. I am just sick of this stupidity. I can't count how many bullets went flying past my head today." I said as I dried off my hands after washing them at the scrub sink. Davia just stood there watching me, as if she was waiting for something.

I started to cry. I stopped and stared at the wall for a few seconds while Davia stayed in place.

Out of the corner of my eye I saw someone in one of our uniforms appear. Davia looked at that person and shook her head side to side. "Not now," she said quietly. "Christian, I know this is hard on you. In fact I think it is hard on you most of everyone. You worked with Jen for seven years; and outside the office I know that you cared about her and loved her very much. I am trying to understand myself why she shut us all out.

PARAMEDIC M.O.S.

I wish there was something I could do to help or make it better. I wish that I could bring her back. I am here if you ever need to talk, it doesn't matter what time of day or night it is, you know that. You are not alone in your pain, but that in no way lessens the blow." Davia said this while keeping her eyes locked on me.

My eyes were now puffy as I wiped the tears with my upper arm sleeve.

"AJ has been so good to me," I said as I rubbed my eyes. "She has looked out for me in a way that I never knew possible. I guess I just feel like my insides are blank now. To see such a beautiful life snuffed out, whether by her actions or not, just goes right to the core of me. I knew that something was up, but there was nothing ever pronounced about her actions. I talked with her that night before, and everything seemed like normal. I feel guilty for not being there to stop her and I know that there was no way I could have been there. I didn't know that she was holding a gun to her head."

I cried more.

"I didn't know that Jen was in so much pain; and I wish I knew so that I could have stopped the pain. I would have done anything to make her feel better. How do you say goodbye chief, how?" Davia inhaled deeply and I felt her remorse. She knew that I would carry this with me for years to come, and she also knew that whatever she said over the next few minutes could be absolutely critical.

"You know," Davia started in, "we see death and destruction every day, and sometimes it is more horrible than others. To try and put a feeling or description on what you have seen is one of the most difficult things to do. I have no great words of wisdom, except to say that I care about you, and I know you are going through a tough time. Let AJ steer for a while, she will take great care of you. She loves you very much and only wants the best. If you feel that work is getting too much, let me know. We can take it one day at a time. I am unsure if you are seeking any outside counseling, but I would suggest it. I am not telling you to go through the counselors that EAP (Employee Assistance Program) provides, as that may be too close for comfort. I do however think it would be good to keep your head clear."

I looked at Davia and composed myself, "I gotcha, and I will take care of that. We are all going to be out of service for awhile, our buses are covered in blood." I said very business like.

Davia patted my back and said "No prob, see you out there. I gotta go deal with this idiot Captain and get to the bottom of his malfunction. Wish me luck."

I smiled and Davia did the same as she disengaged from the wall.

"Chief, look I'm sorry that I laid into the Cap." I said with puppy eyes.

"Don't be! Like I said he is an ass and I will deal with him later. I am just glad that you let him have it here instead of holding it in." Davia smiled and patted my right shoulder again. "When you get back to the station, use my office to call AJ. Take a few minutes." Davia smiled, and the mention and thought of AJ made me smile too.

As I walked out of the scrub area to retrieve my paperwork to write this mess up, I heard it: " Hey, Hey, Hey, WADEE WHAT THE, NO NO NO ,, STOP,,,OOOOOOOOWWWWWWWWWW..... Damnit!"

Joaquin got his Foley. I guess my IV's weren't so bad after all.

PARAMEDIC M.O.S.

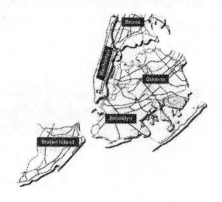

C.B. Garris

Chapter XXIII:

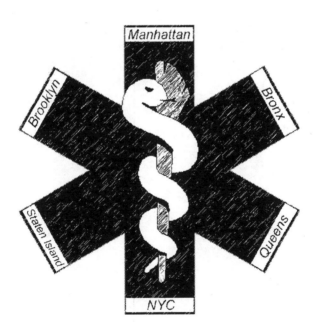

PARAMEDIC M.O.S.

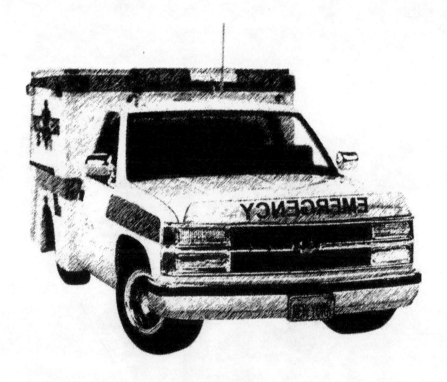

Danny and I drove back to the station down 2nd Avenue. The lights of the city were glaring in a soft rain that began to fall. Rain, that meant car accidents or as we tend to call them "pin jobs" as someone is always getting trapped in the vehicle. When we returned to Station 11, Danny restocked the vehicle while I went up to Davia's office and proceeded to dial AJ.

"Hey," I said gently.

"Hey you, are you okay?" AJ replied knowing that if I am calling her up in the middle of my tour, something must have gone wrong. I told her the story about the shootout and my words with the Captain.

"You actually chewed him out in the middle of Bellevue's ER?" She said giggling hysterically.

"Well it wasn't really in the middle, it was more toward the back of the room." I said joking as best I could.

By now AJ was cackling she was laughing so hard.

"Oh honey, you need to come home." Those were the best words I could have heard.

"I am looking forward to that, and I like being able to call you my home." I said as I got a little bit serious.

"Well Mr. Christian, you are my home and don't you ever forget it." AJ said this as I knew she was aware today was Jen's birthday. I know she was not avoiding the topic, rather she was waiting for me to bring it up. If I didn't bring it up now, I knew that we would discuss it when I got "home."

"You okay?" AJ asked concerned.

"Yeah, as soon as I get outta here I'll be better. I guess I really don't want to be here right now. It's not the same, it feels strange." There was silence, but I know that AJ was listening attentively. She didn't want to stop me in mid sentence and if I was going to break down, she was ready for it.

As I sat there collecting my thoughts she said, "I know that you are going to be okay, it is going to take time so try not to beat yourself up. I know the urge to do so is there, but you don't have to. You have taken enough of a beating lately." I shook my head in silence, and I know that AJ heard it.

"I got a call from both Taylor and L'eeann today and they both could not stop saying how wonderful they think you are. They want us to come back to Los Angeles soon and spend more time with them. They got

PARAMEDIC M.O.S.

a real kick out of you. They also were not afraid to tell me that it was a good thing that you are in my camp, or they both would have taken turns with you."

If ever I could use something to raise my spirit, there was nothing like a genuine compliment.

"Wow, thank you. Please do tell them I say hello when you talk to them next. If it is okay by you, I'd like to get Taylor, Leeann and Miko presents to say thank you for their hospitality." I said with affection.

"Oh honey," AJ replied, "that would be so sweet of you and I am sure they would greatly appreciate that. They would love anything you sent to them. That's what I love about them, they, like me, love the small things. Well, okay only in the area of presents." AJ said as she giggled.

As I was about to start my next sentence, a key entered the door and it was Davia. She looked in and smiled at me sitting in the darkness on the phone with AJ. She waved and her hand told me to take my time. Her office was kind of cool, it overlooked the area of the station where we do roll call. She could watch the crews come in and out of the station behind tinted windows. Even when I was standing at attention for roll call, I could always feel her presence checking out the crews.

I told AJ that I would be at her place after my tour and she sent me kisses through the phone, informing me to be ready for the real thing when I got home."

I walked out of Davia's door as she was coming back up the interior stairwell.

"How's AJ doing? Davia said as she smiled.

"She's a keeper, boss." I cracked a faint smile.

"I am very glad that you and AJ hooked up. You two really have something there."

I smiled as my radio squalked, "I need 10X for a cardiac, 10X." There was a sense of heightened sensitivity in the dispatcher's voice.

As I pulled the radio to answer it, Davia reached to her hip and turned the volume up on her radio.

"10X, go with it Joel," I said letting him know that we were ready for action.

"10X, PD calling for a forthwith on an adolescent with chest pains, Pitt and Delancey, right near the bridge."

"10X, were in the wind, send it over." I didn't even look back at Davia as I slid down the vertical stairwell by placing my boot tips on the railings.

I leaped the last four steps and yelled across the garage, "DANNY, let's rock, Pitt and Delancey!"

Danny shot out of the office behind me as we made for our bus. We took off out of the station like a bat out of hell as I read the job. "Looks like a 14 year serious chest pains, PD drove up on it." We were only about six blocks from the call as Danny went up Clinton Street to East Broadway and as we made a left on Pitt, we saw two NYPD sector cars in the makeshift parking lot. They were waving us in ferociously, and that was a bad sign.

We pulled in and there was about a fifteen year old boy sitting up, being supported by a civilian adult. I got out to examine the kid while Danny went for equipment.

"How ya doin," I said with an much caring enthusiasm as I could.

The kid looked strange, kind of pale and lethargic.

"Sir, what happened here?" I asked the person holding the kid up as I gloved up and check his conjunctiva. The conjunctiva is the inside portion of the bottom eyelid, and when it is dark out it may be hard to determine paleness in skin color, we can check the conjunctiva for perfusion. Pink means good, white means shock.

"Man I don't know, I just found him wandering the street over there and he was acting all crazy, and he kept saying his chest hurt."

While I contemplated the whole "I-found-him-walking-like-this" theory, I knelt right down to the adolescent.

"Son, what's your name," I said in the darkness. We were under the Williamsburg Bridge, right around the corner from the local precinct. I took out my flashlight and saw blood marks on the chest part of the kids clothing.

"Oh shit!" I said slightly out loud.

I pulled his shirt up and found the reason why this kid had chest pain. He had several deep stab wounds in his right chest, above the nipples.

"Danny, it's a stab!" I said hastily to get Danny's full attention.

The NYPD on scene quickly grabbed the civilian and started questioning him, trying to determine if he was a suspect. This kid was going down the toilet quick. I did lung sounds on him and I could hear only air slightly moving in his left upper lung.

"Danny, get me the board, I'll tube him in the bus!"

This kid had no palpable blood pressure and his pulse was fading. In mixture of darkness, flashlights and revolving and strobing emergency

PARAMEDIC M.O.S.

lights; it appears the kid had multiple bruises on his chest. I was afraid he got worked over somewhere else and dropped here by one or more people. Placing him in full c-spine precautions rapidly, we hauled him into the back of the bus as Anita and Connie rolled up in their bus. They saw the rear doors of our ambulance wide open.

Danny was tossing IV bag wrappers all over the back of the ambulance to start as many lines as fast as he could. As I positioned myself to intubate the kid, I saw Ani running up to the back of the bus; Connie was right behind. Ani took a flying leap into the bus, grabbing the IV bag that Danny was fumbling with and said, "Start it, I'll get this."

Danny thanked her and just as I was securing his tube, we all smelled this horrible odor. This kid just defecated all over himself. That was the one sign I hoped wouldn't happen. In major trauma, it is indicative of the body to release before it dies. Thus he defecated, went into hypoxic seizures (from a lack of oxygen), and subsequently full traumatic cardiac arrest. I re-secured the tube after he stopped seizing and told Ani to start hauling ass towards Bellevue. Although Danny has an almost perfect IV initiation rate, tonight would be a bad night. This kid must have bled so much in his thoracic cavity that he had no vasculature left. I told the NYPD officer who was with us in the back to glove up and then give me a pre-filled syringe of Epi in the cabinet in front of him. Connie was doing CPR compressions and I just had this bad feeling that this kid was not going to make it. He was so young and perhaps if we had been called earlier, maybe. But now I am unsure. When I checked the lung sounds, something didn't sound right, it was like I was trying to inflate an already overfilled football.

I dropped an Epi and Atropine down the tube while Danny fought for an IV anywhere. I had the officer sit in my seat and continue ventilations every five compressions. Danny got venipuncture in the kids left jugular vein, and I decided to attempt a needle decompression. I was concerned that a big air bubble caused by the stab wound trapped the air that I should have heard ventilating in and out of his lungs. It could have been air in there or worse blood.

Either way it had to come out. I knelt down as Ani took a right on 1st Avenue and swabbed his left chest in the ribs area with betadine. Betadine is that purple-looking stuff you see on the Discovery channel before an operation. It is a great anti-microbial. I wanted to keep him as aseptic (sterile) as possible.

C.B. Garris

I attached the 14 guage angiocath to a syringe and located the 2nd and 3rd intercostal space on his left side. This area is the empty space between your ribs. I lined up the angle of the catheter and punctured the pleural space. With the catheter still gripped between my thumb and forefinger, I held it in place to allow blood and air to drain. I had Connie stop compressions for a moment and he was still exhibiting asystole (flat line) on the monitor. As Connie continued with compressions, I heard Ani calling communications for the trauma stand-by request at Bellevue, as she simultaneously maneuvered us through traffic with pinpoint precision. As Connie compressed on his chest with focused concentration and sweat, another wave of blood poured out of the catheter all over my chest and boots.

No sooner did that happen did the lung sounds finally not only clear, but we even got electrical activity back in his heart. He was now in v-fib (ventricular fibrillation), so I grabbed the paddles and charged them to 200. I told Connie to grab me two separate pre-filled syringes out of the cabinet, one of Epi and the other Lidocaine. If I don't get this kid back, I was going to drop another Epi down the tube to help jump-start his heart. If I got him back, the Lidocaine will hopefully prevent him from suffering irregular heartbeats leading back to cardiac arrest.

As Ani cut the corner on 28th Street into the Bellevue Campus, I shocked him out of fib into a sinus tachycardia (slightly rapid heart rate) with a pulse. He was showing ectopy (those funny little beats) in an array of sizes. We call these multi-focal PVC's. I dropped 1 mg of Lidocaine down his IV tubing and watched some of those beats normalize.

What was killing me was that I knew that if I was able to drain all that blood out of his chest with needle decompression, when they crack his chest open in the trauma slot, he may be holding onto more blood in his chest cavity. As the back doors opened to the trauma team, I took his blood pressure and noticed that the systolic (the beat the heart makes when it pumps) and the diastolic (the beat of the heart relaxing) were closing in on each other. I did it again and knew that this was it.

"He's tamponoding, let's move." I said as doc Pete looked at my chest full of blood.

"How many stab wounds is it?" Pete asked me as I grabbed the IV's and handed them to the officer who came with us. As I did this, the kid arrested again.

"Damnit!"

PARAMEDIC M.O.S.

I put my heels up on the upper bar of the stretcher and held on as everyone automatically wheeled while I held on and did compressions.

"Pete," I said counting compressions, "3,4 5, I found two in the right chest above the nipple. 3,4,5, and then nothing else. He has multiple contusions, 1, 2, 3, 4, and 5, everywhere. We think he got worked over and somehow found his way back to the site or was dropped there... 3, 4,5."

We rounded the corner to the ER Trauma slots, as everyone in the ER heard all the commotion. There must have been about fourteen people working on this guy between my crews, and the trauma team. We slid into the slot and I continued compressions until they transferred him off of our stretcher.

"1, 2, 3, 4, 5, He's had two Epi's, 3, 4,5, 1 atropine, 4, 5, and 100 mg of Lidocaine."

Barbara Franklin, a trauma nurse, looked up at me to get my attention to make the CPR switch. She knew that I was a mess and that she could take over. I was covered in blood and she was a fresh body.

"Ready; 3, 4, 5 and switch," I said as Barbara stepped up and got her placement on his chest without stopping the pace. I stepped away from the table while they took out a surgical tray. Pete was now on the kids right side, leaning at a forty-five degree angle, with his feet in a horse stance. He knew I already betadine'd the kid, so he didn't waste anytime. He took out a small but effective scalpel and made a clean horizontal incision from this kids armpit to his floating ribs. As he reached in to find where he was going to place the rib spreader, about one liter of blood spilled all over the floor. Danny, Ani, Connie and I just stood there silent.

"Aw Christ, get me some suction in here and those spreaders." When they completed cracking his chest open, Pete looked at his heart to do open carotid massage. This is essentially open heart CPR. When Pete got his hand inside, he said, "Forget this, let's get him to OR now!"

The four of us backed up as two nurses swung the door open, and the bed with all the trauma surgeons, nurses and equipment went flying down the hallway towards the operating room.

What was a nicely sterilized room not more than ten minutes ago, looked like the scene of a quadruple homicide. There was blood throughout most of the back portion of the room, and we all kind of walked in quiet, inconsistent circles. We knew how horrible this was. I took off my shirt immediately and made for the scrub sinks.

"Just another night at work," I thought to myself. I began to scrub up and the officer walked around the corner.

"Check out the name on this kid." The officer said to me as showed me his license.

"Anthony Dellilugi." I said to myself as I read his drivers license. I knew that name, but my head was cluttered. I asked the officer to show me the address again, and he did.

It was at this moment I felt my heart sink as low as it could go. I had this burning sensation in my digestive track now. This was the child of one of our Lieutenant's and even worse, it was Davia's godson. The last time I saw this kids father, Pino, was when he showed up at Erin Dericky's delivery.

"Oh my god." I said slowly.

"What's up, you know this kid?" The officer said to me.

"I know his father and Godmother, they are both MOS's and they're on the job."

"You gotta be kidding me," the officer said surprised.

"I wish I was. Damnit!" I slammed my fist down on the counter, loud enough for all of the staff at the workstation to be startled.

"His father should be working at Station 46," I told the officer. "I'll give you the number. I'll call his Godmother now, she's downtown at my station." I said whipping out my notepad.

"Is he likely?" The officer asked concerned.

"They are doing everything they can, you better just get him here." I said to the officer quickly. I knew that this kid would need a miracle just to make it up to surgery.

After drying off my hands I went right to the nurse's station. I called Davia's office line and she answered.

"Chief Battieri." She sounded very official.

"Hey," I said as gently as I could. "I need you to sit down while I tell you this and then I need you to come up to Bellevue as fast but as safely as you can." I said not knowing where to go with this. I was about to tell her that her godson was about to die, if not already dead.

"Are you okay? What's up?" Davia said as I could hear her putting away whatever she was doing.

"No, but I'm not the concern here. Dav," I paused, "we just brought Anthony into Bellevue and I need you to get up here now." I couldn't say it, and she knew this was bad.

PARAMEDIC M.O.S.

There was a moment of silence and then, "Christian, what happened?" Her voice then became very monotone.

"Davia, he was stabbed multiple times in the chest and beaten pretty bad. He is headed up to surgery now."

"WHAT?" She replied. I felt the shock go through her. I stared at the nurses station, void of any good feelings. One of the nurses looked at me and got up to put her arm around me.

"Dav, come up and I'll fill you in. Midtown South is calling Pino now."

She didn't waste time to say goodbye, as the phone hung up and I knew she was running for her department vehicle.

I called Lenny Washington up at communications.

"WHAT?" he replied in total shock. I asked him to send a couple of patrol bosses our way to help Dav however they could. No sooner did I finish talking with Lenny that I heard sirens pulling up outside. Davia came walking in very fast. As she walked towards me I went to get away from the nurses' station because it was right next to the bloody trauma slot where Anthony was brought into. As I did this, a member of the cleanup crew opened both doors as she looked into the trauma room. Davia looked at me and saw that my shirt was off, exposing my bulletproof vest. She put two and two together seeing the floor of the room.

She stopped and put her hands over her mouth and nose, as I got right up to her. I felt her knees buckle, so I caught her and helped her to a chair. She was crying now.

"Was that him in there?" Davia asked through the tears she was fighting.

I just looked at her, and finally nodded yes once. I knew that I had a stern face as I was clenching my teeth. I wasn't sure which one of us was going to fall apart. Ani came around the corner and saw Davia in tears and me holding her. Ani didn't know what to think.

"Christian, what's going on?" Ani said as she knelt down to Davia putting her arm around her.

"Ani that patient we brought in was Davia's godson." Ani's eye opened wide, as did her mouth since we both were pretty certain he would be pronounced dead by now.

"Oh my God," Ani said quietly as she rubbed Davia's back gently. Ani kept looking at me for something to say, and I dreaded the thought of the trauma surgeon walking out to give us all bad news.

Within a few minutes, not only did several patrol supervisors show up in the ER, but four EMS chiefs, including Chet Williams, the Chief of Operations walked in. All came over to us, as were we taking care of Davia.

Chet walked right over to me and extended his hand. We shook as Chet was trying to size up the state of affairs of everyone in the immediate vicinity. Chet surveyed each person individually as he took extra notice that Ani and I still had evidence of blood on our uniform pants, boots and our arms.

"How's she doing?" Chet asked quietly.

"Chief, she's holding up, but I don't have to tell you how horrible this is. She loves that kid like her own. We did everything we could for the little guy, everything."

"I know you did, and he couldn't have been in better hands." We stood there silently for a minute just breathing, feeling the tremendous weight in the room.

"Shit," Chet said under his breath.

"Okay look, there are enough of us here. Why don't you and Ani go scrub up and get your units back to shape. I know that you and Davia are close, so why don't you get your bus down to the station and come back up to stay with her."

I nodded in approval, "Thanks boss. We'll get outta here and I'll see you in a bit."

Chet patted me on the back, "Don't worry about communications, I'll call them. You just worry about getting cleaned up and getting back up here. I'll page you if anything breaks."

With that we shook hands again, and I knelt down to Davia to let her know where I would be. I gave her a hug and held her for a moment, and then made for the scrub sinks. After I scrubbed up, I called Anjoline to let her know what happened.

"Oh my God," AJ said as I delivered the news. "Want me to come down?"

Without even thinking I replied in agreement, "Hun, I think that would be great. She looks pretty fragile right now."

AJ took a breath, "I will get out of here now, and I should be there or near, by the time you get back to the ER."

"Babe," I said, "You are the best, and I'll see you in a bit. Drive carefully please."

PARAMEDIC M.O.S.

"You know I will," AJ said softly.

Ani and I cleaned up and with our respective partners left Bellevue for our station. We made it back in record time and very little if anything was said. Danny knew that I was about over my limit and that my mind was strictly on getting back up to the ER. As we pulled into the station Danny looked over at me, "You okay man?"

I nodded "Yeah, I just cannot believe how things have gone, and I hope that Davia's godson makes it through surgery."

Danny put the vehicle in park.

"Dude," Danny said, "I'll take care of the bus, you get back up to Bell."

I patted Danny on his right arm, "Thanks man, much appreciated."

"De natha," Danny said as I opened my door to exit.

AMBU came running up to me and she stopped to nudge my thigh. I think she knew something was wrong. She walked slowly next to me, watching the ground in front of my like a century on patrol. I walked into the office to drop off my narcs and radio. As soon as I entered John turned around from the file cabinet and immediately addressed me.

"Hey, how you doin and how's the kid?"

"I'm a lot better than the kid is," I began, "but he is still in surgery. He got really jacked up out there."

John closed the file cabinet with his elbow, and as I locked the narcotics cabinet he placed his cupped hand in my shoulder.

"Look, no matter which one of us got that call, it would have sucked. That kid is lucky that you, Danny, Ani and Connie were the ones to show up. He now has a fighting chance."

Clenching my teeth together, I nodded slowly and looked at John right in his eyes. He knew that I had been emotionally beaten up over the last month, and that this, like all else, would sit heavy on my shoulders if Davia's godson died.

"I hear ya boss, I better get back up there; I want to be there either way."

"You're a good man Chris!" John smiled proudly.

I knelt down to give AMBU a few pets and a kiss on her head. She made sure she got a lick in on my right ear. I made for the door without even going upstairs to my locker.

C.B. Garris

Chapter XXIV:

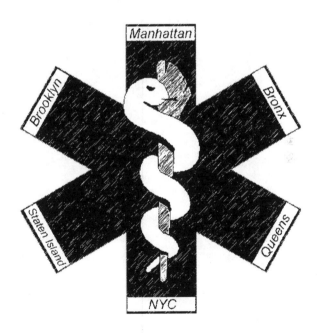

PARAMEDIC M.O.S.

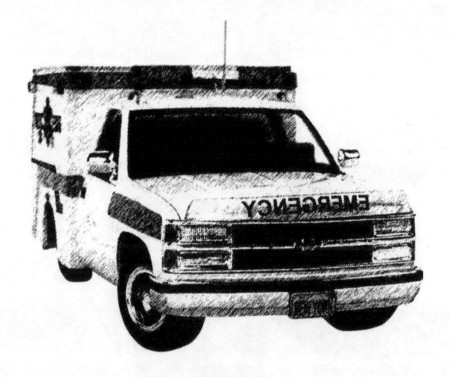

C.B. Garris

I finally woke up late the next evening. Anjoline and I had kept the vigil in the ER until about 7:00 am, when the trauma surgeon walked out informing us that Davia's godson was in critical but stable condition. I almost passed out. I don't know how they did it, but he was alive. As the doc said his statements he pulled me aside.

"I just want to let you know that you made one hell of a call on that needle decompression. That is the only thing that kept this kid alive."

I nodded at the doc, unable to smile. I had been standing close to Anjoline, with Davia sitting down right next to me. As soon as Davia heard that he was alive, she leaped up out of her seat and wrapped her body around me, crying intensely. The thrust of it made me drop my coffee, but I wrapped my arms around her and held her. As the water flowed from Davia's eyes all she kept saying was, "Thank you Christian, thank you, thank you."

She even kissed my cheeks. We all knew that she was on complete emotional overload. After about five to ten minutes of crying and hugging, I was able to sit Davia back down. Anjoline winked at me and went to get Davia a large cup of water from the nurse's lounge.

According to the doc, and, as we already knew, Anthony had lost a tremendous amount of blood, but as the doc put it, "due to the absolute rapid intervention and quick thinking of the crews that brought him in, he now has a fighting chance."

Davia looked at me with nothing but adoration as she held onto and squeezed my hand. I felt this strange connection to everything around me at that moment. Pino reached down to place a firm grip on my shoulder without saying a word. I know that he was holding onto all he could, hoping his son came out of the surgery alive. We treat patients day and night, never knowing them or their families long enough to be connected like this. Here is a situation where I knew someone very close to the patient, and have the chance to see the end result.

"You know Dav," I interjected, "Danny, Connie and Ani were all apart of this too."

Davia was in some altered mental state. She kept running the back of her fingers up and down my cheeks as she smiled at me painfully. Tears were still flowing down her face like a well-titrated intravenous line. As Davia stared at me she lipped, "Thank you," to me again. I just sat there holding her other hand. Anjoline came back with a huge cup of water and a box of tissues, sitting down on the opposite side of Davia. Davia thanked

PARAMEDIC M.O.S.

her and blew her nose several times. Clenching the tissue with one hand, she used her other one to take a big gulp of water from the cup.

"You gotta be exhausted," I said to Davia. "I already spoke with the AOD and she cleared it to have a bed put in his surgical ICU post-op room for you. I talked to Chet and food will be brought to you. Why don't we get you upstairs and settled. AJ and I will go by your place and get some fresh clothes for you. Your husband is already on his way back from his mother's in Florida," I said to Davia with a smile.

"You guys," Davia slipped in, "you guys are the best."

With that we walked Davia upstairs to the post op surgical ICU room. Her godson was a mass of tubes, bandages and IV's. If he makes it, I know it will be a long recovery.

After AJ and I went to Davia's home in the Brighton Beach section of Brooklyn to retrieve her clothes and toothbrush, we returned to Bell and dropped her belongings off. We both then went back to AJ's to collapse. We must have returned home about 11:00 am.

When we awoke it was about 8:00 pm in the evening. AJ had rolled over and wrapped her body around mine. I loved when she did that. I admired her incredibly glowing tan. I found it even more appealing that she had no tan lines.

"What a night," AJ said to me as she pressed her full lips on mine.

"Could you do that again?" I said to her with a smile.

She did without hesitation. In fact she did it for about twenty minutes.

"I love you babe," she said to me as her hair fell in my eyes, immediately darkening the room.

"I'm hungry, how bout you?" I asked AJ.

"I am famished." AJ said as she tickled me. "I know what I really want, but I think we should both indulge in some serious food before our systems go whacko first."

"Hmmm," I remarked, "okay. How about we try to get into The Matsui House for some teppan, and then we can have each other for dessert."

AJ's face lit up, "Oh BABE, you're on." AJ gave me another kiss and we both made for a quick shower, this time without too much frolicking. I called the restaurant and spoke to Tommy Shikonawa, the host who knew AJ and I by name. We usually visited the establishment every few weeks, sometimes even more. Tommy said that they were full, but they were never too full for us. He told us to come right in and he would seat us.

C.B. Garris

When we arrived, Tommy and his hosting staff greeted us with huge smiles. Showito, a very statuesque Japanese woman who was about Anjoline's height, gave both AJ and I hugs, Tommy did the same. We were ushered right past the line of about fifty waiting customers. We were placed with a full table of six other people. The teppan range was already warm; evidence that it had been used numerous times since the 5:00 pm opening time. AJ and I sat in a sort of quiet solace. We were both completely whipped, emotionally and physically.

We were thinking of all that happened, and glad that we have each other. As AJ and I sat quietly holding hands, it was as if the other couples admired our intimate silence. One of the males in the group eyed us for few seconds, and then reached over and hugged and kissed the woman with him. When our chef arrived, the zucchini, onions, bean sprouts, and scallions hit the range with an aromatic sizzle. AJ and I feasted on the veggies, and for her the hibachi chicken and shrimp, while I went for the Chef's Choice: Filet Mignon and Lobster tail.

Our bodies were full by the end of the meal, which was topped off by a strange but tasty Green Tea sorbet. The meal was spectacular as always, almost as sumptuous as an Anjoline kiss.

AJ awoke for her regular tour of 0700-1500. I was actually glad that she woke up extra early this morning. There was something so peaceful about holding her in the darkness and quiet. We almost fell back asleep, but let our bodies stay enough in tune to remain tactile. After she finished showering, dressing and giving me my morning goodbye kiss, she was off. I slept in and caught up on much needed rest. I was due in for 15:00 and made it in by about 13:00. I did my ceremonial walk with AMBU. When I pulled up, she was out by the Oxygen tanks, chasing a ball. It always amazed me how attached we all were to her and she to us. She was our family.

On my return from FDR Park with her, Danny was pulling up. As he placed his car in park, he rolled the window down and stuck out his hand. We shook, and then AMBU jumped up to give him a lick. He said he would be a few minutes, so I went up to get changed. I had hoped that AJ would be arriving as I was walking downstairs but when I stopped in at the Borough Command office, Erin told me she not only got a late job, she was on the phone with telemetry on a messy cardiac arrest. That meant she would definitely not be getting back anytime soon, even if they pronounced on the scene, something neither she nor I liked to do.

PARAMEDIC M.O.S.

Unless it was an obvious mortal injury, I preferred to at least transport the patient. If for nothing else, it would help keep the family from having to remember that so and so died on their bed or floor or in the tub. If they were pronounced dead at the hospital, that is where they "died." Therefore, anything that happened leading up to the pronouncement was people doing all they could to save that person.

Danny and I hit the street on time today. We had a few back-to-back calls that we were cancelled from, and then we had one that just set the record for the month. The assignment came in as an "UNKNOWN," which I truly hated. That usually meant that the call receiving operator could not disseminate the information provided, there was a language barrier, or worse, we were about to walk into a crime scene.

Today it was choice number three. We arrived at the address, in a very wealthy, well known apartment complex on the West Side. The building stood about forty stories, and when we arrived there were no obvious signs of trouble. There was no smoke, fire, muzzle flashes, explosions or people jumping. I wondered if this could have even been a prank.

Danny and I exited the vehicle and noticed that not even the doorman was approaching us. On past occurrences where the building has a doorman, the tenant usually calls down ahead to let them know they called 911 and to expect us. They usually try to corral us to the service elevator, out of fear that it will look bad if an EMS crew is seen in the building. We generally just walk right in the front door, as time is of the essence to us, and we really could care less about appearance. As Danny and I grab the essentials for this "unknown" call, a drug bag, Lifepak, Airway Bag, Trauma Bag and suction unit, we make for the front door.

The doorman greets us with a Brooks Brothers nod as we enter the structure. I kept having this peculiar feeling about this call though. Low and behold, as we walk through the foyer, the elevator opens and a man in his 50's runs towards us covered in blood.

"You have to help me!" He screamed frantically.

I dropped the equipment off of my shoulder to stop him. As I made my best attempt to both calm him down, and also check him for any stab wounds, Danny picked up his NYPD radio and notified them to expedite the officer's enroute.

Chester, the man now in my hands told me that his nephew's friend took Chester's wife hostage in the apartment, stabbing both Chester and her. He was unsure if she was even alive. It turns out that his wife was the

Ambassador to a foreign country. As soon as I heard that, I knew what kind of a circus this was about to turn into. Within a half hour, Danny and I found ourselves on the 32nd floor, the floor below the apartment where this couple lived. We were deployed in the stairwell, while S.W.A.T. teams from the NYPD and FBI coordinated hostage negotiation efforts and hostage rescue efforts with themselves respectively, along with attaché's from the CIA, State Department and the Secret Service. On the first reconnaissance mission, the NYPD S.W.A.T. team members found a note stuck to the door that said,

"Stay away from this door. Anyone who tries to enter will be burned with scalding water and other assorted weapons of choice."

"You've got to be shitting me," Danny said to me as I passed the finding along.

"Dude," I said to Danny while we both sat on our stretcher, "You know we are going to be here for awhile."

Danny sat back with his head against the concrete wall, "Yeh, just what I was hoping for."

This stand off went on for almost eight hours and it included helicopters, and officers rappelling from the top of the structure to use cameras for a better look. There were uniformed and plainclothes law enforcement agents going up and down the stairwell every few minutes; all had their weapons out in case this turned into a shootout. Because of obstructions, all the rappelling officers could visualize was the view of a female laying face up on a floor. She hadn't moved in hours and that was enough for them.

We were moved to the incident floor and awaited our orders. We all had our radios against our ears, waiting for the "GO" word. When they gave it, what must have been about eight S.W.A.T. officers ran through the front door with a thunderous BOOM – evidence of the use of their battering ram. I didn't hear any shots go off, so I peeked around the corner to find a scene from the keystone cops. It turns out that when the S.W.A.T. teams hit the door, the assailant was bending down in front of it on the other side. When the door came down, it did so on top of him, and about seven officers stepped on top of the door. Obviously he was no longer a threat; in fact he was incapacitated. The officers searched the room with their infrared night goggles, but they didn't realize that the assailant was under the door. So I had a pretty good chuckle when they figured it out and placed him in cuffs. The wife it turns out was a smart cookie. She acted as if she was dying from the moment she was stabbed.

PARAMEDIC M.O.S.

Her wounds were pretty superficial, so the back up crew took care of her. I was hoping that the NYPD would have transported this nut bag, but since our vehicle was in the best position, and they figured he was nuts, we were asked if we would take him. I demanded that officers be on board without their weapons. I figured with four officers and me on board, we could handle this idiot. The officers at first wanted him to be face down on the stretcher, at which I told them no way. I also then educated them on the fatal results of doing that from a few recent experiences, that other departments have encountered lately.

They got my drift, and we set the subject up on the stretcher face up. When we had him sit on the stretcher, he kicked an officer straight in the groin. I pushed two officers aside and with a flying leap into the rear of the ambulance, placed my boot in his neck while grabbing the lever at the head of the stretcher to slam him down flat.

"Look you fuck," I said as I slammed the head of the stretcher down, causing our patient/perp to realize that he was suddenly in a bad way.

"You are going to lay hear silently and nicely. One more move like that and this will be the longest vehicular ride you will ever take, and it may be your last. You got me? These gentlemen in blue are police officers, and certain laws and regulations bind them. When you are in this ambulance, you are in my world; and I am not bound by the same restraints these officers are. Now stop fuckin' around."

That said, we all enjoyed a nice, quiet ride to Bellevue, while our patient/perp kept the look of absolute fear in his eyes as I watched him with a direct and stern stare; my boot firmly placed near his throat for the duration of the ride.

Since this one call took up our entire shift, Danny and I left Bellevue, picked up a few cold drinks and made our way back to Station 11. As we approached the Station and were about to turn in, I thought I saw something fly out of the station gates. Unfortunately, I did and it was AMBU. Somehow and for some reason she ran out of the station. I screamed for Danny to stop, and while the vehicle was still moving I opened my door to leap out and capture her. She had a head start on me and before I could get to her I heard a horrendous screech, followed by a thump. Next thing I know, AMBU was lying on the ground motionless in front of the car that hit her.

"AMBU," I screamed as Danny blocked off traffic.

The driver of the car got out totally upset and a few medics ran out of the station. AMBU was breathing, but she was badly hurt. I could tell that she probably broke her hip and had who knows what other kinds of injuries. I told Danny to get a backboard, and I picked up the NYPD portable.

"EMS Paramedic 10X central!"

The PD dispatcher halted all radio traffic and informed me to go ahead.

"EMS Paramedic 10X Central, I have a Member of the Service down at South and Clinton Street; it is an EMS K-9 unit and I need the FDR shut down now. We are heading up to 60th and 1st (The NY Animal Hospital)."

Without any questions or further explanations needed, within about three minutes the NYPD came through and shut down the entire FDR Drive by placing sector cars at all exits and entrances northbound. This bought us enough time to get AMBU in an ambulance, and to get several lines started on her. We couldn't backboard her like a human, but she would be best treated by us, we are her family. This was the day that I was so glad that I volunteered for a Pet Rescue. My time in their facility taught me not only the anatomy of different species, but also how to treat the various traumatic injuries and how they differ from humans. I was able to establish IV's in AMBU's cephalic (front leg) and saphenous (hind leg) veins with eighteen gauge catheters. Unlike humans, in this case I used Lactated Ringers for AMBU's traumatic injuries and potential blood loss issues.

With the entire FDR shutdown, and five ambulances in tow, we all shot up the FDR to the 60th Street Animal Hospital. I must say that when the Veterinarians saw the flood of emergency vehicles, they didn't know what to think. Even more surprising to them was when the back doors to my ambulance swung open and there we were bringing out a large dog; they were extremely perplexed.

As the lead Vet began to ask questions, he looked down at AMBU's necklace, which contained her shrunken EMS shield on it, #K011; he then knew it was our station mascot. We went into the trauma room with her, and the Vet was amazed that I got a few lines established on her already, and 60 cc's of blood as well. As they prepped her for X-rays and eventually surgery, I would not leave her side. AJ paged me several times, but I couldn't let go of AMBU for fear that she was going to die at any moment. She wouldn't move, but every once in awhile she would shift her eyes to me with this look of incredible fear. I was crying now, hoping that she would

PARAMEDIC M.O.S.

make it. I stood at the head of the gurney, making sure that when they weren't taking x-rays, that she was covered with a blanket and comforted. I kept petting her head gently. When she went in for X-ray, I called AJ.

"How bad is she?" AJ said to me with great concern. I told her everything I knew so far, and that I was staying around until we knew what was going to happen. I told her that if she were in stable enough condition to make it to surgery, I would be home later.

AMBU had been sedated after X-ray's to take some of the pain away. I was petting her head when Janet, the other lead Vet walked in.

"I still can't believe that you actually brought her here in an ambulance. I think that is great."

"Doc," I said non-chalantly, "she is a member of the service and there is just no other way."

"Well, here's the deal, she definitely fractured her pelvis, but it occurred in a way that we can repair it and probably with great success. The rest of her injuries seem to be superficial. This hip surgery gets really expensive, so you have to decide whether or not you want to go through with it or put her down."

I looked up at her without even a break, "Doc, AMBU is as much a part of our station as anyone of us. If you are telling me that you can perform a successful surgery on her and that she will not be in pain as a result of it, we will get the money for the surgery."

"Very well," the doc said.

Once AMBU was sleeping soundly in prep for her surgery, I gave her a gentle kiss on her head and made for the door. I returned to the station, returning the vehicle keys, radios and standard equipment for a tour's end. By the time I arrived at Anjoline's house I was whipped and AJ was sleeping soundly. I put my gray book bag down near her dresser as I stepped into the shower to rinse the day off. I did all that I could to be quiet. When I returned to the bedroom, AJ was all wrapped up in her covers, smiling. She opened one end of the covers for me, "Don't bother putting anything on, just get in here next to me," she said confidently.

"How is AMBU," AJ asked as I wrapped my arms around her, feeling the intense warmth that her body always provides.

"She will be going for surgery shortly. The Vet thinks that it will be successful."

AJ ran her hands over the back of my head, intensifying her grip as she got to my neck.

"AMBU got lucky," I said as I sank into the feel of AJ's fingertips against my neck.

"I'm so sorry that you had to witness her getting hit, but I am sure that she was happy you were there."

I shifted in the bed to have AJ lay her entire body on top of me.

"You smell quite freshly showered," AJ squirmed her way to position herself just right, so that she could place her head on my chest. Her eyes read me in a fashion unlike anything I ever knew or hoped for, and there was no way to hide all that I was thinking. She knew I was tired and emotionally drained. In fact, we both were.

"Turn over and let me give you a massage," AJ said as she moved herself off of my chest. Once on my stomach, I listened to the silent vibration that AJ's body always gives off. I felt her well-manicured nails gently reach my back as she swayed them up and down, back to front. She kissed me gently on my shoulder and then I must have fallen asleep.

PARAMEDIC M.O.S.

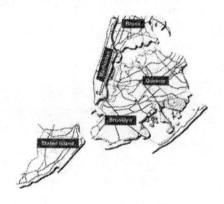

C.B. Garris

Chapter XXV:

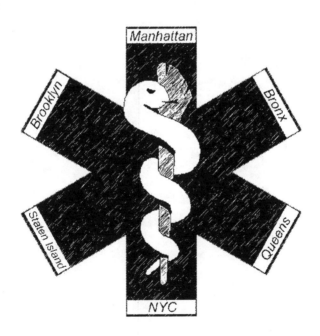

PARAMEDIC M.O.S.

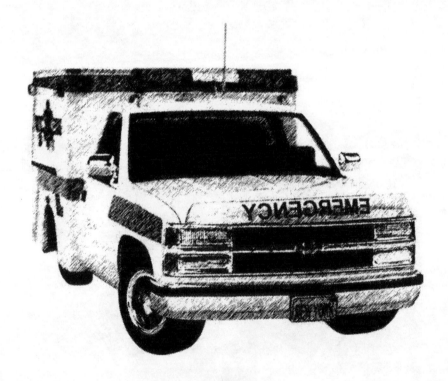

C.B. Garris

All of a sudden I realized I kept hearing those words I last heard before my accident echo in my mind.

"Holy shit, hold on!"

The words got louder and louder until I came to in present time.

When I opened my eyes, I realized I was still in the hospital bed, AJ next to me asleep in the bed they provided for her.

It would be almost a month of in-hospital stay after the accident that put me here, with trauma physicians visiting me three times a day like clock work. It seems that I must have struck a number of things hard enough to bend the shock plate in my vest, which could have been my spine in the rear. They said I had spinal shock and almost everything shutdown, which is why I had to be tubed as I stopped breathing. They were checking into some funky pictures of my back and neck, including the CAT-Scans, MRI'S, and the nuclear isotopic procedures they put me through. It seems I had compression fractures in the thoracic region of my back and I herniated my five lower discs in my back. To top that off, I had one hell of a concussion. Because of the lumbar displacement, any surgery would be very risky. AJ was reassigned to the detail of keeping vigil over me and it was approved on Release Time. The nurses were kind enough to move a bed in next to me so that she could stay with me.

"Hey sweetie," AJ said as I opened my eyes again.

"Hi," I said with as much energy I could find. I felt strange, as if I didn't even know myself. I could have been killed, but then I would have never forgiven myself for leaving AJ.

I tried to sit up, but just as I did, something in my back wrenched me to the bed.

"Damn!" I said as AJ made for my side.

"What's wrong," AJ asked trying to console me.

"I don't know. I tried to sit up, but everything in my back just pulled me to the bed," I said with frustration.

"Your body got badly whacked in the back of the bus Hun. Try and take it easy. This is going to be a bit of a road for you for awhile." AJ remarked affectionately.

"Does anyone know exactly how Danny was killed in the accident?" I asked AJ as I could see she didn't want to answer.

"Babe, what I am going to tell you is really hard, even for me." She paused a few seconds and took a breath. I felt my heart sink.

PARAMEDIC M.O.S.

"The driver who hit your vehicle was doing they estimated about 65 when he connected with your bus. He hit your vehicle so hard that he forced the rear doors open, causing Danny to fly out of them on impact, and since the driver was so drunk, he still had the car in motion. When Danny hit the pavement, the drunk driver ran over him, dismembering him. They worked him, but there really wasn't anything to work with. I am sorry babe." AJ's voice crackled as she began to cry.

I took a bunch of deep breaths and just looked at AJ with a dead stare, as I held her hand firmly. She didn't even try to push me to say anything. I felt like I had been beaten, but not physically. I felt as though all my energy had been expended, as if I don't know where my life force had gone. I kept picturing what AJ told me, and I eventually had her sit me up as I began to vomit. Since I was on only IV fluids for a few days, all I brought up was green bile.

AJ went to the bathroom to get me a damp towel to help wipe my face. I was in full traction and even basic functions that I was normally capable of were near impossible. AJ helped me out of the gown I had on, since I vomited all over it, and began to give me a sponge bath. It had been a few days since I had even a shower; and in my position I was unable to stand or bathe myself. AJ was so gentle to me, and I felt as if I was a garden that she was cultivating. She had this serious look in her face. It was one that I had not seen before. Somewhere as she slowly but carefully sponged my legs, I realized the look was her fear that she could not speak. She was speaking very little, making this a very visceral experience. I lifted my head up gently a number of times and looked at her. She was now in a zone. I felt protected and cared for. I wasn't even sure when I would walk again, but something said to me that regardless of the outcome, Anjoline will be there with me. She was caring for me like I was all that she had left.

Tonight would be my first night of solid food since the accident, and also getting used to the fear that I may never go back to the street as a medic. The charge nurse carefully took me out of traction so that they could sit my bed up. I saw the food tray and wondered what kind of mystery meal I would be starting off with. Just as the food was brought in, one of the other ward nurses walked in with two big batches of flowers, a teddy bear and balloons.

"Here, Mr. Popular, these are for you." Denise Wellan, the ward nurse tonight sat these two huge bouquets of multi-colored roses and tulips down on the nightstand next to me.

"Babe, who sent those?" I asked AJ as she searched through the Baby's Breath for the cards.

"Well, Mr. Famous, these are from Taylor Frentworth and Miko. They send you their love and hope you are back on your feet in no time." I sat there in appreciation of the flowers, still realizing that my entire world has been turned upside down.

"Wow," AJ continued, "They really are fabulous." As I sat up, AJ opened her bag, removing a dark blue Yankees baseball cap. She knew they are my favorite, so she placed it on my head gently.

I looked at the floral arrangements and smiled.

"It's not every day that someone in the hospital receives flowers from one of the world's most famous celebrities. That was really nice of her." I said with a note of flattery in my voice.

AJ stepped away to cut the flowers properly and feed them. She came back in a few minutes from the bathroom with big smiles.

"Well sir, it looks like you did make a big hit with my friends back there." AJ smiled an electric smile, which momentarily made me forget the intense, stabbing sensation I had in my middle back.

PARAMEDIC M.O.S.

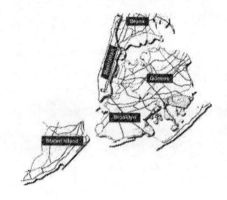

C.B. Garris

Chapter XXVI:

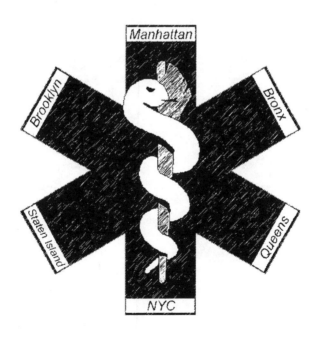

PARAMEDIC M.O.S.

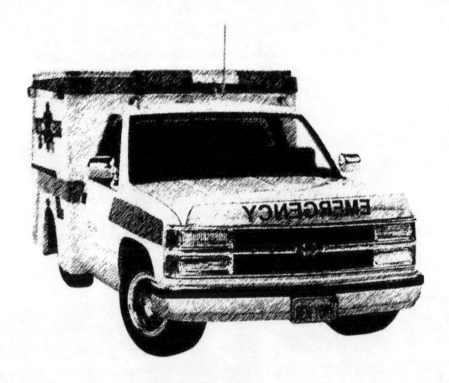

C.B. Garris

After the physicians were content that enough pressure was off of my spine so that I could at least attempt to go home, I was released. I did go through periods in the hospital where I had no appetite, and I got bored so easily. I was in physical therapy three times a week, which would continue once I went home. I was told that AMBU made it through surgery fine, and she too was released from the hospital. Davia took her home for about two weeks for rest before she returned her to the station.

AJ was a real dream to me, as she spent each waking moment with me when she was not at work. She always made sure that there was plenty of food in her home, and that I got to physical therapy on time three times a week. I know that it must have been very trying on her, but she took it all in stride. As I went through the different modalities of my physical therapy with my therapist, Alexandra, I would be introduced to Electrical Muscle Stimulators, Ultrasound, therapeutic massage, and exercises. I lost about fifteen pounds in the hospital from all of the times I was placed on N.P.O (nothing permitted orally) orders from the doc. I became extremely insecure of my body and the way it looked.

It was bad enough that I was to be placed in a specialized spinal brace called a Knight Brace, but I must have looked pretty frustrated. I never really had to work out to maintain my body, because work was my workout. We lifted, carried, acrobated, and used our agility to maintain great shape. Now things were beginning to change. I was atrophying and would have to wait sometime before I could even work out again if ever. My neurosurgeon wanted to cut me open, shave down my facet joints, and remove lots of scar tissue, but that procedure was very risky. I had this thing against someone taking a Black & Decker shaving tool to my spinal cord.

AJ made sure that there were plenty of movies in the house for me to watch, and she would stop to pick up any books I wanted to read. I was being paid by a new program instituted by the agency called LODI (or Line of Duty Injury). The one thing that sucked about this is that I was one of the first medics seriously hurt to have to use this. Unfortunately, it was initiated before anyone really had a clear understanding of what it entailed. Thus, I would routinely hear from the accountant at my physical therapists office that the City lost my file, had no record of my accident and stuff like that and therefore stopped paying my medical bills.

AJ fought tooth and nail with these fools, even when they threatened to stop my benefits because they lost my file. I was only a few months past

PARAMEDIC M.O.S.

the accident, and my entire torso was being held up by a brace. I could move around only gingerly, and required routine physical therapy. I told Davia what happened with my LODI benefits and how they were giving me a hard time. Davia immediately cleared her calendar and drove down to headquarters to have a few words with people in that division. Davia called me later to tell me that she solved the issues, but that she wanted to talk with me in person later on. She also wanted to make sure that AJ would be home. I gave her directions to AJ's and paged AJ so that she knew. AJ said she would be home about 5 p.m.. Davia let me know she would be up and around 6 p.m. and I told her not to eat; AJ will pick something up.

I sat and wondered what was it that Davia would want to tell me like this. That scared me. I was able to get back to the couch, adjusting a few straps on the brace for comfort.

AJ had stopped at Hunan Garden down the street and picked up a feast of food: BBQ'd pork fried rice, beef with broccoli and brown sauce, cashew chicken, Moo Shoo turkey, and some Lo Mein for Davia too. AJ looked very strange when she walked in the door. Something was very out of place, as there was no smile, and her soul seemed elsewhere when she walked in. She opened the front door and made for the kitchen right away. This was out of place for her since she always came to me first, no matter how many bags she had in her hand. I heard her put the bag down and it seemed as though she was banging the pantry closed several times. I worked to get off of the sofa, but it did take a little bit of effort with the brace on. Just before I got to my feet, she appeared in the doorway.

"You, okay?" I said with a lot of apprehension in my voice.

AJ just stood in the doorway as if she was wrapped up in a force field. Now that she stepped into the light it was apparent that she was crying recently.

"Babe?" I said softly, "what's wrong?"

AJ made her way off of the wall and over towards the sofa, sitting down in one lump. Since I had never seen her like this before, I remained absolutely still. I was very unsure if she wanted to be touched, held, admired, caressed or just heard.

Her silence was deafening, as I was reading signs from her that were all bad. I joined her. AJ was looking straight ahead when she began to speak.

"I can't take all this death and destruction." She said softly, although to me it was louder than an elephant running through the room.

I adjusted my body so that I could face her profile completely. "Did you have a job go south on you today?"

AJ sniffled and sighed. Another wave of tears came on.

"I was driving home on the Deegan," she started slowly and quietly, almost as if she was completely removed from herself, "and I pulled up on an accident. One of the cars was crushed, and the other was not much better. I was the first one there, so I jumped out and grabbed my bag. When I got to the passenger side of the crushed vehicle, an adult male and female had been ejected and they were both DOA. The male was under the car and cut in two pieces. When I looked harder, I could look right down into his colon, as his upper torso was completely separated from his body. As for the female, she was ejected and her head was open all over the highway shoulder."

AJ remained poised sitting straight up without moving.

"As for the driver of the other car," she paused, "that fucker was drunk and he didn't have a mark on him. He just sat on the side of the highway singing to himself."

We both sat there inhaling and exhaling. I knew now what this had to do with – her parents. I reached for her hand slowly, hoping she wouldn't pull away. She didn't.

"That sonovabitch bastard killed those two people, and they probably had children." There was escalation in her voice, as if I thought she was going to scream.

"I bet he doesn't even care that he now left some children parentless," her voice continued upward and her crying began mixing in with her next statement, "and I miss them so much!" She let out this intense cry in her words. I didn't know how I could be anything at that moment.

I adjusted on the couch once again and pulled her toward me gently. AJ fell into me without a fight, except for the tears that just kept flowing.

I rocked back and forth gently while holding her, telling her to "Let it out." She certainly did not need any prompting from me, as it came with what seemed without end. We must have sat there on the couch for about twenty minutes saying nothing more. As I had my arms wrapped around AJ, she had both of her hands firmly placed on my forearms, supporting her position. In both hands she held tissues, and I had a few on backup next to me. I felt as if she had reached her limit, and this was something I rarely saw in her. We heard a car pull up and AJ made to her feet. We knew it was Davia, and AJ went to the bathroom to freshen up a bit.

PARAMEDIC M.O.S.

Davia came in as I greeted her at the door.

"Hey, you don't look so hot," she said as she took a long look at my eyes.

"AJ just stopped at a DUI accident on the Deegan coming home. She found an adult couple DOA; one was transected in two at the torso. The accident appears to be the fault of the DUI driver." I was just finishing when AJ walked down the stairs.

AJ and Davia hugged, as AJ reached her hand out and placed it on my rear flank, squeezing gently. She took a long stare at me as AJ asked "Ya'll hungry?" We broke out the food and I adjusted my brace about fifteen times trying to get comfortable on the couch, as AJ and Davia dished out the food. Davia began sharing her experience with the LODI unit and then told me some of the lighter points of what had been going on at the station.

Davia put her plate down and took a swig of her glass of water.

"You are sorely missed at the station, I have to tell you." Davia said as she smiled.

I thanked her while trying to keep everything in perspective.

"The reason I wanted to see you tonight in the company of AJ," Davia said as she took a huge breath and let it out, "is because I had a conversation with Conner Anderson, the agency Deputy Medical Director." She sighed.

"He carefully reviewed your hospital records to date and while we have cleared up the entire problem you had with LODI, Conner suggested that you consider doing your physical therapy elsewhere. Because, of this merger, if you are still on the LODI list when it comes to fruition, the new agency has mentioned something about getting rid of all injured personnel altogether; this has yet to be figured out. Conner said that he can get OPS to authorize all eighteen months of pay and your benefits and care paid for, but if you are still on LODI at merger time, they could just toss you. The trade is that you would have to resign from the Service to get the benefits, kind of like a buyout with bennies.

My greatest fear had just come true.

AJ put her plate down slowly. I just sat there in a dead stare. I guess I had always hoped that there would be a way for me to remain in the Service, and that I would never be faced with having to leave, even if it was in my own best interests. Even after a month of hospitalization, and three months of being at home in a brace, it wouldn't sink in. That is because I would not let it.

"Under the LODI plan, you have the eighteen months of pay coming to you, after that it falls back on the state." Davia said this with complete frustration.

"You mean that's it, just like that? That's the best offer they can make?" I asked with sadness in my expression.

Davia breathed in, "Christian, it's not that you aren't valuable, you're the best one on my staff. With the likelihood of this merger going through at anytime, they are taking a really hard line on anyone who is presently on the injured list, whether or not they will eventually go back to duty; it is so totally screwed up and personally, I don't think those that are forcing this upon us have a fucking clue what they are doing. With the possibility of the agency dissolving at anytime, they are taking a real hard line on anyone who isn't medically or physically clear. I hate to be the one to tell you this, and actually I didn't want it to come from me, but I didn't want one of those administrative bastards to be the one to say anything."

I put my plate down and sank into the couch as AJ moved closer. I looked at the floor for a while. Davia's beeper went off and AJ handed her the phone. There was a four alarm fire brewing in the Bronx and getting bigger. Since she was in Westchester and the fire was on the Bronx/Yonkers line, she was the duty chief assigned.

"Christian, I am sorry and I hate to leave like this, but we will finish this conversation later. With that, we all shared hugs goodbye, and as Davia turned on her department issued unmarked vehicle, she lit up the entire block with her undercover lights. Davia's siren wailed in the background.

As the sound of the siren dissipated, and my frustration shot straight up, I sat with AJ as we talked about what just happened. AJ placed her body against mine as we rested on the couch. In between her touches were my tears.

"I'm not really sure what to say anymore, except I keep feeling like I must have really pissed someone off in the universe," I said solemnly.

"Christian, I have to say that I was scared this day would come. When I walked in and found you in the ER after your accident, I saw the mass of tubes you were connected too, and I thought to myself "this is it." AJ firmed her touch on me.

"I am never going to be one to tell you what to do, but I know this is just one major blow after the other. I put a call into Taylor yesterday and asked her about a great sports medicine rehabilitation center in Santa

PARAMEDIC M.O.S.

Monica. She was in a bad accident four years ago, and the people there did incredible work on her. Aside from being a sports rehab facility, it was also an alternative medicine wellness center, with sports Rehab specialists, acupuncturists and eastern medicine physicians on staff as well. I am unsure how the timing of this next comment is going to feel, but babe, maybe this is the signal that you should make a change." I was looking at AJ's eyes, as I know she really wanted the best for me.

"Are you suggesting that I go out there for awhile for treatment? I don't want to be away from you, and besides the City will never pay for a provider in Los Angeles." I said to AJ as I felt myself get dizzy.

"Actually honey, I was thinking more along the lines of us leaving here all together and moving to L.A. I can easily buy a house there and we can figure out all of the logistics once we are there." AJ sighed. "I am tired of all this toxicity that seems to be going on at work; it is unhealthy and it damn near killed you. I want you in my life and in a much less threatening line of work if possible. I saw how much different you were in Los Angeles, and I think that could be something permanent."

I cried for what seemed like an eternity. AJ just held me, wishing she could stop the pain. I was unsure if I was crying for finding out that I was being taken off the job, or that I have someone next to me that cares for me like Anjoline.

After what must have been more than an hour I looked at AJ and commented, "Wow," as I adjusted into a somewhat less painful position. "I don't know what to say. I know that Taylor said she could find me a job somewhere and..." AJ cut me off.

"And first of all Mr., you won't be working until you are well enough too. First order of business is to get you back to full health, and besides I talked with Taylor today and she said when you are well enough, you will be taken care of."

"I am a little scared, I mean moving so far away and all these recent change, but then I know you are there and I will be fine." I said as I contemplated all of my options. "But my therapy babe, I know the City will give me so much shit to get the bills paid."

AJ looked at me very clearly and said "Don't you worry about what the City will or won't do, if need be, I will pay for your therapy. You will get back to health and you will have the best. I won't have it any other way."

AJ hugged me and held on for a long time. She then helped me out of my brace, and excused herself to the bathroom. She reappeared with a long hot, moist towel, and told me to turn on my stomach. She rested the towel on my back, which provided much needed relief for my muscles that were continuously in spasm. She gave me as firm a massage as I could stand. So much of me wanted to turn over and make love with her, but I knew that my back was in no shape.

As she worked on my back there was silence. The silence was deafening, as AJ knew that I was running my years as a medic through my mind. She knew how hard this decision was for me, even though it appeared the Service already made the decision. I took a number of long breaths and turned my head to the side, still resting on my forearms.

"I guess we are going to Los Angeles then," I said as I turned over to see AJ's smile.

"I was hoping you'd see it my way," AJ said as she brought her lips up to mine. AJ ran her hands over the back of my head, "babe, we will be fine, I know it."

PARAMEDIC M.O.S.

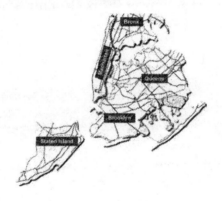

C.B. Garris

Chapter XXVII:

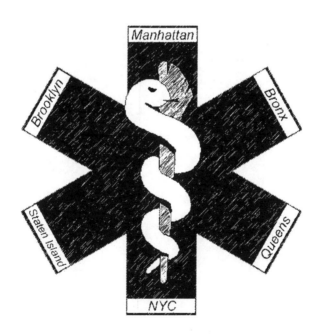

PARAMEDIC M.O.S.

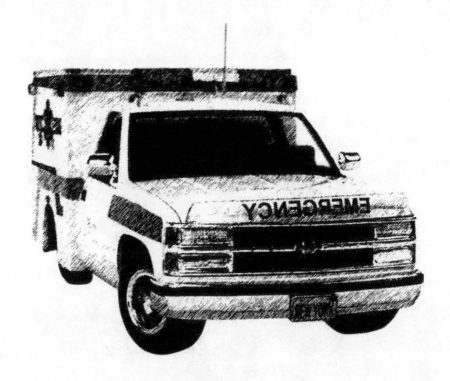

C.B. Garris

AJ and I spent the next week packing up things that she wanted to ship to Taylor's for storage. She gave her two weeks notice of resignation, and as much as she enjoyed being a medic also, I could see that the recent events really wore her down too. It wasn't something that showed in her beautiful face, but her spirit was badly damaged and now it needed time to heal. I was fortunate that I would be able to be a part of that healing. There were times that when we hugged, nothing was really said, yet it was all about the transmission of closeness between. We really didn't know what the future would bring, but we knew we could count on each other. The phone rang as I reached over the sofa to answer it.

"Hey there," Davia said to me in a moderate tone, "How are you feeling?"

"I feel like my whole world went upside down," I replied.

"How's the back?" Davia said as she stopped typing on her computer.

"I have my days, some good, some pretty foul. I am not going to begin to take all of the pain meds my neuro-surgeon prescribed, though there are times I wish I would." I said with a grimace, fixing my brace.

"That bad, huh babe?" Davia said affectionately.

"Sometimes. I try not to think about it, but they say this could take years to recover from."

Davia sighed really hard. I know it was hard for her to hear me speak such words, even if I didn't believe them. Months before, I was fine and in great shape. Now I was atrophying and having to settle in what could be a lifetime of pain and suffering.

"I talked with AJ out at the Academy the other day and she mentioned that you two were thinking of some alternate plans. How are you feeling about that?" Davia said in an extremely caring tone.

I thought for a moment.

"I guess that my choices are rather finite, but because of my experience, once I get back to health, and damnit I will get back to health, perhaps there is a new life for me elsewhere."

Davia sighed again.

"So you are considering a move to Los Angeles?"

I shook my head as I said, "Actually, yeah."

There was the sound of a pen tapping a desk in the background as Davia interjected.

PARAMEDIC M.O.S.

"Christian, as much as I have loved having you under my command, and as hard as it is for me to see you go through all that you have been for months now, I am kind of with Anjoline on this one. I know she loves you dearly and in a fashion that I have never seen another love someone before. If you two can find a life together, and you can heal and even maybe find a profession that will be rewarding enough for you, I need and want you to know that you have my absolute blessing." She was silent.

"I will miss seeing your face here at the station as I already do, and the street will be so much different without you there. Even though I am the Commanding Officer of this borough and a senior officer for the Service, I always feel something missing with you gone. No matter how much rank and pull I have out here that helps me get my job done; nothing made me feel safer than knowing you were out there somewhere. I always knew that if I needed you, you would come running faster than the wind. In fact, I knew that you would know I was in trouble before I did, and that kind of care is nearly impossible to come by. Honey, they broke the mold when they made you and AJ for that matter." The silence found its way back into the conversation.

"I will speak with LODI Division today and ensure that you continue to receive your paychecks, and we will find a way to clear your move to California as special rehabilitative circumstances. Given the circumstances, the Service will want your shields back. I know how much they mean to you and I hate to be the one to tell you that too."

I started to cry. Hearing how much Davia felt about me as a person, a medic and as a friend seemed to bring on a rush of emotions that I could not describe. I knew I had to let go but I did not know how. The Service and those in it consumed so much of my life. I had so much time invested, so much care, and so much that I wanted to see happen. The agency would dissolve soon, so I knew that everything would change. Maybe it was time.

"I will write a letter to the Executive Director and inform him what day I will be handing over my shields." I wiped tears from my eyes as AJ sat down next to me.

"AJ is going to LA next week to start looking for houses, and when she returns I will be going back with her. So that I do not have to do a lot of moving around, she has already arranged for me to stay with her friend Taylor until she gets back from packing up the house."

"Christian, you so deserve her and she you. I am glad if nothing else at this point, that you have each other. I truly admire how she looks out for you and how she recognizes who you are. I am equally as glad that you see her for all that she truly is and I cannot wait to visit you two in Los Angeles." Davia said in a way that I knew that she was smiling.

"You mean you will come out to see us?" I said inquisitively.

"Of course. My honey and I are already planning to be there in a few months once you get settled. If you look over at AJ and see a silly smile on her face, she will be acknowledging the fact that we had a secret meeting about that already."

I turned to AJ who had that silly smile on her face.

"Chief, now that I am resigning from the Service I think it is time for me to tell you something that I have always felt and I speak this as a friend. I love you very much and I always have. We have shared a bond that made my world nice and made me very glad that you were the person whose command I was assigned too. My experiences with you will forever be etched in my mind." I took a long breath.

"Well Mr. Christian, I have always loved you as well. You are just one of those people that makes the world a better place. AJ is the same way and that is why I am not only so glad that you two hooked up, but that we all are connected this way. Hun I gotta get going, I have an OPS meeting in an hour at HQ."

We said our goodbyes and I hung up. Somehow I was a little better with all that was going on. Having Davia's blessing and understanding meant the world to me. If I could only get this damn brace to stop jabbing me in my sides now, I'd be much better.

PARAMEDIC M.O.S.

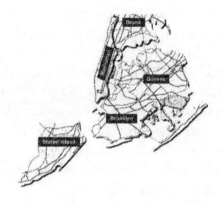

C.B. Garris

Chapter XXVIII:

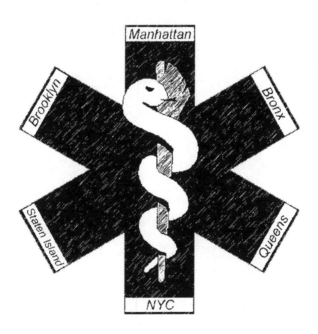

PARAMEDIC M.O.S.

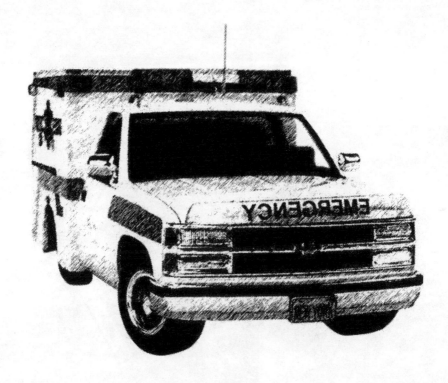

C.B. Garris

AJ drove me down to headquarters on a rainy Thursday afternoon. It would be just a few days before I was to leave for Los Angeles. I walked into Technical Services or what we call the Quartermaster's unit reception area. Jim Blahey was behind the desk.

"Hey Chris, what's up?" He noticed something strange in my look.

AJ walked in behind me with my Service issued Medic bag, department turnout coat and helmet. She rested the equipment on the desk and squeezed my arm gently, kissing me on my cheek.

"I'll wait outside," she said softly.

I was grasping a tight hold onto my shields.

I stood so many times behind these small pieces of metal, knowing what they stood for and how they protected me. They in fact helped me do my job. They gave me the ability to use the gifts I was given, and talent I had as a medic, while presenting a platform of authority that anyone outside of a hospital emergency room had to listen too and abide by at all times. If someone got out of line, threatened me, one of my partners, or the life of a civilian in my presence, that shield helped me effectuate the proper legal remedies on that person, by having the respect of the NYPD. I worked hard for those shields, perhaps harder than I ever have before, and they meant the world to me.

Judgment day arrived and I now have to turn them over.

"Chris, are you resigning?" Jim asked absolutely surprised.

"Unfortunately man, yes. With this new merger looming overhead, the new agency may try and toss out anyone on LODI, even before they heal. One of the conditions of the resolutions they have worked out regarding me is that knowing that they will release me from the Service at the end of the LODI period, they will grant the remainder of my LODI pay and my seeking medical care elsewhere if I relinquish my shields. I am going to be going away to a special sports rehab facility in southern California, and in fact I am moving there permanently."

"Wow, man I don't know what to say. I take it that was AJ who was just here?"

"Yeah, and she is the reason as to why I am still standing at the moment."

Jimmy studied me for a minute, and he heard me clanking my shields together in my right hand.

I saw him take a deep breath and the look in his eye said he placed himself in my position for a moment. The Service meant the world to

PARAMEDIC M.O.S.

those of us who put our life, blood and sweat into it; and separation from the Service was a very lonely day for anyone faced with it.

"You okay, man?" Jim asked as I stood there in quiet contemplation.

I fought off tears as best I could, rocking back and forth. Jimmy's civilian assistant came around the corner to ask him a question, and he scooted him off with a hand gesture.

"What are you going to do in Los Angeles?" Jim asked as he began to process my equipment, though not asking for my shields yet.

"Once I get back to full strength," I said leaning over the counter, "I have a few situations that I am eligible for in a much less threatening environment. I'll see how it goes; it is a much different world out there."

I took a long look at Jim and felt the pit of my stomach start to deepen. I placed my shields on the counter, and they hit with what felt like a tremendous thud. Although they were smaller than the palms of my hands, the sound of them being relinquished echoed in the caverns of my mind.

I stared at my shield number, 2015. I saw my entire career go in front of me and round the back too. Jimmy reached up to secure them, but first extended his hand to me.

"I wish you the best in everything man, and we will miss you around here. Thanks for making the job what it is supposed to be."

I exhaled deeply and we shook hands tightly.

"Thanks Jimmy, I'll drop you a line when I get to L.A."

Jimmy picked up the shields, "You better man, or I'm coming out there to find you." Jimmy smiled and I made my best attempt at one.

I turned to leave and as I almost made the door, Jimmy called me again.

"Yo, buddy. You forgot something."

As I looked up I saw something shining in mid air. My reflex went to catch it with my right hand. It was one of my two shields.

I looked at Jimmy confused for a second.

"You earned that. As far as inventory is concerned, I must have lost one during processing. Never forget man, once a Member of the Service, always a Member of the Service."

I smiled a bit, feeling the shield in my hand and looking over at Jim I commented gratefully.

"Thank you, I am glad I had the chance to serve here."

Jimmy smiled a bright smile, "You have always been on the good team 'round here."

With that we acknowledged our admiration of our just being good-natured people who love what we do; and I exited to a car with a beautiful woman waiting for me.

I stepped into AJ's car and she slipped her right hand over my thigh.

"I will be okay, I just need some time. We will be fine," I said as a tear ran down my face.

"I know we will", she said, "I know."

PARAMEDIC M.O.S.

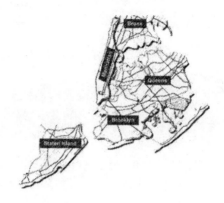

C.B. Garris

Chapter XXIX:

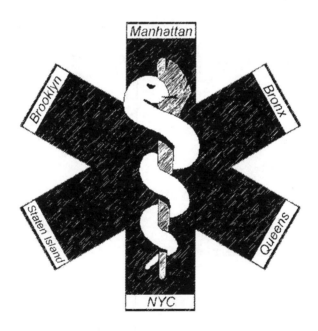

PARAMEDIC M.O.S.

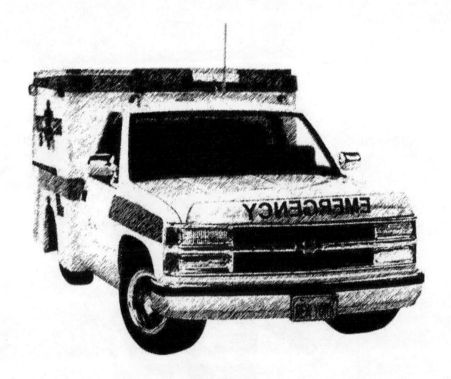

C.B. Garris

It would be a few days before we could assemble all of the things I would need in Los Angeles. AJ set up a surprise going away party for me, which yielded about two hundred people. All of my old academy mates came, partners, commanders, students and people I had touched in some way.

As we talked, laughed, ate and smiled, I looked around the room admiring this group of people. I began to cry during the party and seemed to do so off and on for about four hours. There were hugs, kisses, handshakes, presents, cards, more hugs, thank yous and more genuine affection than I knew what to do with.

These people were my family for years. We worked alongside each other, and saw the best and worst of New York City. We were there at shootings, stabbings, heart attacks, suicides, murders, fires, bombings, terrorist attacks yielding over one thousand patients – nights, days, evenings, riots, plane crashes, train and subway crashes. We were the medical backup for law enforcement when they served warrants or searched for fugitives, all in the name of caring – the very premise of being a Member of the Service.

When the party ended and the last of the MOS's departed, I was absolutely emotionally exhausted. I fell asleep on the couch with AJ draped over me like a blanket.

The following morning she helped me pack my clothes and told me how Taylor was getting an entourage together out there to ensure I got the physical therapy at prescribed times. She told me not to worry and not to feel funny having people take care of me.

"Babe, you have spent a lifetime caring for others selflessly, and you have lost more sleep than anyone I know. You need to take time to heal and someday it will feel okay when someone wants to help you. You are the most independent man I know and you are incredibly talented in so many areas. Miko will be arriving back from Kyoto when you arrive, and she will be watching out for you too. Did I mention that Miko and Taylor both love chess and backgammon, your favorites. Miko said she was practicing against her yacht staff to be ready for you."

I was listening to AJ, although she knew that my head was everywhere.

I kept envisioning all the things I had done, all the places I had been in the Service, all the wacky and outrageous situations I walked away from with my life when I shouldn't have. I was separating from a part of me, but I didn't know how.

PARAMEDIC M.O.S.

We both curled up in bed, with my packed bags on the floor downstairs, ready to go. I had called all of the people I wanted too so that they knew what was happening and where I would be. It felt weird to be leaving.

"You know," AJ, said as she placed her head right above mine, "I know you are scared and it will be a lot of changes to come, but I want to see you happy."

I kissed her gently.

"Sometimes," she continued, "everything is not what it seems and it takes time to weed through difficult situations."

I sighed and looked at the ceiling for a moment.

"I know," I interjected, "but it is such a feeling of being a fish out of water. I am sad that this is the way things have become, as far as me leaving; but I know it is the right thing in order to preserve myself. So many things seem to be wrong here and I think that is why people are dying. Whether they are dying by accident, suicide or medical reasons, something is askew here, and I need to see what more there is to life before I become more of a casualty than I already am of the job."

I felt AJ lower her head against my chest as we lie there silently. I knew that 7:00 a.m. was approaching fast, and I wanted to try and get some rest before I boarded the plane.

I slept for all of two hours during the night. AJ woke up early to find me awake. I got up and showered, preparing myself for the flight. Airports being what they are, when I put my brace on which was made of pliable metal encased in canvas, I knew I would set all kinds of alarms off when I went through security.

AJ spent extra time in the shower today, and when I peeked in she looked as beautiful as ever. She leaned her face out and gave me a warm and gentle kiss.

She knew that I was overwhelmed with change at this point. I was glad she was going with me. As I was checking through one of my bags downstairs, the doorbell rang. Our limo that AJ called for was waiting for us. The driver, who name was Ted, took our bags two at a time. Most of the things would be shipped, but I took about three suitcases of things, and AJ four. We got into the car and it took me a few minutes to adjust my brace to where it was comfortable sitting in the seat. I took a look at the house through the window, dazed with all the thoughts going through my mind.

"What time is our flight babe?" I asked AJ as I looked at her beautiful eyes.

AJ smiled, "Not until 2 p.m.. You feel like you want to make a stop, don't you?"

She asked this question as though she had already planned for me to have a need to make a stop.

"Yeah, I do. Let's have the driver stop over on Corona and a hundred and 8th street. I'd like to get some flowers and make a side trip."

AJ looked at me and smiled. She knocked on the partition, which dropped mechanically. She informed the driver and he acknowledged with absolute respect.

"I'd like to get some flowers for her too," AJ said.

I was comforted that she knew what I was thinking. We found a nice flower shop right at the intersection, and after I picked up a dozen mixed roses and a dozen mixed lilacs, tulips and assorted colorful flowers I gave the driver directions to a cemetery.

We pulled in slowly, and I felt my stomach sink several notches. My eyes sank low as I adjusted to the horrible sight of where I was. It was cloudy out and appeared like it could rain but the precipitation was being good to me.

The car stopped and I sat there for a moment. AJ was staring at me softly. I looked at the floor and sniffed the air around us. I scratched my head and the driver opened AJ's side of the vehicle. She stepped out slowly, and I shuffled out, something I had to do so the brace didn't cause me to fall back in the vehicle. I looked down five plots to where Jennifer was laid to rest and I just stared. AJ put her arm in mine and we walked gently over to her stone. I stood there looking at her name and the dates. I wanted to scream and swing. I felt all of my anger and frustration creep up through my feet, to my hips, and chest and into my throat. I wanted to vomit.

AJ laid the flowers she picked for Jennifer down over where her casket had been placed.

She said out loud, "I miss you very much."

AJ squeezed my arm gently and walked back to the limo, facing me when she got there. I looked around at how peaceful this was for Jennifer now. I ran all the years of our friendship through my mind as I made a declaration to her out loud.

"If you only knew how much I miss you. I remember the first day we met at the academy. You were so cute and funny. You were a best friends,

PARAMEDIC M.O.S.

best friend. We all decided to go down to the Rockaway's to barbeque, and while I searched for firewood for the bonfire, you made it a point to come over to me and spend time with me. You knew that I was alone and troubled. You were so soft to me and gentle just the same. I knew that you had just broken up with someone and it was of no consequence, since I felt your friendship everywhere. We sat there and revealed things about each other that we had never told anyone before. That night before you left to go home, I remember standing on Rockaway Blvd and Beach 86th St. off the pier, laughing with you until three in the morning. I felt so cared for and admired, and we had only just met. I miss you so much. I miss your smile and late night pages to make sure I was having a good day, or if I just needed a hug. We beat the system on thinking that everyone who admires each other like we did had to be involved. Having your care and love was something that meant the world to me; and I wish there was something, anything I could have done to help you and stop you from killing yourself. I am so sorry for that."

I stopped for a minute and cried, falling to my knees. AJ started to walk towards me, but I gestured that I was okay. She stayed right by the car.

"You always had a way of making me feel appreciated when I didn't feel it. You were always there for me, damnit why didn't you let me be there for you?"

I stopped to breathe for a moment.

"I can't ask you these questions face to face and will have to wait until my time comes to ask you. I hope you are at peace Jennifer, because you were the best partner and friend I ever had. The job was never the same without you and wouldn't you figure that no sooner than when you died, I was in a bad accident. I am moving to California with AJ and I won't be back for a while. Because I will be elsewhere does not mean that I won't think of you everyday, and when I need to think of the love we shared for each other, I will call on it. I am forever grateful to have learned what I should expect from others from you. You taught me that my heart was pure if I ever had a question, and to follow it, using my head as the compass. I wish I could hold you and tell you everything is going to be okay. You touched so many lives and you were so beautiful. I try to put out of my mind what I saw when I was last in your apartment, as that is far too much to fathom even for me. You had such an intoxicating laugh that permeated all of me. I know that "Mister" forgives you, and he is safely in the hands of your family right now. You had such warmth and such a touch. Some other place is blessed with you now, and I don't really know how life will be without you in it. I am still getting used to the fact that you aren't here. I wanted to protect you from the things that haunted you, that's what friends are for, and that is what you did for me."

Tears were running like a stream down my face now.

"You are irreplaceable in this world," I continued. "I hope you will forgive me but I have been unable to look at your pictures for awhile. Jen it hurts too much. The pictures are safely secured, and I want you to know that AJ will take great care of me. I know that I will always carry your spirit with me wherever I am, and I will always respect you for the person you were in my life, the amazing medic that you were, and the woman who guys would trip over everywhere. Someday I hope to see you again."

I took a long breath.

"I love you Jen-Jen. May the angels hold you safely, as you are one of them."

I placed the flowers alongside AJ's.

I walked back to the limo and AJ opened her arms. We hugged for a while as I cried hard. AJ said nothing, as nothing needed to be said. This was something I had to do.

As we made our way back towards the Long Island Expressway, AJ kept a firm eye on me. I was looking ahead and down. My biceps were pumping from all of the emotions going through my body.

I looked at AJ for a long while and smiled through my tears. AJ slid over next to me and placed her left hand in my right. Resting her nose tip on mine, she placed her fingers on my face, as I got a wonderful delivery of her perfume.

"We're going to be fine babe." AJ said affectionately and then kissed me.

Looking back at her heart-stopping eyes I acknowledged, "I know we will. I know."

Placing her right arm around me, AJ rested her head on my chest as I ran my fingers gently through her hair. I inhaled deeply and felt all of my senses activate at the scent of her perfume. I looked out the window for a moment and quietly acknowledged the large green sign just off the Van Wyck Expressway that said WELCOME TO JOHN F. KENNEDY INTERNATIONAL AIRPORT.

PARAMEDIC M.O.S.

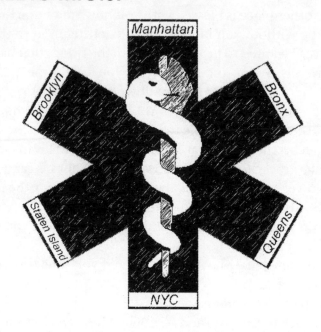

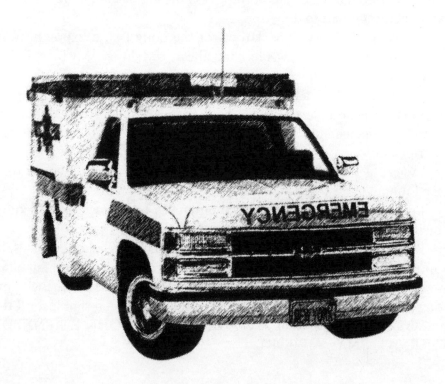

Printed in the United States
By Bookmasters